The Treatment of Drinking Problems

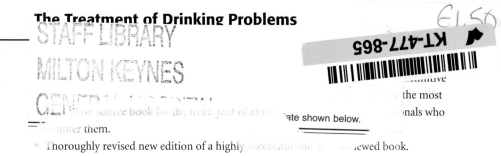

£1.50

KT-477-865

...itive

...ive source book for the treatment of alco... ...ate shown below. ...nals who

...the most

...unter them.

- Thoroughly revised new edition of a highly successful and ... ...iewed book.
- New chapters include an account of the historical development of treatment over the last 300 years, and the latest evidence on the psychiatric co-morbidities which often go with drinking problems.
- Modern trends in relation to psychological and pharmacological interventions are fully covered and the role of self-help groups reappraised.

Griffith Edwards is Editor-in-Chief of the international scientific journal *Addiction*, Professor Emeritus of Addiction Behaviour at the University of London, and Honorary Consultant at the Maudsley Hospital, London.

E. Jane Marshall is Consultant Psychiatrist and Senior Lecturer at the South London and Maudsley NHS Trust and the National Addiction Centre, London.

Christopher C.H. Cook is a Consultant Psychiatrist and Professor of the Psychiatry of Alcohol Misuse, Kent Institute of Medicine and Health Sciences, University of Kent at Canterbury.

From reviews of the previous edition:

'... the best overview on the subject for practitioners who wish to understand and help people with alcohol problems ... a unique perspective ... elegant and succinct prose ... highly readable ... an absolute must to read.'
  The Lancet

'This text continues to be a *must* for anyone working in the field of alcohol misuse.'
  Addiction Biology

'... highly readable ... an invaluable resource ... authoritative ... contains a wealth of readily accessible information on drinking problems and is therefore essential reading for all workers in specialist drug and alcohol agencies.'
  Drug News

The Treatment of Drinking Problems

A guide for the helping professions

Fourth Edition

Griffith Edwards
CBE, DSc, DM, FRCP, FRCPsych (Hon), F Med Sci National Addiction Centre, London

E. Jane Marshall
MRCP(I), MRCPsych, National Addiction Centre, London

Christopher C.H. Cook
MD, MRCPsych, Kent Institute of Medicine and Health Sciences, Canterbury

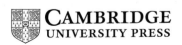

CAMBRIDGE
UNIVERSITY PRESS

PUBLISHED BY THE PRESS SYNDICATE OF THE UNIVERSITY OF CAMBRIDGE
The Pitt Building, Trumpington Street, Cambridge, United Kingdom

CAMBRIDGE UNIVERSITY PRESS
The Edinburgh Building, Cambridge CB2 2RU, UK
40 West 20th Street, New York, NY 10011–4211, USA
477 Williamstown Road, Port Melbourne, VIC 3207, Australia
Ruiz de Alarcón 13, 28014 Madrid, Spain
Dock House, The Waterfront, Cape Town 8001, South Africa

http://www.cambridge.org

First published 2003

Printed in the United Kingdom at the University Press, Cambridge

Typefaces Minion 10.5/14 pt. Formata and Formata BQ   *System* LaTeX 2$_\varepsilon$ [TB]

A catalogue record for this book is available from the British Library

Library of Congress Cataloguing in Publication data
Edwards, Griffith.
    The treatment of drinking problems : a guide for the helping professions / Griffith Edwards,
E. Jane Marshall, Christopher C. H. Cook. – 4th edn.
        p.   cm.
    Includes bibliographical references and indexes.
    ISBN 0 521 01714 9 (pbk.)
    1. Alcoholism – Treatment.   I. Marshall, E. Jane.   II. Cook, Christopher C., M.D.   III. Title.
RC565 .E38   2003
616.86′106–dc21   2002073459

ISBN 0 521 01714 9 paperback

This book is dedicated to

Sue, Daniel and Rose

François, David, Grace and Matthew

Joy, Andrew, Beth, Rachel and Jonathan

Contents

A note on the fourth edition

In its fourth edition, *The Treatment of Drinking Problems* represents the further development of a highly successful text which has been acclaimed internationally and has appeared in six translations. The unique feature of the book remains its ability to address the frontline realities of clinical practice in an informed and empathetic manner while grounding this approach in critical scientific review. The authors provide an overall revision and updating of their previous material, and they have added important new chapters dealing, respectively, with the history of treatment in this field and with the very topical issue of co-morbidity. Case vignettes are used to illustrate a range of common clinical dilemmas and their solutions, and boxed statements highlight key points. *The Treatment of Drinking Problems* will be of value to every type of professional who seeks to help people with drinking problems, and to those responsible for commissioning and designing treatment services. Besides noting its competence, incisiveness and authority, many reviewers have praised the accessible style in which this book is written – it is a teaching text *par excellence.*

Acknowledgements

Richard Barling and Pauline Graham of Cambridge University Press have given valued editorial support. Helpful comments have been received from Francis Keaney and Mark Turner. Annette Malaure provided much valued editorial assistance. Overall administrative back-up on the production of the typescript came from Patricia Davis, for whose unfailing skills and inexhaustible patience we are much indebted.

Statement on interests

The authors at times received fees or support from the manufacturers of several drugs mentioned in this book. No subsidies towards the production of this book have been offered or accepted from any source.

Introduction

When first opening any text, the reasonable expectation of the reader is that the authors should declare what purpose the book in question aims to serve, while also providing a signposting of the chapters to come. These are the matters which this introduction will now address.

A book intended to enhance clinical skills

This book is intended for anyone, generalist or specialist, whose responsibilities imply that they will sometimes or often be encountering people with drinking problems. It is written in the hope that it will be instrumentally useful in enhancing diagnostic and treatment skills in the alcohol arena for this wide variety of professionals. We have also tried to convey a sense of why this kind of work is so perpetually intriguing and worthwhile. We have employed the generic word 'therapist' to describe the person who does the helping and hope that the text will be equally relevant to the needs of psychiatrists and other medical practitioners, nurses, clinical psychologists, social workers, occupational therapists and counsellors. Different professions have their specific skills and roles, but in dealing with drinking problems there is much to be learnt which is relevant across all professions. We intend this book to be of multidisciplinary appeal, but Chapters 3 and 10 deal with matters which inevitably require a technical exposition in biological and medical language

As for the question of how to refer to the person who is given the help, we have used the words 'patient' and 'client' as having much the same meaning. We have as far as possible eschewed the term 'alcoholic', feeling that this designation no longer has scientific meaning and too easily invites stereotyping and alienation, but we are aware that others (particularly members of Alcoholics Anonymous) still find this word useful. We prefer the phrase 'problem drinker' or 'person with a drinking problem', and more specifically and restrictively 'person suffering from alcohol dependence'. The term 'alcohol misuse' will, for ease of communication, now and then be employed, but within a stricter scientific framework we would argue that 'use' and 'misuse' of alcohol are not categorically separate behaviours.

A teaching text

As well as its being of interest to established practitioners, we hope this book will be found useful by students in the many relevant helping professions. It is intended for generalist courses and for specialists in the making, and we want it to engage, hold attention, challenge and inspire, as well as convey information.

Service providers

Besides one-to-one issues of individual treatment, this book is concerned with questions relating to how treatment is most effectively and cost-effectively to be delivered to populations in need. We want it to be useful for people responsible for design and commissioning of services.

Bridging the research and clinical worlds

The clinical position taken in this book is rooted in what science today has to say about the causes of drinking, the nature of alcohol-related problems and of alcohol dependence, and the demonstrable efficacy of different treatment approaches. In staying close to the format of a clinical text, we have felt that the right balance is struck by appropriate review and referencing of key statements, while not diverting into academic review for its own sake.

Internationalism

The way in which alcohol problems are defined and responded to is to an extent shaped by culturally and historically determined beliefs and by national health care provisions, and the pattern of problems encountered and the appropriateness of different types of response must often be different as between poorer and richer countries. There is much need for strengthened international support in training, technological development and sharing of information. While hoping that this book will be useful in many different national settings, we are aware that 'translation' of this kind of text into other cultural environments will require critical scrutiny and close local judgement by our readers.

An interactive endeavour

The preparation of successive editions of this book has been facilitated by a great deal of valued input from colleagues who have written to us, people met at conferences, students taught, patients seen, and books and articles read. We will be immensely grateful for further generous input of that kind – Griffith Edwards (spjepad@iop.kcl.ac.uk) is happy to act as portal.

Plan and content

The chapters of the book are grouped into two sections. Part I is headed 'Background to understanding' and comprises Chapters 1 to 13, and Part II puts together Chapters 14 to 22 under the heading 'Screening, assessment and treatment'.

Part I: Background to understanding
The history of treatment for drinking problems *(Chapter 1)*

This history is relevant to present-day practitioners in terms of insights offered towards understanding the genesis of our current assumptions and the likely directions of new and continued development. History, this chapter argues, vitally teaches lessons.

Causes of drinking problems *(Chapter 2)*

Heavy drinking and alcohol-related problems arise as a result of multiple and interacting influences upon the individual. This chapter provides an overview of environmental factors, genetic predisposition and psychological mechanisms which may lead to the development of drinking problems.

Alcohol as a drug *(Chapter 3)*

A knowledge of the biological effects of alcohol is basic to understanding many of the problems that arise from its use. This chapter brings together information on the absorption and metabolism of alcohol, its effect on several body systems, and in particular its action on the brain. The language is, of necessity, technical, but we hope that the non-medical reader will find it of value.

The alcohol dependence syndrome *(Chapter 4)*

Carrying on from discussion of alcohol as a drug with dependence potential (Chapter 3), this chapter describes the psychobiological basis, profile and clinical significance of the alcohol dependence syndrome. The question is discussed of whether dependence is one syndrome or a group of syndromes.

Alcohol-related problems *(Chapters 5–10)*

If alcohol dependence is one important dimension defining the concerns of this book, alcohol-related problems constitute a second and equally important dimension. Contributions deal in turn with drinking problems and the family (Chapter 5); social complications of excessive drinking (Chapter 6); drinking problems as a cause of neuropsychiatric disorder (Chapter 7); drinking problems and psychiatric co-morbidity (Chapter 8, a very important chapter new to this book); alcohol and other drug problems (Chapter 9); and physical complications of excessive drinking (Chapter 10).

Women with drinking problems *(Chapter 11)*

Alcohol problems are still a source of shame to women, and women are under-represented in treatment settings. The reasons for this situation are discussed, as are the risk factors for women across the life course.

Some special presentations *(Chapter 12)*

This chapter again seeks to emphasize the clinical orientation of the book and identifies some of the special presentations which may be encountered in the clinic on any working day – the young drinker, the patient with violent propensities, the 'very important patient', and so on.

Drinking problems and the life course *(Chapter 13)*

Rounding off Part I, the perspective developed in this chapter is fundamental to the stance taken throughout the treatment section which follows. It is argued that alcohol problems can only be understood as happenings within an ongoing life course, with treatment needing to be fashioned so as to support natural processes of recovery.

Part II: Screening, assessment and treatment

Screening and history taking *(Chapters 14 and 15)*

These chapters open the second section of the book. Case identification and screening are dealt with in Chapter 14 in terms of both laboratory and questionnaire approaches, followed by a discussion in Chapter 15 of how history taking is to be accomplished and used as an initiation of therapy. Separate sections of Chapter 15 describe the assessment interview with patient and spouse, and an approach to case formulation is outlined.

Withdrawal states and treatment of withdrawal *(Chapter 16)*

Detoxification is an important and necessary prelude to the further treatment of the dependent drinker. This chapter covers the scientific and clinical basis of such treatment, and it will also guide the non-medical reader as to the principles underlying the management of alcohol withdrawal. The diversity of withdrawal states, the choice between community and in-patient settings, and the proper use of medication are addressed.

The basic work of treatment *(Chapter 17)*

Here it is argued that what happens in the interactions between patient and therapist is often as important as the formalities of treatment. Attention is paid to such issues as the therapeutic relationship and the likely structure and content of a therapeutic interview.

Alcoholics Anonymous *(Chapter 18)*

AA is an international self-help organization which has helped millions of people with drinking problems. This chapter offers an introduction to its basic tenets, and the essential processes by which it operates. The importance of effective co-operation between treatment professionals and AA is emphasized. The 'Minnesota Model' and its relationship with AA are described.

Special techniques *(Chapter 19)*

Chapter 19 provides a discussion of a range of special techniques, with a particular focus on cognitive–behavioural and pharmaceutical treatments which have proven efficacy. It emphasizes our belief that treatment must be research based.

Working towards normal drinking *(Chapter 20)*

For patients who are not significantly alcohol dependent, normal drinking can, with caution, be a feasible and preferred goal. Criteria for supporting this choice are identified and relevant treatment approaches discussed.

When things go wrong, and putting them right *(Chapter 21)*

Underlining once more the book's commitment to a practical, clinical orientation, Chapter 21 deals with a series of work-a-day situations in which treatment can run up against difficulties, and considers how the therapeutic processes can then be unblocked and got on course again.

Treatment settings, professional roles and the organization of treatment services *(Chapter 22)*

This chapter describes the diversity of treatment settings encountered, and the varied contributions that different professions can make, in the treatment of drinking problems. The aim is to show the ways in which such varied settings and differently trained professionals all have a valuable role to play in helping the drinker. The need for co-operation between agencies and effective organization and planning of services are stressed.

We would, of course, be happy if this book is seen as having a useful place on library shelves. Our pleasure would be even greater if we found it lying around dog-eared and well-used in out-patient clinic rooms, ward side-rooms, nursing stations, doctors' offices and surgeries and other places where treatment actually happens. The best use of this text will be if the reader is willing to move backwards and forwards between its chapters and that rich reality of clinical experience where the greatest learning is always to be done.

Background to understanding

The history of treatment for drinking problems

What professional assistance could a man or woman suffering from a drinking problem have expected to receive in the distant or more recent past? A look at that question may help towards understanding the origins of present ideas and practices in the alcohol treatment arena. It is the history of ideas as much as of practices which needs to be examined – the underlying assumptions make what happens in the clinical encounter.

The structure of this chapter is as follows. The pre-history of treatment is first briefly considered. The roots of formal medical intervention probably developed at the end of the eighteenth and beginning of the nineteenth centuries as products of the European enlightenment, and certain founding texts from that era are examined. From then onwards, there is the evolving history to be told of ideas shaped by their age, and practices shaped by those ideas.

Alcohol problems and the pre-history of treatment

There were over time two historically distinct disease movements in the alcohol field. Those authorities who separately in the nineteenth (Kerr, 1887; Crothers, 1893) and then in the twentieth century (Jellinek, 1960) championed the idea of alcoholism as a disease, in each instance saw the concept as opening the way to benign and scientifically based treatment of the drinker. They tended to contrast the modernism of their formulations with the dark previous centuries during which excessive drinking had been deemed a sin, and had been the province of moralism and the clergy.

Such dismissiveness sold too short the ancient role of the Church in dealing with drinking problems. Over those earlier centuries Christianity gave Europe an all-inclusive framework within which to comprehend and respond to aberrant human behaviour. Unsurprisingly, drinking problems found themselves located within that general frame.

Thus drunkenness was from the days of the early Church preached against and denounced as sinful, with that view fully congruent with the governing images of contemporary life. It was within the power of the sinner to repent and stop sinning without recourse to a doctor. Self-determined change was demanded of the individual and prayed for. The Church developed graded scales of penance to be meted out according to the degree of drunkenness and the position of the drinker within the Church hierarchy – laymen were let off relatively lightly and drunken bishops fared the worst (Edwards, 2000).

The dark days were in fact far from pitch dark, and the Church's response to drunkenness had within it psychological principles of some sophistication. The recent burgeoning of research interest in natural or spontaneous recovery (Klingemann et al., 2001) may help towards a reappraisal of the influence which Christianity and other religions may exert on drinking norms and drinking behaviour. Traditional Jewish mores have been very effective in curbing drunkenness (Snyder, 1958), while Islam has prohibited alcohol (Baasher, 1983).

A brave new dawn

Benjamin Rush (1743–1813) was an American physician who had attended Edinburgh for postgraduate studies. In 1790 he published a pamphet entitled 'An Inquiry into the Effects of Ardent Spirits . . .' (Rush, 1790). He was a signatory to the Declaration of Independence. In 1804, Thomas Trotter, an Edinburgh-trained doctor who served as a ship's surgeon and in his spare time wrote poetry, published an essay on drunkenness (Trotter, 1804). The ideas which these two men developed were congruent with the thinking of the Age of Reason. Drunkenness was for them not a sin but a habit to be unlearnt. As Trotter pithily put it, 'The habit of drunkenness is a disease of the mind.' The key terms employed in that statement had meanings somewhat different from their modern usage. But the message that sin was out of the equation, drunkenness a rationally explicable behaviour, and that medical interventions were to derive from explanations of cause, transcends language and time. This was revolutionary thinking.

BOX 1.1
The habit of drunkenness is a disease of the mind.
Thomas Trotter (1804).

Here is a passage from Rush which shows that idea being taken through to practice:

Our knowledge of the principle of association upon the minds and conducts of men, should lead us to destroy, by other impressions, the influence of all these circumstances, with which recollection and desire of spirits are combined...Now by finding a new and interesting employment, or subject of conversation for drunkards, at the usual times in which they have been accustomed to drink...their habits of intemperance can be completely destroyed.

This is Trotter purposively distancing himself from the religious past:

The priesthood have poured forth its anathemas from the pulpit, and the moralist, no less severe, hath declaimed against it as a vice degrading to our nature. Both have meant well...But the physical influence of custom, confirmed into habit, interwoven with the actions of our sentient system, and reacting on our mental part, have been entirely forgotten.

Rush achieved greater contemporary fame than Trotter, and his *Inquiry* was taken up as a founding text by the Temperance movement. Trotter was, however, the more sensitive clinician, and his *Essay* deserves recognition as the first significant text on the treatment of drinking problems to be published in the English language (it was originally presented in Latin as an Edinburgh MD thesis).

Temperance movements

There is no evidence that Rush's or Trotter's clinical teachings were in their own time ever taken up on a large scale by practitioners. Over most of the nineteenth century the old religious approach continued to operate, with many denunciations from the pulpit still heard. However, over this period the Temperance movement came into being (Blocker, 1989). Temperance was a lay movement which had alliances at times with most of the Christian denominations and particularly strong connections with the Free Churches. It is remembered today for its mass teaching of abstinence, but help was often given to the individual drinker. The reformed drunkard was the show piece at public meetings. Vividly presented accounts of drunken degradation and eventual salvation could be the best show in town (Crowley, 1999). Within the movement, the former inebriate could expect to find esteem and a new identity.

The Washingtonian Temperance Society, founded in Baltimore in 1840, had within it a strong element of self-help and has been seen as the forerunner of Alcoholics Anonymous (Maxwell, 1950). This is the pledge which the six founding members of the movement took one evening in a down-town Baltimore tavern:

We, whose names are annexed, desirous of forming a society for our mutual benefit and to guard against a pernicious practice which is injurious to our health, standing, and families, do pledge ourselves as gentlemen that we will not drink any spirituous or malt liquors, wine or cider.

The Baltimore tavern-keeper was soon complaining about the loss of some of his best customers. The power of mutuality in aiding recovery from alcohol dependence had been discovered – that phrase 'a society for our mutual benefit' was crucial. The clergy, however, objected that reformed drunkards were usurping the leadership of an organization which properly belonged to the cloth, and the Washingtonians flourished only for a few years as a distinct organizational entity.

Another variant of nineteenth century, lay help for the individual drinker, can be seen in the work of the Salvation Army and the writings of its founder, William Booth (Booth, 1890). Booth was a Christian social reformer and acutely aware that much of the rampant drunkenness of Victorian cities was the product of the appalling living conditions of the urban poor. He described alcohol as 'the Lethe of the miserable'. Evangelical Christianity was one important ingredient of the Salvationist approach to the man or woman in the gutter, but there was also a strong emphasis on giving practical help and on environmental remedies. The drunkard might very literally be offered a way out of the drink-sodden urban trap, a place in a Harbour Light home, or a ticket to a Farm Colony overseas.

Institutions find favour

In the 1870s a vigorous movement was launched in America which pressed for the establishment of inebriate asylums to which troubled drinkers were to be admitted for anything between 5 or 10 years and life. This model was advocated in a manifesto put out by the American Society for the Study and Cure of Inebriety (Crothers, 1893):

> ... the great centres of pauperism and criminality will be broken up. This will be accomplished by the establishment of work-house hospitals, where the inebriate can be treated and restrained. Such places must be located in the country, removed from large cities and towns, and conducted on a military basis ... They should be military training hospitals, where all the surroundings are under the exact care of the physician, and every condition of life is regulated with steady uniformity.

If secure institutional separation from drink was to be the major part of the later nineteenth-century cure plan whatever the social class, the well-heeled would receive the added benefits of tonics, steam baths and faradic stimulation – the logic for these physical treatments was vaguely stated in terms of toning up the nerve cells. Even leeches might find favour. For the professional classes there would probably also be daily prayers, supervised country walks, musical evenings, and access to a library and a billiard table.

The institutional movement was medically led, but, despite the talk of medicine and science, it was for the working classes considerably more punitive than anything the Church would have favoured in the supposedly dark past. In the private homes, moral regeneration was intrinsic to the plan. In short, medicalization and stark moralism at this time often went nicely hand in hand. The psychological subtlety of the Rush and Trotter analyses had gone.

The institutional treatment formula had become discredited by the time of the First World War. Not enough clients could be found for the private retreats and the state reformatories were proving to be ineffective and expensive, and were becoming clogged with irrecoverable cases. The inebriate institutions were congruent with the disease theory, with fear of degeneration, and with belief in the validity of incarceration as a response to perceived social threats of various different kinds.

From that era two books remain as prime enshrinement of medical thinking on the institutional treatment of inebriety. Crothers (1893) produced the authoritative American text, while Norman Kerr (1887) wrote an encyclopaedic British text which went through three editions. Kerr was the first president of the British Society for the Study and Cure of Inebriety, which has come through to the present as the Society for the Study of Addiction, while the Proceedings of the Society go forward as the journal *Addiction*. The American Society and its journal had their *raìson d'être* removed by Prohibition. The twentieth-century experts who later promulgated the new disease concept were to an astonishing degree amnesic to those nineteenth-century events.

By 1900 — so far, what?

Choosing the turning of centuries as the markers for this analysis is to an extent arbitrary. But by 1900 the Western world, with its deep background of a sin model and the religious response to the drunkard, had accumulated 100 years of experience with variants of a disease model, and the medical claim to ownership of the problem. Certain major stands in the allegedly post-sin response to inebriety had begun to emerge (see Box 1.2).

BOX 1.2 **Some major strands in the history of treatment for drinking problems**
- Demarcation of case from not case
- The problem as habit
- The enthusiasm for physical treatments
- Institutions much advocated
- Treatment never a medical monopoly

- Not every excessive drinker had automatically become a suitable case for medical treatment. The legitimate medical cases were the drinkers who suffered from an imprecise disease state which was designated *inebriety*, and which was a brain disease with a hereditary element in its aetiology. Common drunkenness was not the doctor's business.
- A view of the problem as habit and treatment as the breaking of habit – the forerunner of the cognitive–behavioural analysis – had been put on offer at the beginning of the century, but did not appeal to the Victorian disease theorists.
- Physical treatments, often of a blindly empirical nature, were being employed.
- Doctors had become champions of institutions and of a milieu approach. They also often became directors or owners of these institutions.
- People who were not doctors were, through the Temperance movement, a continuing part of the response system.

To a remarkable degree, those five strands which had emerged in the nineteenth century were carried through, explored and re-explored as the dominant themes of the twentieth-century treatment endeavour. We will use them as sub-headings for the next section.

The twentieth century and five themes carried forward

Defining who and what needed treatment

For Trotter there was no term available to differentiate case from not case – his essay was on 'drunkenness', rather than on a specific type of diseased person. Come the latter part of the nineteenth century, experts in both the USA and the UK employed the word 'inebriety' to identify an overarching condition, with sub-types defined by the substances involved. Inebriety was thus for Kerr (1887) and Crothers (1893) a generic term roughly equivalent to today's DSM-IV (American Psychiatric Association, 1994), or ICD-10 'dependence' (World Health Organization, 1992). At that time, the word 'addiction' still had only limited currency.

Come the early decades of the nineteenth century and the word 'alcoholic' was quite often being used by medical authorities, but not with any great precision (it had first been introduced as *alcoholismus* by Magnus Huss, a Swedish physician, in 1849). There had been a slow lead-up to that position, but the definitive confirmation that the new nomenclature had won came in 1960 with the publication of E.M. Jellinek's *The Disease Concept of Alcoholism* (Jellinek, 1960). Alcoholism, according to Jellinek, could have its sub-types which were either disease or not disease. But in common medical usage from 1960 onwards, the disease of alcoholism separated the domain of medicine and the worthy sick person from the wasteland of common and unworthy drunkenness. Alcoholism was a disease and a progressive disease (Jellinek, 1952) and the only way for the sufferer to arrest its progression was to espouse life-long abstinence. Jellinek's disease of alcoholism was, however, never operationally defined.

Why worry about words? The word 'alcoholism' mattered because it came to imply that, within this new deal, the only problem was the patient experiencing loss of control over their drinking – the person who had severe withdrawal symptoms, the advanced case, the one stereotype. This 'alcoholism' concept gave an entry to medical treatment and to insurance cover for many people who previously would have been given no help at all, and it was benign in many of its consequences. But at the same time it invited a tunnel vision. The boundaries of the treatment effort and service provision, and of the public health response, were dictated by the one potent word. The person who was drinking enough to harm their health or social well-being, but who did not conform to the stereotype, was left off the helping map. Help had always to be an intensive business, conducted at the start most often in an in-patient setting, but with the help of Alcoholics Anonymous (AA). Aftercare also had to be intensive, with continued AA attendance seen as mandatory. We return to the history of AA shortly.

When survey research began to show that there were particulate problems with alcohol which were widely disseminated in the population and did not conform to the picture of the disease state (Room, 1977), treatment services in some countries began to broaden their focus, with a new emphasis on brief or early intervention in the primary care (Wallace et al., 1988) or general hospital setting (Chick et al., 1985). In North America, that re-focusing has not been so apparent as in Britain and Australia. The American treatment service discourse is still largely about 'the alcoholic' and the provision of specialist care for the dependent drinker (Galanter, 2000).

In 1977 a new conceptual framework was promulgated by the World Health Organization (WHO; Edwards, 1976), which has since won a good deal of international acceptance. This entailed a two-dimensional framework for understanding troubled drinking, with alcohol dependence conceptually distinguished from alcohol-related problems. Within that view the suitable case for treatment becomes anyone who wants help with their drinking, whether or not they are dependent on alcohol. The concept of alcohol dependence was sufficiently specified to allow operationalization (Stockwell et al., 1979).

The habit and treatment as the breaking of habit

Given the clear enunciation of a habit formulation by Rush and Trotter those years ago, it is surprising that the idea should have taken so long to come circling back again. The first re-awakening of interest in that kind of perspective occurred in 1930 when Kantorovitch, working in Russia, described an aversion therapy which employed painful shock as the unconditioned stimulus (see Voegtlin and Lemere, 1950, for a review of the early literature on this topic). In the 1940s Voegtlin and Lemere, at the Shadel Sanatorium in Seattle, began to treat alcohol problems with aversion therapy (Lemere, 1987). Their approach was consciously derived from Pavlov. The conditioned stimulus (smell or sip of alcohol) was to be paired with an unconditioned stimulus (nausea induced by injection of emetine), with the intention of setting up a conditioned aversion to alcohol. A large number of patients were treated at the Shadel. In 1950 these authors reported on a series of 4096 subjects, with a claimed 60% abstinence at the 1-year point (Voegtlin and Lemere, 1950).

With the increasing deployment of psychological principles to the treatment of neurosis, it was a natural extension to apply behavioural and then cognitive methods to the treatment of drinking problems (Sobell and Sobell, 1973, 1976). A large body of research developed exploring the clinical application of the idea of bad drinking as a habit, which with suitable psychological input could be unlearnt (Heather and Robertson, 1981). Relapse was reformulated as a cue-engendered behaviour which could, with training, be extinguished (Marlatt and Gordon, 1985).

Two centuries after Trotter and Rush first signalled these ideas, cognitive–behavioural approaches to the treatment of the drinking habits are today strongly established elements within the treatment repertoire. The extent to which the theoretical underpinnings satisfactorily explain treatment effectiveness is still an open question, but the 200-year-old concept of excessive drinking as habit of the mind has proved to be an enduring and productive contribution to scientific thought, with fruitful follow-through to clinical practice.

The history of physical treatments

As seen with the traditional medical response to many other intractable conditions of unknown aetiology, before modern therapies and controlled trials came onto the scene every imaginable physical treatment was at one time or another thrown by doctors at drinking problems (Edwards, 2000). Here are a few examples of that kind of empiricism in action. Amphetamine sulphate, LSD, cannabis and maintenance doses of diazepam have all appeared in the literature as advised treatments for excessive drinking. Patients have been injected with their own serum to which whisky has been added. Carbon dioxide or oxygen injections have been given subcutaneously as a cure for inebriety. Electroconvulsive therapy (ECT) has been administered to the point of confusion. Brain operations have been performed as a cure for addiction to alcohol and other drugs. The prize for unsubstantiated enthusiasm might go to Shilo (1961). He devised a treatment regime involving the patient's consumption of precisely 231 lemons taken over an exact 29 days.

> **BOX 1.3 The Lemon Cure**
> To stamp out craving for alcohol take 231 lemons over 29 days precisely.
> *Shilo (1961)*

Interest in the pharmacotherapy of drinking problems took a new turn with the introduction of disulfiram (Antabuse) to clinical practice in the 1940s (Hald and Jacobsen, 1948). Its launch pre-dated the dominance of scientific rules set by clinical trials, and disulfiram can perhaps be seen as a drug which rode at the tail-end of the age of empiricism rather than being a treatment timed to arrive at the forefront of rigorous controlled trials. A current appraisal of the place of disulfiram in therapeutics is given in Chapter 19. The new anti-craving drugs such as acamprosate and naltrexone (Chapter 19) are products of a different clinical and scientific era than the lemon cure.

Without negating the value of recent advances, history must suggest that therapists in this arena will do well to remember the uncomfortable past. Drug cures for the drinking habit are much to be welcomed, provided their worth is not talked up into being the simple and conclusive cure for a highly complex condition.

How the institutional treatment theme was carried forward

Astley Cooper (1913), medical superintendent and licensee of the Ghyllwood Sanatorium in Cumberland, stated in his textbook that 'Without fear of contradiction ... we say that for the thorough treatment of inebriety, the special sanatorium stands alone.' Until well into the second half of the twentieth century, Astley Cooper's assertion was unlikely to have met with medical dissent. The treatment of inebriety in Europe and the USA was for many years still built on the teaching and practices of the 1870s, although the reformatories had been got out of the way. Treatment was offered to private patients in the traditional pleasant surroundings, while those without financial resources would find themselves shut away in state mental hospitals or asylums. Treatment of the disease of inebriety was for all comers still co-terminus with institutional care.

With the arrival following the Second World War of the concept of alcoholism as a disease, new impetus was given to institutional care. A mix of private and public provisions supported this intention. In the UK a crucial influence was exerted by the alcoholism treatment unit which had been opened within the National Health Service by Dr Max Glatt at Warlingham Park Hospital in the early 1950s (Glatt, 1955). A substantial in-patient stay was at first advocated as the routine, with patients bussed out to attend AA. This model was enthusiastically taken up by the British Department of Health with the intention that units of that kind would be established throughout the UK, as the lead element in response to the now needy and deserving person suffering from the disease of alcoholism (Thom, 1999). The emphasis on group therapy was new, but otherwise what was seen as the therapeutic cutting edge was in fact to a large degree a recapitulation of earlier keenness for the institutional treatment of the inebriate.

In the USA, a development occurred from the 1970s onwards which emphasized a mix of in-patient care, milieu therapy and a Twelve Step (AA) approach, within what came to be referred to as the Minnesota Model (see Chapter 18). This regime rested squarely on the disease concept of alcoholism. From the late 1980s onwards, the popularity of this model was cramped by questions concerning cost-effectiveness, and by the imperatives of managed care (Galanter, 2000). Whatever the country, it is probably the economic imperatives rather than a change in theoretical orientation or the weight of research evidence that in today's treatment world have damped the ancient enthusiasm for the institution as remedy which stands alone.

Evolutions in the non-medical contribution to treatment

The twentieth-century evolutions in the non-medical contribution to the treatment of drinking problems have gone so far as to considerably change the face of the modern treatment enterprise.

A dominant influence of this type was seen in the evolution of AA from its small beginnings in 1933 as an off-shoot of the Oxford Group (an evangelical Christian sect) to an organization at present with a world-wide membership of over 2 million people (Kurtz, 1991). The influence of AA on shaping twentieth-century approaches to the treatment of alcohol dependence has been vast in terms of both setting ideas and determining practice (Edwards, 1996). It is a lay organization which has succeeded in powerfully shaping professional assumptions as to the nature of the condition being treated and the kind of treatment required – and all this although AA's primary and continuing impact is exerted through its group meetings and the help given to the next individual walking through the door.

Several historical strands can be seen as coming together in AA. Christianity is back in the picture, but without the clergy, and for some members of AA also without God. The ancient role model of 'reformed drunkard' is now the AA sponsor or the person who can capitalize on their experience to gain employment as a counsellor in a Twelve Step facility. The best show in town has been muted to become the still often gripping centrepiece of any AA meeting, the recovering alcoholic 'telling their story'.

If AA as transmitter of the ancient themes of repentance and redemption and salvation through faith has been one force shaping twentieth-century treatment, another powerful influence in the latter part of the twentieth century was the reincarnation of rationality seen in the influence of behavioural and cognitive psychology (Gossop, 1996). When dependence is viewed as habit to be unlearnt, it is evidently the psychologists who should be called on as experts in that kind of work.

Thus today's highly important overall non-medical contributions to the treatment of drinking problems derive from traditions which enshrine historically very different views on the nature of the problem and the help which the inebriate needs.

History — what significance for today's clinic?

History is relevant to any and every modern practitioner in this field, in terms of the invitation it makes to ask oneself certain questions. Others may see different questions as salient, but here is one tentative list of ideas on what history might give to some reflections while waiting for the next patient to arrive at today's clinic.

- In what way do today's facilities define the suitable case for treatment? What overt or latent assumptions, administrative fiats or historical influences set the rules? Are they optimal?
- What rationality, productive contradictions, muddling through or historical lumber set the therapist's personal model of understanding as to the nature of the condition which will today be treated? Have we really worked that question out in our minds? What do we do with sin, free will, habit, disease and other conceptual legacies? Is that model shared with our fellow professionals or patients?
- In a historically changing scene, what is the contribution which any specific professional skills are best likely today to make? How do our efforts fit with the larger, ever-shifting totality of the professional and lay effort to help the person with a drinking problem?
- How congruent are our professional beliefs with the background cultural beliefs of a multi-ethnic society, with how anyone watching tonight's television is likely to understand human behaviour?

Perhaps also, if we have time after the clinic to look in the library at some of the founding texts, we may find that today's work can be enriched by a sense of fellowship with clinicians who sat waiting for their patients more distantly. Let's close this chapter by again going back to Trotter (1804):

When inebriety has become so far habitual that some disease appears in consequence ... it is in vain to prescribe for it till the evil genius of the habit has been subdued. On such an occasion it is difficult to lay down rules. The physician must be guided by his own discretion: he must scrutinise the character of his patient, his pursuits, his modes of living, his very passions and private affairs. He must consult his own experience of human nature, and what he has learnt in the school of the world. The great point to be obtained is the confidence of the sick man; but this is not to be accomplished at a first visit. It is to be remembered that a bodily infirmity is not the only thing to be corrected.

Then Trotter gives that absolute summing up of his understanding, with the italics found in the original:

The habit of drunkenness is a disease of the mind.

REFERENCES

American Psychiatric Association (1994) *Diagnostic and Statistical Manual of Mental Disorders,* 4th edn *(DSM-IV)*. Washington, DC: American Psychiatric Association.

Astley Cooper, J.A. (1913) *Pathological Inebriety: its Causation and Treatment.* London: Baillière, Tindall and Cox.

Baasher, T. (1983) The use of drugs in the Islamic world. In *Drug Use and Misuse, Cultural Perspectives*, ed. Edwards, G., Arif, A. and Jaffe, J. London: Croom Helm; Geneva: World Health Organization, 21–34.

Blocker, J.S. (1989) *American Temperance Movements: Cycles of Reform.* Boston, MA: Twayne.

Booth, W. (1890) *In Darkest England and the Way Out.* London: International Headquarters of the Salvation Army.

Chick, J., Lloyd, G. and Crombie, E. (1985) Counselling problem drinkers in medical wards: a controlled study. *British Medical Journal* 290, 965–7.

Crothers, T. (1893) *The Disease of Inebriety from Alcohol, Opium, and other Narcotic Drugs, its Etiology, Pathology, Treatment and Medical–Legal Relations.* Arranged and compiled by the American Association for the Study and Cure of Inebriety. Bristol: John Wright and Co.

Crowley, J.W., ed. (1999) *Drunkard's Progress. Narratives of Addiction, Despair and Recovery.* Baltimore, MD: The Johns Hopkins University Press.

Edwards, G. (1976) Alcohol-related problems in the disability perspective. A summary of the consensus of the WHO group of investigators on criteria for identifying and classifying disabilities related to alcohol consumption. Eds Edwards, G., Gross, M.M., Keller, M. and Moser, J. *Journal of Studies on Alcohol* 37, 1360–82.

Edwards, G. (1996) Alcoholics Anonymous as a mirror held up to nature. In *Psychotherapy, Psychological Treatments and the Addictions*, ed. Edwards, G. and Dare, C. Cambridge: Cambridge University Press, 230–9.

Edwards, G. (2000) *Alcohol: the Ambiguous Molecule.* London, Penguin Books.

Galanter, M., ed. (2000) *Recent Developments in Alcoholism.* Volume 15. *Services Research in the Era of Managed Care.* New York: Kluewer Academic/Plenum Publishers.

Glatt, M.M. (1955) Treatment centre for alcoholics in a mental hospital. *Lancet* 1, 1316–20.

Gossop, M. (1996) Cognitive and behavioural treatments for substance misuse. In *Psychotherapy, Psychological Treatments and the Addictions*, ed. Edwards, G. and Dare, C. Cambridge: Cambridge University Press, 158–72.

Hald, J. and Jacobsen, E. (1948) A drug sensitising the organism to ethyl alcohol. *Lancet* 255, 1001–4.

Heather, N. and Robertson, I. (1981) *Controlled Drinking.* London: Methuen.

Huss, M. (1849) *Alcoholismus chronicus eller chronisk.* Stockholm: Alkolssjukdom.

Jellinek, E.M. (1952) Phases of alcohol addiction. *Quarterly Journal of Studies on Alcohol* 13, 573–684.

Jellinek, E.M. (1960) *The Disease Concept of Alcoholism.* New Brunswick, NJ: Hillhouse Press.

Kerr, N. (1887) *Inebriety, its Etiology, Pathology, Treatment and Jurisprudence.* London: H K Lewis.

Klingemann, H., Sobell L., Barker, J. et al. (2001) *Promoting Self-change from Problem Substance Use.* Dordrecht, The Netherlands: Kluewer Academic Publishers.

Kurtz, E. (1991) *Not-God: a History of Alcoholics Anonymous.* Center City, MN: Hazelden.

Lemere, F. (1987) Aversion treatment of alcoholism: some reminiscences. *British Journal of Addiction* 82, 257–8.

Marlatt, G.A. and Gordon, J.R. (1985) *Relapse Prevention.* New York: Guilford Press.

Maxwell, M.A. (1950) The Washingtonian Movement. *Quarterly Journal of Studies on Alcohol* 11, 411–15.

Room, R. (1977) Measurement and distribution of drinking patterns and problems in general populations. In *Alcohol Related Disabilities*, ed. Edwards, G., Gross, M.M., Keller, M., Moser, J. and Room, R. WHO Offset Publication No. 32. Geneva: World Health Organization, 61–8.

Rush, B. (1790) An Inquiry into the Effects of Ardent Spirits on the Human Body and Mind, with an Account of the Means for Preventing and of the Remedies for Curing Them. Eighth Edition 1814, Brookfields: E Merriam. Reprinted in *Quarterly Journal of Studies on Alcohol* (1943–44) 4, 325–41.

Shilo, B.F. (1961) O lechenii limonnym sokom khronicheskikh alkogolikov (On the treatment of chronic alcoholics with lemon juice). *Zdravookhr Beloruss* 7, 54–5.

Snyder, C.R. (1958) *Alcohol and the Jews: a Cultural Study of Drinking and Sobriety.* Glencoe, IL: Free Press.

Sobell, M.B. and Sobell, L.C. (1973) Alcoholics treated by individualized behavior therapy: one year treatment trial. *Behaviour Research and Therapy* 11, 599–618.

Sobell, M.B. and Sobell, L.C. (1976) Second year treatment outcome of alcoholics treated by individual behaviour therapy: results. *Behaviour Research and Therapy* 14, 195–215.

Stockwell, T., Hodgson, R., Edwards, G., Taylor, C. and Rankin, H. (1979) The development of a questionnaire to measure alcohol dependence. *British Journal of Addiction* 74, 79–87.

Thom, B. (1999) *Dealing with Drink.* London: Free Association Books.

Trotter, T. (1804) *An Essay, Medical, Philosophical, and Chemical, on Drunkenness, and its Effects on the Human Body.* London: T.N. Longman and G. Rees. Facsimile reproduction 1988 with an introduction by Roy Porter. London: Routledge.

Voegtlin, W.L. and Lemere, F. (1950) Conditioned reflex treatment of chronic alcoholism: a review of 4096 cases. *Quarterly Journal of Studies on Alcohol* 11, 199–204.

Wallace, P., Cutler, S. and Haines, A. (1988) Randomised controlled trial of general practitioner intervention in patients with excessive alcohol consumption. *British Medical Journal* 297, 663–8.

World Health Organization (1992) *The ICD-10 Classification of Mental and Behavioural Disorders.* Geneva: World Health Organization.

2

Causes of drinking problems

Why do some people drink so much more than others? Why also are some people able to drink large amounts of alcohol with apparent impunity, while others remain moderate and yet suffer problems as a result of their drinking? This chapter attempts to provide answers to these two questions. However, the complexity of the individual case and the extensiveness of the research literature both indicate that too simple answers should not be expected. Nor should it be imagined that any single factor can provide an adequate explanation. Drinking behaviour and the problems with which it is associated are determined by multiple, interacting factors which concern both the individual and his or her environment.

Drinking and drinking problems

The causes of 'heavy' drinking and drinking problems can only be properly under-stood within the context of an overall view of 'normal' drinking in the population as a whole. This is because there is no clear boundary between normal and heavy drinking, and because drinking problems occur in normal as well as heavy drinkers. A graph demonstrating the typical distribution of alcohol consumption within a population is shown in Figure 2.1. It may be seen that while the majority of people drink 'moderately', a small percentage drink very heavily indeed (a small percentage can mean a lot of people). However, it is quite arbitrary (on the basis of quantity alone) to choose a point at which to draw the line separating 'normal' and 'heavy' drinkers.

Extensive research has shown that the higher the average consumption of alcohol in a population, the higher the population's incidence of alcohol-related problems. This holds true for almost all types of alcohol-related problem – for example, drink driving offences, mortality due to cirrhosis of the liver and crimes of violence may all show such a relationship. This relationship also holds good at the individual level.

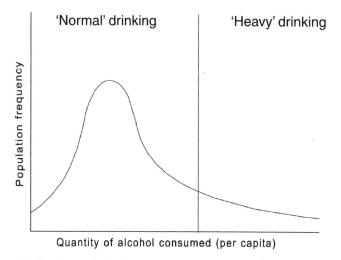

'Normal' drinking   'Heavy' drinking

Population frequency

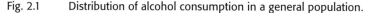

Quantity of alcohol consumed (per capita)

Fig. 2.1   Distribution of alcohol consumption in a general population.

Thus, for example, the risk of sustaining alcoholic liver disease, the risk of developing physical dependence upon alcohol and the risk of breast cancer in females all vary in proportion to an individual's habitual level of alcohol consumption (Edwards et al., 1994). With maximum benefit achieved at a low level of consumption (one to two drinks a day), alcohol can reduce the risk of coronary heart disease among men aged over 40 years and post-menopausal women.

Whilst heavy drinkers are at greater risk of various complications or problems arising from their drinking, Figure 2.1 reveals that (depending upon the arbitrary point at which we draw the line) there are many fewer heavy drinkers in the population than there are normal drinkers. Thus, although alcohol-related problems are relatively rare amongst normal drinkers, the bulk of such problems in the population as a whole may still occur in normal drinkers, not in heavy drinkers. This has been referred to as the 'prevention paradox' because, paradoxically, preventive measures aimed at reducing such problems have to be directed at the whole population of drinkers – not just the heavy drinkers.

In fact, the prevention paradox applies to some types of alcohol-related problems and not to others. The extent to which it applies depends upon the proportion of drinkers affected by a particular problem at each level of alcohol consumption (Edwards et al., 1994). In general terms, the prevention paradox applies to the more immediate social problems such as drinking and driving. In contrast, very heavy drinkers contribute the majority of chronic medical problems in a population (for instance cirrhosis).

The quantity of alcohol consumed is not the only characteristic of drinking which affects the occurrence of drinking problems. Pattern of alcohol consumption is also important. Accordingly, different drinking problems are likely to arise in the woman who drinks four glasses of wine every day as compared with the woman who drinks three bottles of wine in 2 days but who then drinks nothing for 2 or 3 weeks. Whilst the former is at greater risk of damage to the liver, brain and other organs, the latter is at greater risk of marital dysharmony and other social problems. Of course, the episodic or 'binge' drinker may have a relatively modest average consumption over time, and this may offer at least a partial explanation for the prevention paradox.

Political and economic causes of drinking problems

Unsurprisingly, the supply of alcohol within a community responds to demand. Thus, where the desirability of alcohol increases, new sources (legal or illegal) will be created to meet that demand. However, the relationship is not unidirectional. Variations in supply can and do influence demand (Holder, 2000). Within individual countries over time, and in comparisons of different countries at any given time, it has been shown that reducing the real price of alcohol tends to increase the overall consumption of alcohol by a population. Similarly, measures which make alcohol more readily available by reducing restrictions on its supply also tend to increase consumption. Thus major influences upon per-capita consumption in a population include factors amenable to political manipulation – such as taxation, licensing laws and trade agreements. Manipulation of such influences can have enormous impact upon the level of alcohol consumption of a population. Conversely, failure to utilize such controls can allow alcohol consumption to escalate and related problems to reach epidemic proportions (Edwards et al., 1994).

Many of the influences upon the economics of alcohol consumption are not deliberately manipulated, but follow in the wake of social change. Thus, for example, rapid socio-economic changes in Eastern Europe led to increased availability of alcohol, increased consumption and increased drinking problems during the early 1990s. This would suggest that, where possible, policy initiatives should be put in place as an intentional preventive measure, in advance of such changes. Equally, where controls on price and access already exist, they should not be removed for political, ideological or trade reasons, with their public health significance ignored.

The influence of supply upon demand for alcohol indicates that the alcohol supply system (production, distribution, wholesale, import/export and retail sale) will be an important consideration in any analysis of alcohol policy in relation to public health and safety. Many important questions are raised concerning the relationship between a multinational drinks industry and national governments, and the nature, strategy and determination of growth within this industry. In short, policy makers and researchers must ask 'What drives the alcohol supply side?' (Edwards and Holder, 2000). It is important to remember that the supply system operates at a local level as well as at national and international levels. Factors such as the density and distribution of outlets may influence local incidence of alcohol-related road traffic accidents or violence (Gruenewald and Treno, 2000).

Socio-cultural causes of drinking problems

The availability of alcohol and factors which influence availability (such as economic influences) are not the only factors of importance at a population level. Acceptability of alcohol consumption also plays an important part, and this is determined to a large degree by social and cultural values. However, these influences operate at various levels. For example, national and racial, religious, occupational and family influences may all play a part.

Some cultures and societies promote total abstinence, for example Islamic culture or the USA during Prohibition. In these cases, the influence on drinking is explicitly negative, although there may be an associated counter-reaction towards illicit drinking, such that some members of the population still drink and the population as a whole may suffer from the associated criminal activity. At the other extreme are permissive cultures, including many Mediterranean countries, where drinking is actively endorsed. Such countries usually have high rates of morbidity attributable to, for example, alcoholic liver disease. In between these extremes there may be a mixture of cultural influences encouraging or discouraging drinking. In some cases, strongly opposing influences may be found in the same culture. Thus, for example, in Ireland there is a strong temperance movement within a culture that otherwise accepts and encourages drinking as part of the general social order. In Jewish societies drinking is generally socially accepted, but strong negative connotations are attached to deviant drinking behaviour such as public drunkenness. Some would argue that this combination is responsible for the low incidence of alcohol-related problems in Jewish societies (Bales, 1946).

One important element of culture is religious practice. It will be noted that virtually all of the examples offered in the last paragraph have some bearing on this. It has been observed that 'alcoholics' are less likely to be involved in religious practices (Larson and Wilson, 1980) and that religious observance is correlated with lower rates of drinking problems (Koenig et al., 1994). Amongst young people, religiosity and attendance at religious services are associated with more moderate alcohol consumption (Booth and Martin, 1998).

Culture can influence the pattern and context, as well as the amount, of alcohol consumption. Pattern of alcohol consumption may in turn be an important determinant of drinking problems. Thus, in France habitual consumption of wine with meals is associated with a relatively high, but constant, per-capita consumption which predisposes towards chronic medical complications such as cirrhosis and certain cancers. In urban centres in the UK and North America, particularly amongst working-class men, alcohol is more likely to be consumed away from the home and often in relatively large quantities at a sitting. This pattern of drinking to intoxication seems to be more likely to be accompanied by adverse social consequences such as marital dysharmony, accidents, interpersonal violence or drunkenness offences.

Culture may also influence the ways in which people behave when intoxicated. Thus, drunken behaviour may be determined not only by the biological effects of alcohol as a drug, but also by social and cultural expectations as to how people will behave when drinking (MacAndrew and Edgerton, 1970). This may influence, for example, the likelihood of drunken antisocial behaviour.

There is a wide variation in drinking behaviour, and alcohol-related problems, amongst different occupations. To some degree this may be a selection process which affects choice of occupation. However, there is also evidence that occupational environment itself influences drinking. Thus, for example, new employees in the drinks industry are likely to be relatively heavy drinkers, but there is evidence that they further increase their alcohol consumption after working in that industry (Plant, 1979). To some extent, as in this example, this may reflect ready availability of alcohol in a particular occupational environment. However, in different industries and occupations, a variety of other factors are also thought to be important, including, for example, frequent absence from home, lack of supervision, long and irregular hours, social and peer pressures to drink (e.g. business lunches) and high stresses or hazards in the workplace.

Family 'culture' may also be an important influence upon drinking. In addition to any genetic influences, it seems likely that children will 'inherit' heavy drinking patterns by virtue of learning this behaviour, and any associated values or beliefs, from their parents. However, not all heavy-drinking parents beget heavy-drinking children. Where family rituals (including family traditions, ways of celebrating special occasions and daily routines) are not disrupted by parental drinking, and where adult children deliberately establish new rituals when they marry, it seems that 'alcoholism' is less likely to be passed on to the next generation (Wolin et al., 1979; Bennett and Wolin, 1986). The importance of family factors is discussed further in Chapter 5.

Stress and life events

Major life events and everyday hassles both appear to increase the amounts that people drink. This may be explained on the basis that alcohol relieves anxiety and is thus used as a means of coping with stress (the so-called 'tension reduction' hypothesis). There is also evidence that an increased frequency of life events precedes the onset of alcohol misuse (Tatossian et al., 1983). These factors would therefore appear to be an important contributor to the development of drinking problems. However, the research evidence is not consistent and heavy drinking tends to cause further stress in the form of the problems that it generates (divorce, unemployment, ill health, and so on). There is also evidence that alcohol can exacerbate anxiety rather than relieve it. The association between heavy drinking and stress is therefore a complex one and should not be seen as simple cause and effect.

Contextual drinking problems

Drink driving is an important example of a contextual drinking problem. Relatively modest alcohol consumption, which would cause no social, psychological or medical problems in most other contexts, may be the cause of serious injury or death when the drinker is also the driver of a car. Similar considerations also apply to other forms of transportation, as well as to a variety of other safety-sensitive situations, particularly in the workplace. The risk of a person being drowned in a boating accident will increase even with a blood level of 10 mg%, and at 250 mg% the relative risk will be 52 times that of a person with a zero blood alcohol concentration (Smith et al., 2001)

Nature and nurture

Thus far, this analysis of the causes of heavy drinking and drinking problems may appear to indicate that the drinker is a victim of the environment, with individual factors having little part to play. These environmental influences are summarized in Box 2.1. Of course, this is at variance with our experience of the free will that we deploy in making decisions about our drinking, as well as the observation that some individuals in a heavy drinking environment drink moderately, or not at all.

BOX 2.1 **Some environmental determinants of drinking problems**
- Individual and population levels of drinking
- Culture and religion
- Occupation
- Family experience of heavy drinking
- Stress and life events
- Safety-sensitive environments, e.g. driving

What part do individual factors play in the causes of heavy drinking and drinking problems?

It has long been observed that drinking problems tend to run in families (Cotton, 1979). The explanation for this was often assumed to be the effect of the family environment upon its members, tending in some way to produce uniformity of behaviour. There is almost certainly some truth in this hypothesis. However, more recent research has attempted to disentangle the effects of family environment from those of heredity. By studying identical and non-identical twins, and children raised in adoptive families and apart from their biological parents, it is possible to separate the effects of 'nature' and 'nurture'. With only a few exceptions, such studies have tended to confirm that there is a genetic component to drinking behaviour and drinking problems, in addition to the undeniably important influence of the environment (Cook, 1994).

What is it that is inherited, which in some way causes heavy drinking, alcohol-related problems or alcohol dependence? In most cases the answer to this question is not known. However, some clues are available and we may indulge in some informed speculation. For example, in Oriental populations, a genetic variant of one of the enzymes involved in alcohol metabolism (aldehyde dehydrogenase) is responsible for a 'flushing' syndrome which is manifested by an unpleasant physiological response to the ingestion of alcohol. Carriers of the mutant gene tend to drink little or no alcohol, because they feel unwell when they do. This genetic effect, due to a single gene mutation, dramatically reduces the incidence of heavy drinking and thus the alcohol-related problems amongst those affected by it. Similar but more subtle effects may influence the amount that Caucasian individuals drink.

Genetic effects also directly influence the incidence of drinking problems. For example, it would seem likely that particular organ systems (e.g. liver or brain) might be subject to genetic variation in vulnerability to alcohol-induced damage. This hypothesis is supported, for example, by one of the twin studies of drinking problems, which showed evidence for a genetic influence upon both alcohol-induced liver disease and alcoholic psychosis (Hrubec and Omenn, 1981).

There is also evidence of a genetic influence upon liability to alcohol dependence (Cook and Gurling, 2001). The exact mechanism by which this effect is conferred is not yet known. However, alcohol dependence is associated with an increase in the number of voltage-operated calcium channels in the cell membrane and this is affected by gene activation (Harper et al., 1989). One hypothesis could be that there are genetically determined differences in the extent to which the number of these channels is increased in response to heavy drinking. Alternatively, it has been suggested that an inherited state of hyperexcitability in the central nervous system is temporarily corrected by ingestion of alcohol. Such individuals may therefore be predisposed to drinking as a means of obtaining relief, and thus may be at greater risk of developing alcohol dependence (Begleiter and Porjesz, 1999).

A recent, large, multi-centre research project undertaken in the USA applied molecular genetic research methods to the study of alcohol dependence and other drinking problems. In contrast to twin and adoption studies, these methods potentially enable the identification of specific genes or chromosomal regions which show evidence of influencing the incidence of alcohol dependence and other drinking problems. Results so far suggest that a region of chromosome 4 may confer a protection against alcohol dependence in some families. Other chromosomal regions (e.g. on chromosomes 1 and 7) are thought to confer susceptibility to alcohol dependence (Reich et al., 1998).

How, then, can the evidence supporting the importance of both genetic and environmental causes for heavy drinking and drinking problems be brought together? The truth is, of course, that a behaviour such as alcohol consumption cannot be totally understood on the basis of either genes or environment alone, but only as a product of the interaction between a variety of genetic and environmental influences. Thus, one might see an individual as being more or less disposed to heavy drinking, or to particular alcohol-related problems, or to dependence upon alcohol. This level of predisposition determines the risk, or probability of being a heavy drinker, or of suffering from a particular drink-related problem. If a combination of environmental and genetic risk factors exceeds a certain hypothetical threshold, then that individual will drink heavily, or suffer a particular problem associated with their drinking.

We may now understand the enigma of the individual who drinks heavily and escapes harm, or of the person who drinks moderately and suffers various complications. In the former case, the individual may be predisposed to heavy drinking by a combination of heredity and environmental factors. However, at the same time, that person may have a (genetic) constitutional resilience which protects them from liver damage and may learn (from their environment) social controls and patterns of behaviour which avoid public drunkenness, drink driving or other alcohol-related problems. In the latter case, the reverse may be true. Thus, the individual may drink moderately as a result of minimal genetic and environmental predisposition towards heavy drinking and yet be subject to, say, liver disease owing to genetic susceptibility of the liver to damage by alcohol.

Psychological explanations of drinking behaviour

The psychological characteristics of an individual may be seen as a product of their genetic constitution and the environment in which they live and grow. Psychological theories of drinking behaviour have been many and varied, but we can identify at least three main themes here. Firstly, there are psychodynamic theories which explain drinking as a result of early experiences and relationships. Secondly, cognitive and behavioural theories explain drinking as a learned behaviour. Thirdly, it has been suggested that certain personalities are particularly vulnerable, perhaps because of a tendency to use alcohol to deal with stress, anxiety, depression or other problems.

It is often possible to apply all of these explanations to a given case. Take, for example, a woman with a drinking problem talking about her childhood:

> I can't think how I ever took to drinking myself when I remember what I went through in childhood. I hated the smell of the stuff. My father was more often drunk than sober, and my mother was stark terrified of him, would hide us away when she heard him coming home. What do I go and do? I follow exactly in his footsteps. I'm as nasty when drunk as ever my Dad used to be.

This woman may be drinking as a way of coping with the anger that she feels towards her father. She may also be drinking to relieve her feelings of guilt about the way that she treats her own family. As this causes more harm to the family, more guilt is generated and so a vicious cycle is set up, in which guilt leads to drinking which leads to more guilt, and so on. The dynamic therapist might see this as a problem concerning unresolved anger towards her father. However, this scenario can also be understood on the basis of learnt patterns of behaviour copied from her father, or on the basis of a conditioning process whereby drinking is reinforced because (in the short term) it relieves unpleasant experiences of anxiety, anger and guilt. A genetic influence may also be at work.

The theory that there is a specific 'addictive personality' is now largely disproved. In so far as it is possible to separate the consequences of drinking from its causes, it does not appear to be possible to predict 'addictive' personality traits which inevitably lead to alcohol misuse, drug addiction or other problems of an addictive nature. However, some personality traits do seem to predispose to heavy drinking or alcohol misuse. Thus, a tendency to experience anxiety or depression or antisocial traits may increase the risk of heavy drinking. None of these traits inevitably leads to drinking problems, and not all heavy drinkers or problem drinkers manifest them.

In addition to these psychological explanations of the origins of heavy drinking, there is the observation that heavy drinking may be associated with various psychiatric disorders. These disorders may be complications arising from the excessive consumption of alcohol, or they may be the underlying cause of heavy drinking, and often they are both. In such cases, it can be difficult to make judgements as to which problem came first. The relationship between psychiatric problems (including personality disorder) and drinking is explored further in Chapter 7.

The lifetime perspective

'Alcoholism' is viewed by some as a chronic, progressive and, if left unchecked, inevitably fatal disease (Johnson, 1980). Certainly, a review of the life history of a typical member of Alcoholics Anonymous (AA) would appear to support this contention.

John started drinking in his early teens. He soon found that his friends were impressed by his ability to 'hold his drink', and as he grew older his social life increasingly revolved around pubs, bars and clubs. Being naturally rather shy, he found that drinking not only relieved his anxieties about meeting people, but it also 'made him belong' within a social scene that revolved around alcohol. At the age of 18 he was charged with drinking and driving. His girlfriend left him a year later saying that she could no longer tolerate the way that he behaved when he was drinking. Within 5 years he had also lost two jobs because of persistent lateness and poor performance. At the age of 24 years, when attending hospital for a head injury following a fall, he was noted to be severely alcohol dependent.

Such stories illustrate the combination of individual factors (personality, for instance) and environmental factors (social pressures and the 'youth culture') that lead to alcohol dependence, and appear to support the contention that 'alcoholism' is indeed qualitatively different from 'normal' drinking. Yet, as has already been stated, an epidemiological perspective does not appear to support this contention. In fact, many young people drink heavily and experience some of the predictable alcohol-related problems associated with such consumption, yet they do not inevitably progress to more serious or more frequent problems, or to alcohol dependence (Temple and Fillmore, 1985). Indeed, increasing age generally seems to moderate the less-restrained alcohol consumption of youth.

A person's age is, of course, simply another example of an individual characteristic which influences their liability to develop drinking problems. The importance of the lifetime perspective of heavy drinking is further emphasized by the interaction that occurs between age and environmental factors. Drink–driving is a particularly poignant example of this. The young person is relatively inexperienced, both in terms of driving and also in terms of drinking behaviour. At a given blood alcohol concentration, this combination results in a much higher risk of accidents for the younger driver.

A fuller consideration of the life course perspective is given in Chapter 13.

Application to practical contexts

Some of the research described in this chapter remains academic in day-to-day practice. For example, efforts to help the problem drinker may be relatively uninfluenced by the knowledge that he or she has a strong family history of drinking problems. Nor will it be very important in practice to know whether that familiality is determined by genetic or cultural causes. However, neither should it be assumed that such matters are irrelevant to the practical contexts within which policies are made and clinical treatments offered.

Present or future applications of research and knowledge concerning the causes of drinking problems may be identified in the realms of prevention and treatment. Policy making, health and public education, individual and family counselling and drug treatments are all influenced in various ways (Box 2.2).

BOX 2.2 **Levels of application of knowledge of the causes of drinking problems to prevention and treatment**

Prevention
- Policy (e.g. taxation, licensing laws, drink driving legislation, workplace policy)
- Health education (e.g. advising the individual patient on 'sensible' drinking)
- Public education (e.g. promoting public awareness of the nature and causes of alcohol-related problems)

Treatment
- Assessment (e.g. family history, occupational history, spiritual/religious history)
- Matching of treatments to patients (e.g. relapse prevention, drug treatments)
- Family therapy (e.g. addressing family routines and rituals in the 'alcoholic family')

Policy making is most obviously influenced by the wealth of research on the ways in which the availability and acceptability of alcohol within the community influence the epidemiology of alcohol-related problems (Edwards et al., 1994; Holder and Edwards, 1995). Taxation, legislation, service planning and workplace policies are all potentially effective tools of prevention. Such policies are known to be effective because of empirical research support. They are effective in practice because of the ways in which they influence and manipulate the underlying causes of alcohol-related problems.

Knowledge of the causes of alcohol-related problems also influences face-to-face health education in clinical practice and public education in the wider community. For example, the question often arises as to what constitutes 'safe' or 'sensible' drinking. In truth, and as this chapter shows, the answer to this question will vary depending upon a range of individual and environmental vulnerability factors, many of which may be unknown. Because of this uncertainty, general guidelines for sensible drinking have been offered, which are estimated to be appropriate for most members of the population (Royal College of Psychiatrists, 1986; British

Medical Association, 1995; Royal College of Physicians et al., 1995). No drinking is, however, absolutely safe for all drinkers, on all occasions, and in all environments, and advice cannot properly be mechanistic. The child of the parent with a drinking problem, the person who is anxious or depressed and the drinks industry employee are examples of people at particular risk, who may find it difficult to adhere to simple advice in practice, because of either constitutional susceptibility or environmental pressures, or both. A knowledge of the environmental and constitutional factors which make an individual vulnerable to drinking problems is therefore important, both to the professional asked to advise on such matters and also to the individual wishing to make rational decisions about their own drinking.

In relation to the actual business of treatment, the matters discussed in this chapter are relevant to the approach to case assessment that is outlined in Chapter 15. There, it will be suggested that whenever assessing patients, or planning their treatment, the requirement must be to look in detail both at the individuals and their environment and to examine the multiple factors, both remote and current, which may bear on the genesis of their drinking problem. The research discussed in the present chapter gives that assessment approach its scientific underpinning.

It is also likely that in future different interventions will be offered to different groups of problem drinkers. Relapse prevention methods may be particularly appropriate for those people who drink to relieve anxiety. Particular drug treatments may be more beneficial for those with certain types of genetic predisposition (Lawford et al., 1995). However, at present, relatively little is known about how to achieve the optimum match of different treatments with different problem drinkers (Lindström, 1992).

In addition to the population and individual contexts, knowledge of the causes of alcohol-related problems has application to the support and treatment offered to families. Although family therapy or family counselling is often not available as a component of treatment, our knowledge of the ways in which genetics and family environment contribute to the causation of alcohol-related problems would suggest that there is an important place at this level for both information giving and psychological therapy. For example, a knowledge of the way in which family rituals and routines are impacted by alcohol misuse has been used as the basis of therapy for the alcoholic family (Steinglass et al., 1987; see Chapter 5).

Overall, it may be said that a knowledge of the causes of and predispositions to drinking problems is likely to offer a more informed, focused and effective approach to any area of engagement with alcohol-related problems. This is true regardless of whether the professional is working with individuals, groups, families or communities; whether in treatment or prevention; and whether the domain of interest is clinical, educational or political.

REFERENCES

Bales, R.F. (1946) Cultural differences in rates of alcoholism. *Quarterly Journal of Studies on Alcohol* 6, 489–99.

Begleiter, H. and Porjesz, B. (1999) What is inherited in the predisposition toward alcoholism? A proposed model. *Alcoholism, Clinical and Experimental Research* 23, 1125–35.

Bennett, L.A. and Wolin, S.J. (1986) Daughters and sons of alcoholics: developmental paths in transmission. *Alcoholism* 22, 3–15.

Booth, J. and Martin, J.E. (1998) Spiritual and religious factors in substance use, dependence, and recovery. In *Handbook of Religion and Mental Health*, ed. Koenig, H.G. San Diego: Academic Press, 175–200.

British Medical Association (1995) *Alcohol: Guidelines on Sensible Drinking*. London, British Medical Association.

Cook, C.C.H. (1994) Aetiology of alcohol misuse. In *Seminars in Psychiatry: Alcohol and Drug Misuse*, ed. Chick, J. and Cantwell, R. London: Royal College of Psychiatrists, 94–125.

Cook, C.C.H. and Gurling, H.M.D. (2001) Genetic predisposition to alcohol dependence and problems. In *International Handbook of Alcohol Dependence and Problems*, ed. Heather, N., Peters, T.J. and Stockwell, T. Chichester: John Wiley and Sons, 257–9.

Cotton, N.S. (1979) The familial incidence of alcoholism. *Journal of Studies on Alcohol* 40, 89–116.

Edwards, G., Anderson, P., Babor, T.F. et al. (1994) *Alcohol Policy and the Public Good*. Oxford: Oxford University Press.

Edwards, G. and Holder, H.D. (2000) The alcohol supply: its importance to public health and safety, and essential research questions. The supply side initiative: international collaboration to study the alcohol supply, ed. Holder, H.D. *Addiction* 95 (Suppl. 4): 621–7.

Gruenewald, P.J. and Treno, A.J. (2000) Local and global alcohol supply: economic and geographic models of community systems. The supply side initiative: international collaboration to study the alcohol supply, ed. Holder, H.D. *Addiction* 95 (Suppl. 4): 537–49.

Harper, J.C., Brennan, C.H. and Littleton, J.M. (1989) Genetic up-regulation of calcium channels in a cellular model of ethanol dependence. *Neuropharmacology* 28, 1299–302.

Holder, H.D. (2000) The supply side initiative as an international collaboration to study alcohol supply, drinking and consequences: current knowledge, policy issues, and research opportunities. The supply side initiative: international collaboration to study the alcohol supply, ed. Holder, H.D. *Addiction* 95 (Suppl. 4): 461–3.

Holder, H. and Edwards, G. (1995) *Alcohol and Public Policy: Evidence and Issues*. Oxford: Oxford University Press.

Hrubec, Z. and Omenn, G.S. (1981) Evidence of genetic predisposition to alcoholic psychosis and cirrhosis: twin concordances for alcoholism and its biological end points by zygosity among male veterans. *Alcoholism, Clinical and Experimental Research* 5, 207–15.

Johnson, V.E. (1980) *I'll Quit Tomorrow*. New York, Harper and Row.

Koenig, H.G., George, L.K., Meador, K.G., Blazer, D.G. and Ford, S.M. (1994) Religious practices and alcoholism in a southern adult population. *Hospital and Community Psychiatry* 45, 225–31.

Larson, D.B. and Wilson, W.P. (1980) Religious life of alcoholics. *Southern Medical Journal* 73, 723–7.

Lawford, B.R., Young, R.McD., Rowell, J.A. et al. (1995) Bromocriptine in the treatment of alcoholics with the D2 dopamine receptor A1 allele. *Nature Medicine* 1, 337–41.

Lindström, L. (1992) *Managing Alcoholism: Matching Clients to Treatments.* Oxford: Oxford University Press.

MacAndrew, C. and Edgerton, R.B. (1970) *Drunken Comportment.* London: Nelson.

Plant, M.A. (1979) *Drinking Careers.* London: Tavistock.

Reich, T., Edenberg, H.J., Goate, A. et al. (1998) A genome-wide search for genes affecting the risk for alcohol dependence. *American Journal of Medical Genetics* 81, 207–15.

Royal College of Physicians, Royal College of Psychiatrists, Royal College of General Practitioners (1995) *Alcohol and the Heart in Perspective: Sensible Limits Reaffirmed.* London: Royal Colleges of Physicians, Psychiatrists and General Practitioners.

Royal College of Psychiatrists (1986) *Alcohol: Our Favourite Drug.* London: Tavistock.

Smith, G.S., Keyl, P.M., Hadley, J.A. et al. (2001) Drinking and recreational boating fatalities. A population-based case-control study. *Journal of the American Medical Association* 286, 2974–80.

Steinglass, P., Bennett, L.A., Wolin, S.J. and Reiss, D. (1987) *The Alcoholic Family.* London: Hutchinson.

Tatossian, A., Charpy, J.P., Remy, M., Prinquey, D. and Poinso, Y. (1983) Events in the lives of 120 chronic alcoholics: preliminary study. *Annales Medico-Psychologiques* 141, 824–41.

Temple, M.T. and Fillmore, K.M. (1985) The variability of drinking patterns and problems among young men age 16–31: a longitudinal study. *International Journal of the Addictions* 20, 1595–620.

Wolin, S.J., Bennett, L.A. and Noonan, D.L. (1979) Family rituals and the recurrence of alcoholism over generations. *American Journal of Psychiatry* 136, 589–93.

3

Alcohol as a drug

The purpose of this chapter

Alcohol is a beverage which is rich with symbolic significance when used within social, cultural and religious custom and ritual. Its properties have been familiar to countless peoples around the world for thousands of years. However, it is also a drug which has important pharmacological and toxic effects, both upon the mind and upon almost every organ and system in the human body. A knowledge of these pharmacological effects is basic to understanding many of the problems that arise from its use, as well as to a consideration of how we may offer treatment for these problems. There is today considerable excitement among researchers about advances in our understanding of the biological actions of alcohol and we hope that this chapter conveys that sense: much more is known in this field than 10–20 years ago.

What is discussed here will inevitably make difficult reading for people whose expertise is in a discipline other than medicine. Some of those readers may want to move on straightaway to Chapter 4, but others may find it valuable to obtain at least a nodding acquaintance with what is happening at this pharmacological frontline. We are in no way seeking to imply that biological sciences provide the only or key insight into the determinants of drinking behaviour – in this book psychological and social influences on drinking and the genesis of drinking problems will receive very full attention.

Absorption and distribution

Alcohol is rapidly absorbed into the circulation from the stomach, small intestine and colon, and the time to maximum concentration in the blood ranges from 30 to 90 minutes. The rate of absorption is influenced by a number of factors. Higher alcohol concentrations (up to a maximum of 40% by volume) and the presence of carbon dioxide and bicarbonate in fizzy drinks increase absorption. The presence of food in the stomach slows absorption by delaying gastric emptying. A fall in body temperature and physical exercise also reduce absorption, as does the presence of sugar in the alcohol. Peak blood levels are higher if the same quantity of alcohol is ingested in a single dose rather than in several small doses (Agarwal and Goedde, 1990). In women, the stage of the menstrual cycle can influence absorption.

Following absorption, alcohol is distributed throughout the body. It is hydrophilic (water loving), accumulates in tissues with the highest water content, and can cross the placenta into the foetal circulation. Highly perfused organs such as the brain, lungs and kidney show the highest alcohol levels, whereas in tissues with less blood flow, such as muscle, alcohol concentrations are lower.

Blood alcohol concentration (BAC) is very similar to tissue levels in most of the body except fat. The relatively higher body fat in women leads to a higher BAC than would occur in men after an equivalent dose of alcohol. This may explain, at least in part, the increased vulnerability of women to certain types of tissue damage.

Excretion and metabolism

Between 90% and 98% of ingested alcohol is eliminated from the body by oxidation to carbon dioxide and water. Most of the alcohol that escapes oxidation is excreted unchanged in expired air, urine and sweat; elimination by these routes may increase after a heavy drinking bout or at elevated temperatures.

Hepatic alcohol metabolism

The amount of alcohol oxidized per unit time depends on body weight. In the healthy adult, the average rate of metabolism is 120 mg per kg per hour, equivalent to 30 ml in 3 hours (Fleming et al., 2001). Breakdown can be faster in the heavier drinker (see below). Alcohol may undergo first pass metabolism (FPM) in the stomach, but 90–98% of ingested alcohol is metabolized in the liver. The major pathway is oxidation by alcohol dehydrogenase (ADH) to acetaldehyde (Fig. 3.1). Acetaldehyde is highly toxic and is rapidly oxidized by aldehyde dehydrogenase (ALDH) to acetate. Both ADH and ALDH are nicotinamide adenine dinucleotide (NAD) dependent and the oxidations of alcohol and acetaldehyde reduce NAD to NADH. Excess NADH can cause hyperlacticacidaemia, which can contribute to acidosis, reduce urinary excretion of uric acid and lead to secondary hyperuricaemia. NADH also contributes to hypoglycaemia and hyperlipidaemia (Lieber, 1995; see Chapter 10).

The enzymes ADH and ALDH are under genetic control. Five classes of ADH have been described and the class 1 variety is largely responsible for the first step in

ETHANOL

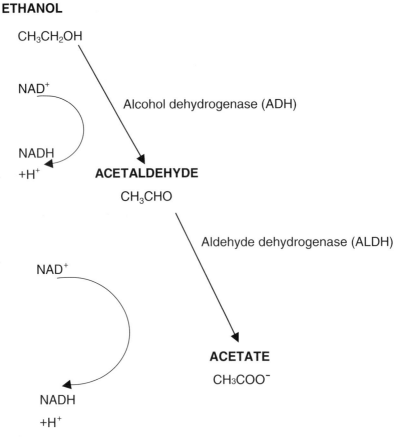

Fig. 3.1   Metabolism of alcohol.

alcohol metabolism in the liver. At least four isozymes of ALDH have been detected in humans. ALDH2, the isozyme largely responsible for the oxidation of acetaldehyde, exists in two forms, one of which is virtually inactive. Low-activity ALDH2, which is common in Orientals, leads to a flushing reaction when alcohol is taken. This reaction is unpleasant; therefore individuals with low-activity ALDH2 are less inclined to drink and are thus less vulnerable to developing alcohol dependence. Low-activity ALDH2 is also associated with a reduced rate of alcoholic liver disease (see Chapter 2). The acetate formed from acetaldehyde is released into the circulation and is largely taken up by muscle and heart for oxidation via the tricarboxylic acid cycle (Crabb, 1993).

Although ADH is the major pathway for the oxidation of alcohol, it can be oxidized by two other enzymes systems, the microsomal ethanol-oxidizing system (MEOS) located in the smooth endoplasmic reticulum (SER), and catalase, located in peroxisomes. The contribution of catalase is thought to be minimal. The MEOS is dependent on the cytochrome P450 system that is located on the SER. It usually plays a small role in the metabolism of alcohol, but this role increases with increased consumption. Chronic alcohol intake enhances MEOS activity by a process of inducing a form of P450 called CYP2E1. The induction of CYP2E1 leads to an increase in the rate of alcohol metabolism and to an increased tolerance to alcohol and other drugs. Induction also leads to an increased production of acetaldehyde which is toxic, and to increases in the metabolism of other drugs such as tolbutamide (an oral anti-diabetic drug), warfarin (an oral anticoagulant or blood thinner), propranolol, diazepam and rifamycins (anti-tuberculous drugs) (Lieber, 2001).

Induction of CYP2E1 can convert many drugs into toxic metabolites, including anaesthetic agents, illicit drugs such as cocaine, other drugs such as isoniazid (an important anti-tuberculous drug), phenylbutazone (a strong anti-inflammatory drug) and paracetamol. Therapeutic amounts of paracetamol can cause hepatic damage in heavy drinkers (Lieber, 1995). Induction of CYP2E1 also results in increased production of reactive radicals and toxic metabolites which contribute to liver injury.

Extrahepatic alcohol metabolism

Extrahepatic metabolism of alcohol (metabolism outside the liver) is low. However, the stomach is exposed to large quantities of alcohol and the gastric mucosa (lining of the stomach) also contains several enzymes with ADH activity (ADH isoenzymes). Class IV ADH (now called σ-ADH or sigma ADH) is present in the gastric mucosa and not in the liver. Class V ADH is present in both stomach and liver. It is now accepted that alcohol is subjected to a FPM by the ADH isoenzymes in the stomach and that this represents some kind of protection against the systemic effects of alcohol (Lieber, 2001). Ethnic and gender differences in the role of gastric ADH in FPM of ethanol have been described. For instance, a large percentage of Japanese people lack or have a low-activity sigma ADH, and their FPM is reduced. Gastric ADH activity is lower in Caucasian women than in men and this diminished activity is accentuated in women with alcohol dependence. This leads to higher blood alcohol levels in women, thus increasing their vulnerability to end organ damage. Women also have a smaller water space. This is discussed further in Chapters 10 and 11 (Frezza et al., 1990).

Gastric ADH isoenzymes work optimally when there is a relatively high alcohol concentration. Thus, for equivalent amounts of alcohol, whisky will be associated with a higher FPM and lower blood level than beer. Fasting also decreases FPM. When alcohol is metabolized in the stomach, it is converted to acetaldehyde, which, because of its toxicity, may cause gastric injury.

Pharmacological effects

Cardiovascular system

The effects of alcohol on the circulation are minor. Moderate doses cause a small, transient increase in heart rate and vasodilatation, especially in the skin, with facial flushing. There is no increase in coronary blood flow. Blood pressure, cardiac output and force of cardiac contractility are not significantly affected by moderate amounts of alcohol. Large doses produce an increase in cerebral blood flow, decreased cerebrovascular resistance and reduced cerebral oxygen uptake.

Body temperature

Moderate amounts of alcohol can lead to peripheral vasodilatation and sweating. Increased sweating can, in turn, lead to heat loss and a fall in body temperature. Large amounts of alcohol can depress the central temperature-regulating mechanism, causing a more pronounced fall in body temperature.

Gastrointestinal tract

Alcohol can stimulate gastric secretion by reflex excitation of sensory endings in the buccal (mouth) and gastric mucosa and by a direct action on the stomach, possibly involving the release of gastrin. Strong alcoholic drinks cause inflammation of the stomach lining and produce an erosive gastritis. Alcohol intoxication causes cessation of gastrointestinal secretory and motor functions.

Kidney

Alcohol itself produces a diuretic effect independent from the increased flow associated with the ingestion of large volumes of fluid. This diuretic effect is proportional to the blood alcohol concentration and occurs when levels are rising, but not when they are stable or falling.

Respiration

Moderate amounts of alcohol may stimulate or depress respiration, whereas large amounts (greater than 400 mg per 100 ml) produce depression of respiration.

Central nervous system

The effects of alcohol on the brain are dependent on dose and the rate of rise in BAC. Driving skill is affected at 30 mg%. Ataxia, inattention and slowed reaction times are evident at levels of about 50 mg%. Mood and behavioural changes occur at levels of approximately 50–100 mg%. At levels of 150–300 mg%, there is loss of self-control, slurred speech and clumsiness. Individuals unused to heavy drinking are moderately intoxicated at BAC levels of 150–250 mg% and obvious intoxication is usually evident at 300 mg%. At BACs of 300–500 mg%, individuals are usually severely intoxicated, and stupor and hypothermia may sometimes supervene. Hypoglycaemia and seizures are occasionally a feature of BACs in this range. Heavy drinkers become tolerant to the central nervous system (CNS) effects of alcohol and may on occasion have BAC levels of 500 mg% without obvious signs of intoxication. However, for non-tolerant drinkers, such levels are associated with depressed reflexes, respiratory depression, hypotension, hypothermia and sometimes death.

Alcohol is a relatively non-specific psychoactive drug which interacts with the major neurotransmitter systems, gamma-aminobutyric acid (GABA), glutamate, dopamine, endogenous opioids and serotonin, as well as second messenger systems (Eckardt et al., 1998; Nutt, 1999). It has been shown that the stimulatory sedative, anxiolytic and reinforcing effects of alcohol occur within different and relatively narrow dose ranges (Grant et al., 1990a). Until relatively recently, it was thought that the CNS effects of alcohol were mediated by its action on neuronal membranes, increasing their 'fluidity and permeability'. It is now thought that neuronal proteins sensitive to alcohol are more important. These include receptor-ion channel complexes and proteins involved in neuronal signal transduction processes. An account of the action of alcohol on the major neurotransmitter systems now follows.

Alcohol and the GABA receptor complex

GABA is the main inhibitory neurotransmitter in the brain. It acts at two receptor types, type A and type B. The GABA-benzodiazepine site on the $GABA_A$ receptor is considered to be the main target for alcohol. When alcohol binds to the postsynaptic $GABA_A$ receptor, it activates the chloride channel and potentiates GABA-ergic neurotransmission. The GABA-ergic system is thought to be hypofunctional in alcoholism and therefore vulnerable to the effects of alcohol.

The GABA receptor is made up of five separate sub-units, of which there are six types (α, β, γ, δ, ρ, ϵ), each existing in a number of different forms, e.g. isoforms, $\alpha1$–$\alpha6$ (Lingford-Hughes and Nutt, 2001). Certain combinations of sub-units seem to be commoner than others and particular combinations mediate different effects. The commonest combination is $\alpha1$, $\beta2$, $\gamma2$, which seems to be particularly sensitive to alcohol. On the other hand, the $\alpha6$ receptor sub-unit, mainly found in the cerebellum, is thought to mediate alcohol-induced ataxia and motor inco-ordination, and is different from the sub-unit mediating alcohol-induced sedation (Lingford-Hughes and Nutt, 2001). The GABA-enhancing actions of alcohol are found at low concentrations (<100 mg/dl). At higher concentrations (>250 mg/dl), alcohol has a direct action on the receptor, causing a prolonged opening of the chloride channel that is GABA independent (Nutt, 1999).

In animals, chronic exposure to alcohol leads to tolerance and dependence which, in turn, results in reduced potentiation of GABA-ergic neurotransmission, reduced behavioural responses and withdrawal symptoms (Lingford-Hughes and Nutt, 2001). The proposed mechanisms underlying these findings are too complicated to discuss here. However, it seems as if chronic ethanol exposure is associated with altered expression of particular GABA-benzodiazepine sub-units. A number of studies have explored the role of GABA-ergic system function in ethanol reinforcement. Reinforcement in this context is the process by which animals or humans seek alcohol because it induces pleasant feelings (positive reinforcement) or relieves unpleasant experiences such as alcohol withdrawal (negative reinforcement). The dopaminergic mesolimbic system is involved in mediating reinforcement and GABA-ergic neurons modulate this system at various points.

As already mentioned, evidence from animal research suggests that the GABA-ergic system is hypofunctional in alcohol dependence. However, there is little supporting evidence from human studies. Human post-mortem studies measuring the level of GABA$_A$ receptors in alcohol dependence are inconclusive. This might reflect the use of different 'markers' (radioligands) or simply that animal models of alcohol dependence differ from human models in the pattern of alcohol consumption, and in the time between the study and last consumption of alcohol. Recent neuroimaging studies in abstinent alcohol dependent subjects have reported decreased levels of the GABA-benzodiazepine receptor in the frontal cortex, particularly the medial frontal region (Gilman et al., 1996; Lingford-Hughes et al., 1998). It is unclear whether these reductions were caused by the alcohol abuse or pre-dated it. However, the regional pattern of GABA-benzodiazepine receptor loss would suggest that only certain populations of receptor are involved in alcohol dependence.

A number of positron emission tomography (PET) studies carried out by Volkow and colleagues lend support to the notion that the GABA-benzodiazepine receptor system may be hypofunctional in alcohol dependence (Volkow et al., 1993, 1995). Newly abstinent alcohol dependent subjects were shown to display abnormal lorazepam-induced responses in brain glucose metabolism compared with controls, as measured by PET and [18F] fluorodeoxyglucose. A later study showed that the relative activity of the GABA-benzodiazepine receptor did not alter during detoxification and early abstinence, implying it was not involved in withdrawal. The study was repeated in healthy male subjects with and without a family history of alcohol dependence. A blunted response was seen in the cerebellum of those with a family history, possibly reflecting a vulnerability to alcohol dependence.

BOX 3.1 **Alcohol and the GABA receptor**

The GABA-benzodiazepine receptor plays an important role in mediating the central effects of alcohol and alcohol dependence. It is thought to play a role in tolerance and reinforcement. There is some evidence to suggest that the GABA-benzodiazepine receptor is hypofunctional in alcohol dependence. It is not clear whether this hypofunctionality pre-dates the alcohol problem (i.e. is a trait) or is a consequence of heavy drinking.

Alcohol and the glutamate receptor

Glutamate is the main excitory neurotransmitter system in the brain. It acts on at least three different types of receptor, but the effects of alcohol appear to be mediated by one of these, the N-methyl-D-aspartate (NMDA) receptor (Tsai et al., 1995). The NMDA receptor sits in the cell membrane and allows the passage of calcium ions (Ca^{++}) into the cell. This channel is usually blocked by a magnesium ion (Mg^{++}). When the neuron is partially depolarized, this Mg^{++} block is removed, allowing calcium into the cell, where glutamate binds to the recognition site on the NMDA receptor. Excessive influx of calcium is neurotoxic. Alcohol acts as a blocker of the NMDA channel, thus opposing the effects of glutamate. Thus, in acute doses it reduces brain excitability.

Chronic exposure to alcohol is thought to result in an increase in the number of NMDA receptors, as the brain tries to counteract the blocking effect of alcohol. This, in turn, increases glutamate function (restores it to normal in the presence of alcohol) – and contributes to the development of tolerance. On cessation of alcohol, blood alcohol levels in the brain fall, there is a relative excess of NMDA function and an associated increase in calcium influx (hyperexcitability of alcohol withdrawal and neuronal death).

As previously mentioned, the calcium channel is usually blocked by a magnesium ion. Alcohol dependence is often associated with magnesium deficiency. Magnesium deficiency, together with an increase in NMDA receptors, puts alcohol dependent individuals in withdrawal at special risk of seizures.

It must also be asked whether alcohol dependent individuals suffer neurotoxicity every time they withdraw from alcohol? Withdrawal episodes treated with benzodiazepines may not adequately ameliorate the disequilibrium at the NMDA receptor. There is increasing evidence that alcohol dependence and withdrawal (including seizures) are mediated by alcohol-related changes at the NMDA receptor. In theory, NMDA should have a role to play in the treatment of alcohol withdrawal.

BOX 3.2 **Alcohol and the glutamate receptor**

Alcohol-related changes at the NMDA receptor contribute to alcohol dependence and particularly to symptoms of alcohol withdrawal. The NMDA receptor appears to play no role in tolerance. It may play a role in the learning of addictive behaviour.

Alcohol and the serotonin (5-HT) receptor

The 5-hydroxytryptamine (5-HT) or serotonin neurotransmitter system has been implicated in the aetiology of alcohol dependence, particularly in the early onset variety. It is hypothesized that low brain 5-HT function is associated with a vulnerability to developing early onset alcohol dependence, also with greater impulsivity and higher levels of aggressive behaviour. In contrast, individuals with late onset alcohol dependence are thought to have high levels of 5-HT function and thus high levels of anxiety. It is postulated that people in this group drink to 'reduce tension'. Abnormalities in the 5-HT system have also been reported in depression, anxiety, bulimia and suicidal behaviour, all of which commonly occur in association with alcohol dependence.

In the brain, the serotonergic neurons are primarily located in the brainstem raphe nuclei. There are a number of receptor sub-types, e.g. $5\text{-}HT_{1A}$, $5\text{-}HT_{2A}$, $5\text{-}HT_3$. There is also a transporter system or reuptake site on the neuron through which released serotonin is removed from the synapse.

Many animal studies suggest that reduced serotonergic function is associated with alcohol preference (an animal model of alcohol dependence). Alcohol-preferring rats have reduced levels of 5-HT in the raphe nucleus (reduced number of neurons). Levels of $5\text{-}HT_{2A}$ receptors are reduced and $5\text{-}HT_3$ receptors are unchanged in preferring compared with non-preferring rats. A number of (but not all) human studies support the view that 5-HT function is reduced in alcohol dependence. This may not be a simple 5-HT deficiency, but a more complex reaction between mechanisms controlling serotonin regulation at the transporter and their interaction with drinking (Johnson and Ait-Daoud, 2000). This effect persists into abstinence and may be a trait not a state marker (Lingford-Hughes and Nutt, 2001). If 5-HT function is diminished in alcohol dependence, medication known to increase 5-HT levels, via reuptake inhibition in selective serotonin reuptake inhibitors (SSRIs) such as fluoxetine, citalopram, or via agonists such as buspirone, should theoretically reduce alcohol consumption. The situation must be more complex, because these drugs do not produce the postulated effect (Le Marquand et al., 1994).

Another area of interest in relation to $5\text{-}HT_2$ receptors is the finding that $5\text{-}HT_2$ agonists are perceived as the same as alcohol in drug discrimination paradigms. This might suggest that $5\text{-}HT_2$ antagonists have a role in helping to reduce drinking.

A population of $5\text{-}HT_2$ receptors is found on inhibitory cortical GABA interneurons where they stimulate GABA release. Reduced $5\text{-}HT_2$ function in early onset alcohol dependence means less cortical inhibition and a predisposition to impulsive behaviour. This relative lack of GABA inhibition may also explain the relative resistance of early onset individuals to sedative drugs such as alcohol and benzo-diazepines (Nutt, 1999).

The 5-HT$_3$ receptor is involved in the expression of alcohol's rewarding effects via interactions between dopamine (DA) and 5-HT$_3$ in the midbrain and cortex. 5-HT$_3$ receptors are located in the terminals of mesocorticolimbic DA-containing neurons. Ondansetron, a 5-HT$_3$ antagonist, has been reported to reduce alcohol consumption in humans, by modulating dopaminergic transmission (Johnson et al., 2000).

BOX 3.3 Alcohol and the serotonergic system

Chronic alcohol use and dependence are associated with reduced functioning in the serotonergic system. This may be more apparent in early onset 'alcoholism', which is, in turn, associated with a positive family history and impulsivity.

Alcohol and the dopamine receptor

Dopamine plays a role in mediating the pleasurable consequences of alcohol (Nutt, 1999; Lingford-Hughes and Nutt, 2001). However, non-dopaminergic pathways are also involved. The mesolimbic DA system (ventral tegmental area → nucleus accumbens) plays a significant role in mediating the reinforcing properties of alcohol. In animal models, alcohol increases the firing of dopaminergic neurons and increases the release of DA from these neurons in the nucleus accumbens. It has been proposed that vulnerability to alcohol dependence is associated with a hypofunctional mesolimbic dopaminergic system.

The activity of the dopaminergic system in alcohol dependence has been studied using neuroendocrine challenges. The growth hormone (GH) response to the DA agonists apomorphine (acts at D$_1$ and D$_2$ receptors) and bromocriptine (acts at D$_2$ receptors) is used as an index of dopaminergic activity. Abstinent alcoholics consistently show a reduced dopaminergic responsivity reflecting alterations within the hypothalamus/pituitary axis in alcohol dependence.

Theoretically, the blocking of DA function in the mesolimbic area should reduce the positive reinforcement induced by alcohol (block the pleasurable effects). Tiapride, a D$_2$ antagonist, performed better than placebo in promoting abstinence, self-esteem and life satisfaction in a randomized, controlled trial of alcohol dependent subjects (see Chapter 19). However, the use of DA antagonists is limited because of their association with long-term neurological side effects. The anti-alcohol action of these drugs is in part related to their increased potency at 5-HT$_2$ receptors.

> **BOX 3.4 Alcohol and dopaminergic pathways**
> Dopaminergic pathways are involved in mediating the pleasurable effects of alcohol
> (positive reinforcement). Reduced function in the mesolimbic dopaminergic system may be
> associated with a vulnerability to developing alcohol dependence.

Noradrenaline

Although there is evidence to show that impaired noradrenergic function is associated with alcohol dependence and that noradrenergic hyperactivity underlies many symptoms of alcohol withdrawal, the system is often overlooked. It is unclear whether reduced levels of noradrenaline (NAd) precede the onset of alcohol abuse and dependence. NAd may also play a role in tolerance to alcohol.

The locus coeruleus is the major noradrenergic nucleus in the brain and is involved in the regulation of attention and activity of the autonomic nervous system. It is unclear whether it is different in alcohol dependence. In alcohol withdrawal, cerebrospinal fluid and urinary levels of NAd and its metabolites are elevated. It also plays a role in tolerance.

Alcohol and the endogenous opioid system

The reinforcing and pleasurable effects of alcohol are mediated, at least in part, by activation of the endogenous opioid system. Alcohol consumption causes activation of the opioid system – specifically the β-endorphin pathways primarily originating in the nucleus arcuatus. This activity leads in the β-endorphin pathways to increased DA release in the nucleus accumbens by: (1) disinhibition of the tonic inhibition of GABA neurons on DA cells in the ventral tegmental area, and (2) direct stimulation of DA cells in the nucleus accumbens. Mu opioid receptor antagonists such as naloxone and naltrexone block these central effects of β-endorphins and have been shown to reduce alcohol consumption in animal models.

Neuropeptide Y

Neuropeptide Y (NPY) is an inhibitory neuromodulator thought to modulate NAd, which may play a major role in protecting neural circuits from excessive stimulation. It has been shown to have an anxiolytic profile in several animal models of anxiety. NPY has a similar electrophysiological profile to alcohol and may be involved in mediating its effects (Lingford-Hughes and Nutt, 2001).

The development of alcohol dependence

Individuals with drinking problems are a very diverse group yet share many commonalities, as is evident to anyone who takes a good drinking history (see Chapter 15).

There is increasing evidence that the evolution of alcohol dependence can be explained in terms of both psychological and pharmacological processes and it appears likely that neuroadaptation changes in the brain underlie the compulsion to drink, increased tolerance, alcohol withdrawal and the other features of the syndrome. Not everyone who drinks heavily becomes dependent. Some may be more vulnerable than others by virtue of constitutional make-up, genetic, personality or impulsivity factors or environmental influences. Hypothetical pathways into alcohol dependence might include the use of alcohol as a stimulant/euphoriant, to relieve anxiety and stress, or for sedation (Littleton and Little, 1994).

Pathways into alcohol dependence

Stimulant/euphoriant effects

Alcohol has traditionally been classified as a depressant drug. The view that it causes stimulation and euphoria, although controversial, is now more widely accepted, though there is still debate as to whether this effect is separate from its anxiolytic or amnesic properties (Littleton and Little, 1994). The putative stimulant effect of alcohol can be explained by its action in the mesolimbic system of the brain, where it causes the release of DA. This effect of alcohol may be mediated by an initial release of opioid peptides, via an action of alcohol on 5-HT receptors, or by interactions with GABA or other neurotransmitters in the ventral tegmental area where the DA neurons originate.

The stimulant/euphoriant effect of alcohol, mediated by increased release of DA, is less than that observed for the CNS stimulants, amphetamine and cocaine. Nevertheless, the positive reinforcement associated with the feeling of euphoria or 'reward' can also explain the development of a psychological dependence on alcohol. Alcohol interacts with the brain's reward system, and this stimulates its continued use. DA function can be blocked by neuroleptics (antagonists at DA D_2 receptors), which reduce alcohol-induced euphoria, but their side-effect profile precludes their use.

Two of the three classes of opioid receptor (mu and delta) also seem to be involved in the reinforcing actions of alcohol (Nutt, 1999). Alcohol consumption increases concentrations of plasma endorphins, thus activating the system. Opioid receptor antagonists such as naltrexone and nalmefene have been shown to reduce relapse and lower alcohol consumption in alcohol dependent subjects (Volpicelli et al., 1992, 1997; O'Malley et al., 1992). They are thought to act by decreasing the euphoric rewarding and/or reinforcing effects of alcohol. This is discussed further in Chapter 18.

Anxiety reduction

Alcohol is a potent anxiolytic agent and is often used at parties and social events to relieve anxiety and promote confidence. This effect appears to be mediated largely by its action on the GABA$_A$ receptor. Alcohol enhances the action of GABA at certain types of GABA$_A$ receptor, reducing the cell's excitability and decreasing anxiety. The anxiolytic action of alcohol is theoretically a 'rewarding' effect, and has the potential to reinforce further alcohol consumption and to contribute to the development of psychological dependence.

Amnesia

The amnesic effects of alcohol are seen after both acute and chronic high consumption. These effects may be due to the fact that alcohol acts as a blocker of the NMDA receptor, opposing the effects of glutamate. When activated by large amounts of glutamate, NMDA receptors allow entry of Ca^{++} into the neuron, where they act as a second messenger, leading to changes in intracellular proteins that result in adaptations which underlie learning and memory (Littleton and Little, 1994). It could be postulated that alcohol-induced amnesia is rewarding in the case of severe depression or in situations in which alcohol is used to 'numb' traumatic memories, e.g. of childhood sexual abuse. The quantities of alcohol consumed in order to obtain amnesia are likely to lead to physical dependence.

Neuroadaptation

Chronic alcohol consumption leads to cellular adaptive changes in the brain. These changes can alter the degree of reinforcement experienced and possibly lead to the development of tolerance, dependence and withdrawal (Hoffman and Tabakoff, 1996; Anton, 1996; Gordis, 1998). Although tolerance is one of the key elements of the alcohol dependence syndrome, the neuroadaptations underlying its development appear to be different from the neuroadaptations underlying the development of physical dependence and withdrawal. This would explain why some individuals manifest alcohol tolerance but not the components of the physical dependence syndrome.

Tolerance

Tolerance is defined as the decrease in sensitivity to the effects of alcohol that occurs as a result of previous exposure to it (Kalant, 1996). Three types of tolerance have been described – acute, rapid and chronic. Acute tolerance occurs within the duration of a single exposure to alcohol. Tolerance to the effects of the second dose of alcohol, given between 8 hours and 3 days after the effects of the first dose have disappeared, is termed rapid tolerance. Chronic tolerance occurs after repeated administrations of alcohol. It is not known whether acute, rapid and chronic tolerance are mediated by the same process. However, there is probably a learned psychological component to acute tolerance (Vogel-Sprott, 1992).

Tolerance shares many of the features of learning and memory and it is thought that both operant learning and classical or Pavlovian conditioning play a major role in its development. Interactions between the serotonergic, glutamatergic and vasopressinergic systems, forming a circuit in the limbic forebrain, are thought to play a central role in the development and maintenance of tolerance.

The alcohol withdrawal syndrome

Neuroadaptation that opposes the action of alcohol and is reversed slowly on cessation of drinking can produce a withdrawal syndrome. This type of adaptation is effective while alcohol is present in the brain, but when alcohol is removed, adaptations are made in the opposite direction, thus producing an alcohol withdrawal state.

Neuroadaptation within the CNS is a complex phenomenon and what follows is an attempt to simplify it for the non-medical reader. A fuller account can be found in reviews by Littleton and Little (1994) and Hoffman and Tabakoff (1996). Neuroadaptation can be divided into 'specific' and 'non-specific' components. 'Specific' neuroadaptation occurs in the transmitter/neuroreceptor system. 'Non-specific' neuroadaptation occurs 'downstream' of receptors and may involve second messenger systems to which receptors are coupled. This form of adaptation is likely to be widespread and can explain cross-tolerance and dependence on other classes of drugs, e.g. benzodiazepines.

Examples of 'specific' adaptation are seen in the NMDA and GABA$_A$ systems. 'Acute' use of alcohol blocks the activation of the NMDA receptor by glutamate and reduces its function. Animal studies show that chronic alcohol use leads to 'upregulation' (increase) of the NMDA receptors in order to compensate for prolonged inhibition. Alcohol withdrawal is accompanied by glutamatergic hyperactivity, which is thought to underlie the various symptoms and signs, including withdrawal seizures (Grant et al., 1990b), and to contribute to cell death and alcohol-related brain damage (Tsai et al., 1995, 1998).

Acutely, alcohol potentiates the effect of GABA at the GABA$_A$ receptor. Here one would expect that the adaptive response would be a reduction ('downregulation') in the number of GABA$_A$ receptors. The situation appears to be more complex, and is influenced by the fact that the GABA$_A$ receptor is present in many isoforms with differential sensitivities to alcohol. Animal studies suggest that the brain can modify its response to alcohol on GABA$_A$ receptors without changing the total numbers of these receptors. Thus it currently appears unlikely that the GABA$_A$ receptor plays a major role in the generation of withdrawal symptoms.

An example of 'non-specific' neuroadaptation implicated in alcohol withdrawal involves voltage-operated calcium channels (VOCCs). Alcohol inhibits the function of the 'L-type' (dihydropyridine-sensitive) calcium channel in the membrane of the neuronal cell body (Littleton and Little, 1994), thus reducing calcium entry and probably neurotransmitter release. Chronic alcohol administration increases the number of these channels in the neuronal membrane ('upregulation'). When alcohol is withdrawn, the increased number of channels and increased calcium entry lead to excessive neurotransmitter release, and this contributes to the alcohol withdrawal state (Littleton and Little, 1994).

Reinstatement

How can we explain the process by which someone with alcohol dependence who has been abstinent for several years develops severe alcohol withdrawal symptoms days or weeks following relapse? This phenomenon is known as 'reinstatement' and is extraordinary because of the way the whole alcohol dependence syndrome re-emerges, as if there is an irreversible 'addiction memory' laid down in the brain.

Future directions

In recent years, neuropharmacological research has helped to uncover the mechanisms underlying the actions of alcohol, 'appetite' for alcohol, and the biological basis of dependence. This has led to a renewed interest in pharmacotherapies for alcohol dependence, already with some promising results. The challenge now is to integrate insights from the neuropharmacology, molecular genetics and clinical science with understanding from other and wider disciplines, particularly psychology. Drinking is a behaviour with multiple determinants and the truly crucial questions will, in the long run, yield only to multidisciplinary (and interdisciplinary) research.

REFERENCES

Agarwal, D.P. and Goedde, H.W. (1990) *Alcohol Metabolism, Alcohol Intolerance and Alcoholism. Biochemical and Pharmacogenetic Aspects.* Berlin, Heidelberg: Springer-Verlag.

Anton, R.F. (1996) Neurobehavioural basis for the pharmacotherapy of alcoholism: current and future directions. *Alcohol and Alcoholism* 31, 43–53.

Crabb, D.W. (1993) The liver. In *Recent Developments in Alcoholism*, Vol. 11, ed. Galanter, M. New York: Plenum Press, 207–30.

Eckardt, M.J., File, S.E., Gessa, G.L. et al. (1998) Effects of moderate alcohol consumption on the central nervous system. *Alcoholism: Clinical and Experimental Reseach* 22, 998–1040.

Fleming, M., Mihic, S.J., Harris, R.A. (2001) Ethanol. In *Goodman and Gilman's The Pharmacological Basis of Therapeutics*, 10th edn, eds in chief Hardman, J.G., Limberd, L.E. New York: McGraw Hill, 429–45.

Frezza, M., Di Padova, C., Pozzato, G., Terpin, M., Baraona, E. and Lieber, C.S. (1990) High blood alcohol levels in women. The role of decreased gastric alcohol dehydrogenase activity and first-pass metabolism. *New England Journal of Medicine* 322, 95–9.

Gianoulakis, C. (1998) Alcohol-seeking behaviour. The roles of the hypothalamic–pituitary–adrenal axis and the endogenous opioid system. *Alcohol, Health and Research World* 22, 202–10.

Gilman, S., Koeppe, R., Adams, K. et al. (1996) Positron emission tomographic studies of cerebral benzodiazepine-receptor binding in chronic alcoholics. *Annals of Neurology* 40, 163–71.

Gordis, E. (1998) The neurobiology of alcohol abuse and alcoholism: building knowledge, creating hope. *Drug and Alcohol Dependence* 51, 9–11.

Grant, K.A., Hoffman, P.L. and Tabakoff, B. (1990a) Neurobiological and behavioural approaches to tolerance and dependence. In *The Nature of Drug Dependence*, ed. Edwards, G. and Lader, M. Oxford: Oxford University Press, 135–69.

Grant, K.A., Valverius, P., Hudspith, M. and Tabakoff, B. (1990b) Ethanol withdrawal seizures and the NMDA receptor complex. *European Journal of Pharmacology* 176, 289–96.

Hoffman, P.L. and Tabakoff, B. (1996) Alcohol dependence: a commentary on the mechanisms. *Alcohol and Alcoholism* 31, 333–40.

Johnson, B.A. and Ait-Daoud, N. (2000) Neuropharmacological treatments for alcoholism. *Psychopharmacology* 149, 327–44.

Johnson, B.A., Roache, J.D., Javors, M.A. et al. (2000) Ondansetron for reduction of drinking among biologically predisposed alcoholic patients. A randomized controlled trial. *Journal of the American Medical Association* 284, 963–71.

Kalant, H. (1996) Current state of knowledge about the mechanisms of alcohol tolerance. *Addiction Biology* 1, 133–41.

Le Marquand, D., Pihl, R. and Benkelfat, C. (1994) Serotonin and alcohol intake, abuse and dependence: clinical evidence. *Biological Psychiatry* 36, 326–37.

Lieber, C.S. (1995) Medical disorders of alcoholism. *New England Journal of Medicine* 333, 1058–65.

Lieber, C.S. (2001) Molecular basis and metabolic consequences of ethanol metabolism. In *International Handbook of Alcohol Dependence and Problems*, ed. Heather, N., Peters, T.J. and Stockwell, T. Chichester: John Wiley and Sons, 75–102.

Lingford-Hughes, A.R., Acton, P.D., Gacinovic, S. et al. (1998) Reduced levels of GABA-benzodiazepine receptor in alcohol dependency in the absence of grey matter atrophy. *British Journal of Psychiatry* 173, 116–22.

Lingford-Hughes, A. and Nutt, D.J. (2001) Neuropharmacology of ethanol and alcohol dependence. In *International Handbook of Alcohol Dependence and Problems*, ed. Heather, N., Peters, T.J. and Stockwell, T. Chichester: John Wiley and Sons, 103–127.

Littleton, J. and Little, H. (1994) Current concepts of ethanol dependence. *Addiction* 89, 1397–412.

Nutt, D.J. (1999) Alcohol and the brain. Pharmacological insights for psychiatrists. *British Journal of Psychiatry* 175, 114–19.

O'Malley, S., Jaffe, A.J., Chang, G., Schottenfeld, R.S., Meyer, R.E. and Rounsaville, B. (1992) Naltrexone and coping skills therapy for alcohol dependence: a controlled study. *Archives of General Psychiatry* 49, 881–7.

Tsai, G., Gastfriend, D.R. and Coyle, J.T. (1995) The glutamatergic basis of human alcoholism. *American Journal of Psychiatry* 152, 332–40.

Tsai, G.E., Ragan, P., Chang, R., Chen, S., Linnoila, M.I. and Coyle, J.T. (1998) Increased glutamatergic neurotransmission and oxidative stress after alcohol withdrawal. *American Journal of Psychiatry* 155, 726–32.

Vogel-Sprott, M. (1992) *Alcohol Tolerance and Social Drinking*. New York: Guilford Press.

Volkow, N., Wang, G., Begleiter, H. et al. (1995) Regional brain metabolic response to lorazepam in subjects at risk for alcoholism. *Alcoholism: Clinical and Experimental Research* 19, 510–16.

Volkow, N., Wang, G., Hitzemann, R. et al. (1993) Decreased cerebral response to inhibitory neurotransmission in alcoholics. *American Journal of Psychiatry* 150, 417–22.

Volpicelli, J., Alterman, A., Hayashida, M. and O'Brien, C. (1992) Naltrexone in the treatment of alcohol dependence. *Archives of General Psychiatry* 49, 876–80.

Volpicelli, J.R., Rhines, K.C., Rhines, J.S., Volpicelli, L.A., Alterman, A.I. and O'Brien, C.P. (1997) Naltrexone and alcohol dependence: role of subject compliance. *Archives of General Psychiatry* 54, 737–42.

4

The alcohol dependence syndrome

Dependence is an important clinical reality, and understanding of its implications is one essential part of the therapists' competence if they are to deal with drinking problems. That should not be misinterpreted as implying that dependence is everything, and many patients with drinking problems are not suffering from the dependence syndrome.

A mechanistic approach to the diagnosis of dependence is insufficient. Dependence cannot be conceived as 'not present' or 'present', with the diagnostic task then completed. The skill lies in being able to recognize the subtleties of symptomatology which will reveal not only whether this condition is there at all but also, if it exists, the degree of its development. What has also to be learnt is how the syndrome's manifestations are moulded by personality, by environmental influence or by cultural forces. It is the ability to comprehend the variations on the theme that constitute the real art.

If therapists cannot recognize *degrees* of dependence, they will not be able to fit their approach to the particular patient, and they may retreat into seeing 'addiction to alcohol' as a fixed entity from which all patients with drinking problems are presumed to suffer, for whom the universal goal must be total abstinence, and with the treatment which is offered universally intensive. The needed skill is the development of a discriminating judgement which is able in each case to sense out the degree of dependence, identify the rational treatment goal for that person, and propose the treatment fitted to that particular individual's problem.

Dependence implies an altered relationship between a person and their drinking. A man or woman may start to drink for many reasons, and when they are dependent, many of these reasons will still pertain and are not necessarily wiped out because of the super-added fact of the dependence. However, the dependence now provides reasons for drinking which are truly super-added, and which may dominate the many preceding reasons for drinking and heavy drinking. Dependence becomes a duress.

This chapter is organized in the following way. First, the clinical origin of the syndrome concept is discussed and its scientific underpinning outlined. A detailed description of the individual elements within the syndrome is then given, followed by a case history to illustrate the picture in the round and its coherence. The question of whether dependence is best viewed as a unitary condition with many and continuous variations, or alternatively as a family of disorders within a typology, will be considered.

The alcohol dependence syndrome: clinical concept and scientific underpinning

Clinical genesis of the concept

The concept of *syndrome* is used in medicine to designate a clustering of signs and symptoms. Not all the elements may be present in every instance, but the picture must be sufficiently regular and coherent to permit its clinical recognition and to allow distinction between syndrome and non-syndrome.

A syndrome is a descriptive clinical formulation which is, at least initially, likely to be agnostic as to causation or pathology. The existence of alcohol dependence has been evident to acute observers for many years (e.g. Trotter, 1804; Kerr, 1888), but in the 1970s a detailed clinical description was enunciated within a syndrome model (Edwards and Gross, 1976; Edwards et al., 1977). It was suggested by Edwards and Gross that clinical observation revealed a repeated clustering of signs and symptoms in certain heavy drinkers. Further, it was postulated that the syndrome existed in degrees of severity rather than as a categorical absolute, that its presentation could be shaped by pathoplastic influences rather than its being concrete and invariable, and that alcohol dependence should be conceptually distinguished from alcohol-related problems. This clinically derived formulation was at that stage designated as only provisional and, within the general research tradition of psychiatric taxonomy, the *validity* of the syndrome had then to be determined.

Alcohol dependence: establishing syndrome validity

Following the original description, research has tested multiple aspects of validity (Edwards, 1986). Studies have, for instance, been directed at determining the internal homogeneity of the syndrome and the degree to which its postulated elements co-occur (Stockwell et al., 1979, 1983; Chick, 1980; Meehan et al., 1985; Feingold and Rounsaville, 1995), and the related issues of construct validity (Heather et al., 1983), concurrent validity (Stockwell et al., 1983; Kivlahan et al., 1989; Caetano 1993) and predictive validity (Hodgson et al., 1979; Rankin et al., 1982). Further contributions to an understanding of syndrome structure has come from large-scale epidemiological studies conducted with standardized instruments or interview methods (Grant et al., 1992; Cottler, 1993; Rapaport et al., 1993; Rounsaville et al., 1993; Cottler et al., 1995). The conceptual separation of 'dependence' from 'abuse' appears to be well supported (Hasin and Paykin, 1999).

The overall conclusion to be drawn from this, by now extensive, body of research is that the syndrome is a reality rather than a chimera of the clinical eye. That is not to say that all elements are in psychometric terms equally well tied into the syndrome. Within a psychometric perspective, some elements may be redundant, and difficulties have been encountered in operationalizing elements such as narrowing of repertoire, subjective change and reinstatement (Cottler et al., 1995).

Alcohol dependence: the neurobiological basis

If the clinical description of alcohol dependence was the first step and the establishment of its validity the second, the third stage in this sequential process must be to determine the nature of the underlying biological and psychological processes which are involved in the genesis, perpetuation and reinstatement of the condition (see Chapters 2 and 3).

What *is* dependence? There has over recent years been progress on many fronts (White, 1996; West, 2001a), but a definitive answer to that question is still not to hand. We have bits of the answer, but the puzzle does not as yet entirely fit together. Although biological and psychological aspects of dependence can usefully be studied in their own right, the larger and outstanding challenge is to delineate the totality of the interactive psychobiological system which underlies dependence (Edwards and Lader, 1990).

At the biological level, the systems which make alcohol behaviourally reinforcing are partly but not completely understood: it is certain that more than one transmitter system is involved (Glue and Nutt, 1990; Nutt, 1999; Littleton, 2001). Withdrawal symptoms are caused by both decreased inhibition and increased excitement. There have been many advances on the genetic front (Ball and Murray, 1994). There is debate as to whether the primary drug effect on the brain is the dominant mechanism which reinforces the alcohol-seeking habit, or whether relief of withdrawal is also a significant reinforcer (Edwards, 1990). The mechanisms which underly acquisition of tolerance and the underlying biology of withdrawal symptoms are much better understood than previously. What is still missing is understanding of the mechanisms to explain why, once a drinker has developed dependence, the condition is so readily reinstated if drinking is started again after a period of abstinence (Edwards, 1990).

At the psychological level, analysis has focused on the identification of cues which trigger craving or alcohol-seeking behaviour and on the alteration in cue-responsivity, which are a feature of dependence (Glautier and Drummond, 1992). The learning mechanisms involved in dependence include both classical and operant conditioning (Greeley et al., 1993; Glautier and Drummond, 1994), and it is also likely that altered expectancies and other cognitive processes significantly contribute to the psychological basis of dependence (Jones and McMahon, 1996; Williams and Ricciardelli, 1996; Jones et al., 2001).

Further insights into the nature of dependence are likely to involve advances in the understanding of relevant biological, behavioural and cognitive processes and, most importantly, their interactions (Edwards et al., 1981; West, 2001b). It is not a condition that can be comprehended within any single-level reductionist model (Edwards, 1994).

The study of dependence thus continues to pose challenges to multiple sciences and provides a classical example of research effort productively harnessed to refutation or confirmation of what was previously no more than clinical intuition. Sight should, however, never be lost of the fact that whatever the science may have to tell, there is still at the centre a core of existential experience – the dependence sensed as unwelcome, foreign, a taking over of self, the duress.

Individual elements of the dependence syndrome

The elements of the syndrome as originally formulated by Edwards and Gross (1976) are summarized in Box 4.1. It is these elements which are discussed sequentially below, rather than only the more restrictive syndromal formulations described in ICD-10 (World Health Organization, 1992) or DSM-IV (American Psychiatric Association, 1994).

BOX 4.1 **The alcohol dependence syndrome: key elements**
- Narrowing of repertoire
- Salience of drinking
- Increased tolerance to alcohol
- Withdrawal symptoms
- Relief or avoidance of withdrawal symptoms by further drinking
- Subjective awareness of compulsion to drink
- Reinstatement after abstinence

Narrowing of repertoire

The ordinary drinker's consumption and choice of drink will vary from day to day and from week to week: they may have a beer at lunch on one day, nothing to drink on another, share a bottle of wine at dinner one night, and then go to a party on a Saturday and have several drinks. Their drinking is patterned by varying internal cues and external circumstances.

At first, a person becoming caught up in heavy drinking may widen their repertoire and the range of cues that signal drinking. As dependence advances, the cues are increasingly related to relief or avoidance of alcohol withdrawal, and their personal drinking repertoire becomes increasingly narrowed. The dependent person begins to drink the same whether it is a workday, weekend or holiday; the nature of the company or their own mood makes less and less difference. Questioning may distinguish earlier and later stages of dependence by the degree to which the repertoire is narrowed. With advanced dependence, the drinking may become scheduled to a strict daily timetable to maintain a high blood alcohol. However, more careful questioning will show that even when dependence is well established, some capacity for variation remains. The syndrome must be pictured as subtle and plastic rather than as something set hard, but as dependence advances the patterns tend to become increasingly fixed and changed (Mundt et al., 1995).

Salience of drinking

The stereotyping of the drinking pattern as dependence advances leads to the individual giving priority to maintaining their alcohol intake. The spouse's distressed scolding – once effective – is later neutralized by the drinker as evidence of a lack of understanding. Income which had previously to serve many needs now supports the drinking habit as the first demand. Gratification of the need for drink may become more important for the patient with liver damage than considerations of survival. Diagnostically, the progressive change in the salience given to alcohol is important, rather than the behaviour at any one time. Patients may relate that they used to be proud of their house but now the paint is peeling, used always to take the children to football matches, but now spend no time with the family, used to have rather conventional moral standards but will now beg, borrow or steal to obtain money for alcohol.

Increased tolerance to alcohol

Alcohol is a drug to which the central nervous system (CNS) develops tolerance (see Chapter 3). Patients themselves report on tolerance in terms of 'having a good head for liquor' or 'being able to drink the other person under the table'. Clinically, tolerance is shown by the dependent person being able to sustain an alcohol intake and go about their business at blood alcohol levels that would incapacitate the non-tolerant drinker. This does not mean that their functioning is unimpaired – they will be a dangerous driver, but because of their tolerance they will (unfortunately) still be able to drive. Acute tolerance which any normal subject will experience in response to even a single dose of alcohol needs to be distinguished from the chronic tolerance which is a feature of the dependence syndrome (Kalant, 1996).

Cross-tolerance will extend to certain other drugs, notably general depressants such as barbiturates and benzodiazepines, which means that the person who has become tolerant to alcohol will also have a tolerance to these drugs and *vice versa*. The rate of development of tolerance is variable, but the heavy drinker who is not dependent can manifest tolerance. In later stages of dependence, for reasons which are unclear, individuals begins to lose their previously acquired tolerance and become incapacitated by quantities of alcohol which they could previously handle. They may begin to fall down drunk in the street.

Withdrawal symptoms

At first these symptoms are intermittent and mild; they cause little incapacity and one symptom may be experienced without others. As dependence increases, so do the frequency and severity of the withdrawal symptoms. When the picture is fully developed, typically the patient has severe multiple symptoms every morning on waking and perhaps even in the middle of the night. Questioning often reveals that severely dependent patients experience mild withdrawal symptoms (which they recognize as such) at any time during the day when their alcohol level falls. Complete withdrawal is therefore not necessary to precipitate disturbance.

Patients often remember rather exactly the dating of the period when they first began to experience withdrawal, and there is no necessary association with a sudden increase in alcohol intake.

The spectrum of symptoms is wide and includes tremor, nausea, sweating, sensitivity to sound (hyperacusis), ringing in the ears (tinnitus), itching, muscle cramps, mood disturbance, sleep disturbance, hallucinations, *grand mal* seizures, and the fully developed picture of delirium tremens. There are four key symptoms.

- *Tremor.* This nicely illustrates that it is *degree* of symptom experience that is essential to the clinical observation, rather than a recording in the case notes simply that the patient does or does not experience withdrawal tremor. Shakiness may have been experienced only once or twice, or intermittently and mildly, or it may be experienced every morning and to a degree which is incapacitating, or with many intervening intensities and frequencies. As well as the hands shaking, there may be facial tremor or the whole body shaking. The therapist has to cultivate an awareness of something equivalent to the Beaufort Scale for wind strength, and look out for the patient saying that they rattle their morning teacup against the saucer. In the extreme case, a drinker may rely on the kindness of the barmaid to lift the day's first pint to their lips.

- *Nausea.* The patient or client who is asked only whether they vomit may well deny it. Their experience, however, may be that if they attempt to clean their teeth in the morning, they will retch; or they may never eat breakfast because they know it would be too risky. A common story is that most of the first drink of the day is vomited back.
- *Sweating.* This may be dramatic: the patient wakes regularly in the early hours of the morning with soaking sweats. At the earlier stages of dependence, they may report no more than feeling clammy.
- *Mood disturbance.* In the earlier stages, patients may phrase the experience in terms of 'being a bit edgy' or 'nerves not too good', but when dependence is fully developed they may use vivid descriptions to indicate a state of appalling agitation and depression. Often the anxiety seems to be characterized by a frightened reaction to loud noises or traffic (sometimes with a phobia of crossing the road), a fear of a friend coming up suddenly from behind, fright at 'the twigs on the trees rubbing together'. The over-sensitivity can be like that of a gouty patient who fears a fly alighting on their toe. An underlying mood disorder may at times exacerbate withdrawal symptoms (Johnson et al., 1991).

Relief or avoidance of withdrawal symptoms by further drinking

In the earliest stages, the patient may be aware that at lunchtime the first drink of the day 'helps to straighten me up a bit'. At the other extreme, a patient may require a drink every morning before getting out of bed, as a matter of desperate need. As with withdrawal symptoms, relief drinking must not be conceived as only a morning event; the patient may wake in the middle of the night for the drink which will abort incipient withdrawal. They may be aware that if they go 3 or 4 hours without a drink during the day, the next drink is valued especially for its relief effect. Relief drinking is cued not only by frank withdrawal, but also by minimal symptoms of subacute withdrawal, which signal worse distress if drink is not taken. The dependent individual may try to maintain a steady alcohol level which they have learnt to recognize as comfortably above the danger level for withdrawal, and to this extent their drinking is cued by withdrawal avoidance as well as withdrawal relief.

Clues to the degree of a patient's dependence are often given by the small details they provide of the circumstances and timing of the first drink of the day, and their attitude towards it. If they get up, have a bath, dress and read the paper before that drink, then dependence is not very advanced. A housewife who finishes her morning chores before having her first drink is at a different stage of dependence from the woman who is pouring whisky into her first cup of tea. Someone engaged in relief drinking may have ritualized the procedure. A man may go to the early-morning pub at 7 a.m., go straight up to the bar where the barman will know immediately to give him his pint of lager, which he will grab at clumsily with both hands and drink down fast. He may go to the lavatory and vomit some of this pint back, but he can then drink the next pint at greater leisure, and he will know that within 20 or 30 minutes of walking into that pub 'the drink will have cured me'. A drinker may relate that they know the exact quantity of alcohol required for this 'cure' and the exact time interval for the alcohol to take effect, and they report also that the 'cure' is repeatedly so complete as to be almost miraculous. Sometimes they describe what is presumably a conditioned effect: the mere fact of having a glass in their hand gives relief.

That the dependence syndrome is a plastic condition rather than something immutable is brought out again by the way this particular element is shaped by social and personal factors. For the building labourer, the idea of keeping drink in the house may be so against sub-cultural expectations that he will always wait for the pubs to open rather than 'keep a drink indoors'. The person of rigid personality may endure considerable withdrawal for some hours rather than take a drink before lunch. To understand fully what the patient reports always requires that these shaping factors are taken into account.

Subjective awareness of compulsion to drink

The conventional phrases used to describe the dependent person's subjective experience are not altogether satisfactory. For instance, awareness of 'loss of control' is said to be crucial to understanding abnormal drinking and patients sometimes say, 'If I have one or two, I'll go on', or 'If I go into the pub, promises don't mean anything', or 'Once I've really got the taste of it, I'm away'. Control is probably best seen as variably or intermittently impaired rather than 'lost'. Although 'loss of control' has been pictured in some of the classic texts as the touchstone for the diagnosis of addiction to alcohol, it is obvious that many so-called 'social drinkers' at times drink too much and are sorry and embarrassed afterwards.

Another complex experience which can too easily be wrapped up in conventional phrasing is the experience of 'craving' (Drummond et al., 2000). The patient may describe it in unambiguous terms – he or she may be 'gasping for a drink'. The subjective interpretation of the withdrawal may, however, be much influenced by environment, and the patient who is withdrawing on a ward may not experience any craving. Cues for craving may include the feeling of intoxication as well as incipient or developed withdrawal, mood (anger, depression, elation), or situational cues (being in a bar or with a drinking friend).

The patient who is in a withdrawal state (or partial withdrawal) may report compulsively ruminating on alcohol and having hit on the strategy of blocking these ruminations by bringing in other lines of thought.

Reinstatement after abstinence

If patients begin again to drink, relapse into the previous stage of the dependence syndrome follows an extremely variable time course. Typically, the person who had only a moderate degree of dependence will take weeks or months to reinstate dependence, perhaps pulling back once or twice on the way. A severely dependent patient typically reports being 'hooked' again within a few days of starting to drink, although even here there are exceptions: on the first day they may become abnormally drunk and be surprised to find that they have lost their tolerance. However, within a few days they are experiencing severe withdrawal symptoms and drinking for relief, the subjective experience of compulsion is reinstated, and their drinking is back in the old stereotyped pattern. A syndrome which had taken years to develop can be fully reinstated within 72 hours of drinking or sooner, and this is one of the most puzzling features of the condition.

A case history

A 45-year-old window cleaner told the following story. He had grown up in a working-class area of his city and identified himself with its culture. He saw the pub as being an essential part of that world, perhaps its centre. Before he had left school, he and his mates were going into pubs, and to brazen out the age question in the face of the barman's suspicions was proof of manhood. He had never worked other than as a window cleaner, and he said that a lot of his trade was picked up at the bar. When it rained, the pub was the place to retreat. He was married with three children and left the management of the home to his wife. Everything therefore was so set up as to enable a man who 'always liked his beer' to sustain a daily intake of 5 to 10 pints as compatible with his pattern of life.

About 6 years before he presented for treatment, he had begun to notice that his hands were a little shaky in the morning – 'not too good for the job'. He started to call into the pub at 11 a.m. and would have a couple of pints, which would relieve the shakiness and generally make him feel better. His daily intake of beer, which had gradually increased over recent years, was now about 15–20 pints each day, but he never took any alcoholic drink other than beer. He was able to identify a transitional phase as occurring 5–6 years prior to presenting for help, and separating his previous lifetime of 'liking the beer' from the last 5 years of 'being bad like I am now'. The experience of withdrawal symptoms had intensified rapidly during that phase.

He had for 3 years experienced severe withdrawal symptoms every morning, and it was the retching and vomiting which worried him particularly – 'All right when I'm lying flat, but as soon as I sit up in bed it starts, have to rush to the toilet, heave my heart out'. He had heavy night sweats. He did not at first directly mention the mood component in the withdrawal experience, and words like 'anxiety' or 'depression' were not part of his ordinary vocabulary. But he 'felt bad, sort of butterflies', and on closer questioning it was clear that each morning he was experiencing unpleasant mood disturbance, although he did not spontaneously differentiate between physical and mental symptoms; it was a matter of 'feeling bad, more than terrible'. Tremor was such that 'I'll knock over the tea pot'. Withdrawal seemed only to be a morning experience, presumably because he otherwise kept his blood level constantly topped up.

Evidence for drinking to relieve withdrawal was present, but here a colouring due to class-related attitudes was to be seen. He never kept drink in his own home, and this was a taboo which, despite the intensity of his dependence, he was unwilling to break. So far as he was concerned, 'bringing drink indoors' would have been a depravity. He therefore tried to stay in bed almost until the pubs opened and would then be in the pub exactly at opening time. His needs were so well known that the barman would have two separate pints of beer drawn and waiting for him. He drank these pints straight down, and during the first hour he would have a third pint. But by the end of 30 minutes he was feeling much better, and within the hour he was 'guaranteed right as rain'.

The increased tolerance to alcohol had existed for many years before this man developed the dependence syndrome; no naïve drinker would be able to drink 5 or 6 pints of beer at lunchtime and then do an afternoon's work (and climb a ladder).

The narrowing of drinking repertoire by the time he sought treatment had become extreme. From 11 a.m. to 2.30 p.m. he was in the pub and drank 8 pints of beer during that time. He came home and slept, returned to the pub at 6 p.m. and drank another 8 pints up to 10 p.m., when he would always go home and take the dog out for a walk. He would get back to the pub later and have a final drink. Sometimes, when he was short of money, his daily intake would fall a little lower and, if he was flush with money, it might be a bit more. There had been occasions when he was ill with influenza and had spent a week or 10 days at home, and he had then been completely off drink, with some mild hallucinatory experience during the first few days.

The salience of drink seeking over other considerations was witnessed by a number of features. Work would now have got in the way of his drinking so he had largely stopped working, and drinking had really become his occupation. Provided he had money for his beer, nothing else mattered. He had previously always prided himself on 'giving the wife a good wage'; she now went out to work, and he took from her whatever money he could by wheedling or demand. He would 'take the rent money' and had cashed an insurance policy. His drinking was also financed by welfare benefits.

The subjective awareness of compulsion was sensed. He contrasted 'the old days' with his present. In the old days, if there was a job to do, he went out and did it, and 'I drank but I didn't have to drink – now I have to drink'. He had recently promised himself to cut down on his drinking and get back to regular work, but, 'It's no good, the beer's really got a grip of me, and if I go into that pub I can't get out again. When I've got a pint, I'm thinking of the next pint'. He did not spontaneously use the word 'craving', but he was aware of his need for the first drink of the day: 'If anyone stood between me and that beer I'd go mad'.

The fact that this man had on occasions been abstinent for 10 days or so because of minor illnesses made it possible to gain information on reinstatement. As soon as he was able to get out of the house, his first walk would be back to the pub. He would tell himself that he 'wasn't going to drink in that bad way again', but full reinstatement of the whole picture nowadays only seemed to take about a week, and within 2 or 3 days of restarting his drinking he was again experiencing severe withdrawal symptoms. He summed things up by saying 'Don't know what's happened really, but the drink's got on top of me'.

Dependence: interpreting the picture

Given an awareness of the basic elements of the syndrome, when confronted with a history such as that given by the window cleaner, there is the task of bringing this theoretical knowledge to bear on the understanding of the individual story. Using this patient's history where appropriate as illustration, the matter can be discussed under a number of headings.

Sensitivity to language

Clinical work is dependent on being alert to meanings of words and nuances of phrase which are partly idiosyncratic to that one patient, but often culturally endowed. There should be a willingness to play phrasings backwards and forwards until there is a flash of mutual comprehension. The possibility of understanding will often be destroyed if such conventional terms as 'craving' or 'loss of control' are prematurely introduced. However, the phrasing which is remembered from one patient's account may, on occasion, seem immediately to reach another patient's experience – for instance, 'drinking one drink and thinking about the next one'.

Assessing the coherence of the picture

The picture which emerges of any patient's experience of the dependence syndrome ought to be coherent. If one element of the syndrome is well established, another element should not be absent. For instance, if patients or clients report that they are suffering from severe withdrawal symptoms, but their regular daily intake of alcohol is only the equivalent of 6 pints of beer (say, 100–120 g ethanol), the story perhaps does not fit properly together. Either part of the information on which the picture is being built is inaccurate (the patients are perhaps under-reporting their drinking), or morning symptoms of some other origin are being interpreted as alcohol withdrawal symptoms. Inconsistencies are therefore valuable observations in their own right. They should alert the diagnostician to making a closer investigation of the case. Co-existent drug taking may distort the picture. A seeming inconsistency may be accounted for by the influence of personality or culture, which are matters dealt with more fully below.

Influence of culture and environment

The picture given by the window cleaner is typical of alcohol dependence as manifested by an Englishman from his social background and of his age. As ever, there were personal as well as social causes for the drinking, but the social factors were in this instance important determinants of the years of heavy drinking which were the prelude to dependence, and these same factors then followed through to shape aspects of the dependence syndrome. For instance, a class-related insistence on not drinking in the house meant that a degree of dependence, which would normally have resulted in drink being kept by the bed for morning relief, was characterized instead by the patient's waiting for the pubs to open. True to class drinking habits, he drank only beer, despite the uncomfortable fluid intake. His stereotyped dependent drinking (like all his previous drinking) was centred round the pub. His whole present drinking pattern can be seen as an extension of 'pub drinking' rather than as something standing completely outside an accepted social pattern. This man's peculiar and makeshift, but real, economic stability (his wife's earnings and the welfare benefits) enabled his dependent drinking to be conducted in a steady fashion.

Influence of personality

Not much has so far been said about this man's personality, but there can be no doubt that there was play between his personality and features of his dependence. His responsiveness to cultural dictates is in itself evidence of a personality trait, and he was basically a conventional person. The flat pattern of his dependent drinking, the rigidity of that narrowed drinking repertoire (the dog faithfully taken for a walk each evening), the exact daily repetition of the ritualized first 2 pints, might all be read as evidence of a rigid element in his temperament, and he had always been a methodical window cleaner. The salience which he gave to his drinking when he had become dependent on alcohol was understandable as an extension of what had always been his detachment from the family; he had never felt that responsibilities went beyond giving his wife a regular cash sum, and now he retreated from that one obligation.

Degrees of dependence

Although one element may be more or less developed than others (sometimes as a result of unexplained variation or sometimes because of the impact of modifying social or personal factors), the coherent picture which emerges should be of a certain *degree* of dependence, with each element more or less in step. Thus, if, as with the window cleaner, withdrawal symptoms are severe and experienced every day, it is to be expected that there will be a well-established pattern of relief drinking. Tolerance will be well developed if severe withdrawal is experienced, although around this stage in the history some evidence of declining tolerance might begin to appear. The narrowing of drinking repertoire reported by this man was commensurate with his other symptoms, and it would, for instance, have been surprising if, with this degree of dependence, he had been drinking much less at weekends than on weekdays. The daily alcohol intake was commensurate and the salience he accorded his drinking fitted in with the total picture. The subjective awareness of compulsion was typical of this degree of development. Typically, the syndrome was rapidly reinstated after a few days' abstinence.

It is not easy to set up absolute rules for grading the severity of dependence, but it would be a fair guide to say that if anyone has experienced withdrawal symptoms on a more or less daily basis for 6–12 months and engaged in regular relief drinking in response to those symptoms over the same period (with other elements congruently developed), they are severely dependent on alcohol. If they have experienced withdrawal symptoms on no more than a few occasions, but have been aware that alcohol usefully brings relief (even without intentionally bringing forward the first drink of the day), an early case of dependence can be diagnosed. Between those two pictures there are many gradations, rather than fixed degrees. A history of an attack of delirium tremens is clinching evidence of severe dependence, but discussion of alcohol-related and dependence-related mental illness is postponed to Chapter 7.

Should dependence be diagnosed in the absence of withdrawal symptoms?

The diagnostic rubric of DSM-IV allows alcohol dependence to be diagnosed in the absence of withdrawal symptoms. That approach will probably catch in the net many people who are drinking heavily, but who are not experiencing the kind of disturbance described in this chapter as constituting the alcohol dependence syndrome. The question is important and not merely semantic (Carroll et al., 1994). In a large American household survey, Schuckit et al. (1998) found that subjects positive for alcohol dependence, according to DSM-III-R, differed markedly according to whether physiological symptoms (withdrawal or tolerance) were or were not present. Those with physiological symptoms drank more heavily than the others and experienced more adverse consequences from their drinking. In another population study, Hasin et al. (2000) found that experience of tremors was predictive of poorer 1-year outcome and chronicity. A syndrome by its nature is a state difficult to differentiate absolutely from non-syndrome, but for clinical purposes it is probably best to restrict the diagnosis of alcohol dependence to patients who have experienced withdrawal symptoms to at least some degree.

The time element

To discuss the severity of dependence inevitably introduces consideration of the time element. The longer someone has been putting themselves through repeated cycles of withdrawal and relief, the more severe the dependence they will have contracted.

However, note has also to be taken of the rapidity or gradualness of the transition between heavy drinking and dependence, and of the age at which dependence developed. The window cleaner had sustained a pattern of heavy drinking for many years before the dependence syndrome started to be seen, and this is perhaps typical of a history in which the determinants of drinking are largely cultural. Why dependence should have become manifest at a certain phase in his life is unexplained. Whatever the underlying causes, it is, however, rather typical for the man with a long-standing heavy alcohol intake to be able to identify a transition period of about 12 months during which the dependence symptoms had their onset and a quickly mounting severity. With other cultures, personalities and patterns of drinking, dependence may arise earlier or later in life, after longer or shorter alcohol exposure, and may advance with greater or lesser rapidity.

In summary, to understand fully the individual's dependence, the present picture has to be related to its evolution over time, and the determinants of that evolution identified (see Chapter 13).

Dependence: the later stages

Patients may continue to drink dependently and at a heavy level for many years, and when one sees them again after a 10-year interval, the account in the old case notes can seem, astonishingly, to be the description of the present – nothing has changed. If, however, they neither die nor stop drinking, sooner or later the presentation is likely to evolve towards the breakdown of the old picture and a more fragmented type of drinking.

There are a number of themes within this evolution which can be identified.

- *Dependence becomes progressively worse.* We are referring here to the dependence disorder *per se* rather than to the surround of alcohol-related disabilities which are likely at this stage to occur with increasing severity. The withdrawal symptoms may have plateaued at the same level for many years or have gradually worsened, but at a certain phase there will probably be a rapidly mounting intensity of morning distress. The patient may, for example, report an appalling experience of shakes or almost suicidal disturbance in mood each morning. The immediate morning drink is a matter of terrifying urgency. Hearing voices, seeing things, frightening half-waking dreams may all be experienced on a come-and-go basis, or the patient may experience attacks of frank delirium tremens.

- *Gross and incapacitating intoxication becomes more common.* Reference has already been made to the late-stage possibility of an actual decline in tolerance. A patient reported his experience in the following terms: 'That last year, whenever I started to drink, I got so drunk that I literally didn't know night from day, just a haze. It would get so I couldn't go into any bar because I was just an embarrassment, and I was falling over in the street, brought home by strangers.'

The loss of tolerance can at the extreme be so severe that the patient is intoxicated after only a couple of drinks. Brain damage often underlies this picture. Gross and repeated amnesia becomes common. Although loss of tolerance and accompanying brain damage are usually the major factors lying behind this 'getting very drunk', other factors may also be involved, such as the fear of withdrawal leading to desperate and misjudged efforts to top up the blood alcohol, or a searching after the good feelings that alcohol used to give but no longer provides.

- *Drinking makes the patient feel very ill.* The drinker finds that they can no longer drink in their previous continuous manner because after a few days of drinking they now feel so ill that, despite the threat of withdrawal symptoms, their suffering forces them to desist. The mounting intensity of the morning withdrawal contributes to this general feeling of distress, but it is likely to be compounded by the consequences of various alcohol-induced physical disorders, for instance gastritis, liver disease or chronic pancreatitis. Concomitant psychiatric disorder may also become more common at this stage.

The result of these various factors is that the patient moves towards a pattern of short, acute and incapacitating bouts, each of them a chaotic and devastating experience. This end-result seems in large measure to be determined by the progression of the dependence itself – by the march of incompletely understood physiological and psycho-physiological processes. However, social and environmental factors must, as ever, also be taken into the analysis: marriage break-up and the loss of every constraint and support can make for further inevitability.

Many variations or a few species? The Jellinek typology

The window cleaner's story provides a history of one particular person's dependence, and it cannot adequately represent the whole range of pictures which can be encountered. There is an infinite number of ways in which the dependence syndrome and its degrees of development can be moulded in their manifestations by secondary factors, and it is not helpful to pick out sub-patterns and accord them the status of distinct 'species' of alcoholism. Setting up a segmented listing of 'types of dependence' would go against the central concept of one clearly identifiable syndrome which is moulded into different patterns by a variety of forces which have in each instance to be understood. Over time and with changing circumstances, an individual's presentation of the syndrome may vary greatly.

The Jellinek typology

To reject the notion of 'species of alcoholism' is, however, to go against the Jellinek typology of alcoholism (Jellinek, 1960). E.M. Jellinek was an American scientist who made profoundly influential contributions to the study of drinking. As usually quoted and simplified, his system set out a five-fold species categorization (see Box 4.2).

> ### BOX 4.2 **Jellinek's typology of alcoholism**
>
> *Alpha alcoholism*: excessive drinking for purely psychological reasons without evidence of 'tissue adaptation'.
>
> *Beta alcoholism*: excessive drinking which has led to tissue damage, but where there is no dependence on alcohol.
>
> *Gamma alcoholism*: excessive drinking where there is evidence of tolerance and withdrawal, a peaky and fluctuant alcohol intake, and marked 'loss of control'. Jellinek saw this as the pattern typical of Anglo-Saxon countries.
>
> *Delta alcoholism*: excessive drinking where there is evidence of tolerance and withdrawal, but with a much steadier level of alcohol intake. Rather than the patient manifesting 'loss of control', they would exhibit what was called 'inability to abstain'. The pattern was seen as typical of France and of other wine-drinking countries.
>
> *Epsilon alcoholism*: bout drinking, or what used to be termed dipsomania.

Jellinek's typology deserves scrutiny. Study of his original writing shows that his views on categorization were more subtle than would be supposed from the oversimplified extracts from his thinking which later became the popular basis for a typology. For instance, the distinction he drew between gamma and delta alcoholism showed an awareness of the need to take into account the shaping influence of culture. When he discussed epsilon alcoholism, he noted that the picture might be the result of the fragmentation of a previous pattern of continuous drinking by the influence of Alcoholics Anonymous (AA) membership. He did not see his five-part typology as exhaustive, but said that all the other letters of the Greek alphabet might be needed in addition, and then some other alphabets besides. Yet, because of its attractive simplicity, it is the typology which is widely known, with Jellinek's insistence on the arbitrariness of a restricted focus on these few patterns usually ignored.

More orderly or more chaotic dependent drinking

Jellinek's contrasting identifications of gamma (loss of control) and delta (inability to abstain) species point to an important aspect of drinking behaviour which shows variation between cases. He was, however, describing extreme types, and today the best use of his insights is to note the dimension of variation to which his ideas drew attention, rather than to accept the notion of contrasting ideal types with nothing in between. The relationship between the constructs of 'loss of control' and 'inability to abstain' has been investigated by Kachler et al. (1995).

Some alcohol dependent patients drink predominantly in a chaotic fashion. When they start to drink they go on to a variable and uncertain upper limit of blood alcohol. Others, although suffering from alcohol dependence of similar severity, usually so order their drinking that they attain much the same high blood alcohol level every day and one with which their tolerance can cope; they do not overshoot the mark, albeit that the mark is an abnormally high one. Although it is possible to meet patients who seem to conform to one or other extreme stereotype (always losing control on the one hand, unable to abstain on the other), more careful enquiry usually reveals that, even with the seemingly clear-cut and stereotyped case, patterns are more varied than first meets the eye. A client who now appears to be drinking in a chaotic fashion is only doing so since they lost their job and their marriage broke up; before then their dependence manifested itself by heavy continuous drinking through the business day, followed by armchair drinking in the evening. Someone who appears to be drinking predominantly in a controlled fashion may reveal that there are patches when their drinking is more peaky and uncertain in its patterning. The true variety of patterns will be missed if all that is available to the diagnostician's thinking is a few pigeon-holes.

Continuous or intermittent drinking

Jellinek picked up another important dimension when he contrasted epsilon (bout) drinking with other types, but again the reality is degrees of variation, rather than an absolute contrast between dependent patients who drink unfailingly every day and those who drink unfailingly in sharply demarcated bouts.

The degree of intermittency which often will be found to characterize supposedly 'continuous' drinking is surprising (Schuckit et al., 1997). Even the Skid Row drinker, who is pictured as someone who drinks with relentless continuity, will usually be found to have several months of more or less voluntary abstinence during any year, even leaving aside the enforced abstinences during imprisonment; they may have abstained because they were 'too sick to drink', because they had temporarily settled in a job, or because they were living in a hostel where drinking was not allowed.

The person who at first presents with seemingly clear-cut bout drinking will often, on closer questioning, give a previous history of dependent drinking cast in a more continuous pattern. That a move towards a pattern of short bouts is common at the most advanced stages of dependence has already been noted, but bout drinking can also emerge as the predominant mode earlier in the drinking career. Remorse, mood swing, physical distress, mounting pressure from a spouse, the need to get back to work, running out of money, the general practitioner's calling at the house, AA friends coming to the rescue, may all mean that a drinker may at any stage begin intermittently to pull out of their drinking. They relapse, pull out again, and hence 'bout drinking'.

The boutiness of the drinking is thus not witness to a patient suffering from a unique *species* of alcoholism, but to the many and complex influences which are moulding the presentation of the core dependence syndrome. The coherence of the dependence picture should be such that the patient who is highly dependent will be able to swing his drinking repertoire only between bouts of heavy dependent drinking and intervening periods of total or near-total abstinence. The less-dependent person will have bouts with hazier edges, and intervening periods of non-dependent drinking which gradually edge again towards the establishment of dependence.

What has been said here about patterns of drinking seeks squarely to meet the complexity of clinical reality as it will actually be found. The task is to describe each individual's drinking pattern as it in reality exists, and then to try as best as possible to identify the influences which shape this pattern.

Other ideas on the typology question

Although this chapter argues that the most helpful clinical perspective is one which conceives alcohol dependence as a single core syndrome with infinitely varied patterning in individual presentation (see also Vaillant, 1994), other authors, particularly in America, favour the idea of typology (Babor et al., 1994). Cloninger et al. (1981) and Cloninger (1987) have suggested a Type 1 versus Type 2 dichotomy on the basis of sex, family history and age of onset. Babor et al. (1992a, 1992b) have proposed a distinction between Types A and B on the basis of vulnerability and severity; Schuckit (1985) has differentiated between primary and secondary alcoholism; Johnson et al. (1998) have developed a typology based on relative genetic and environmental loading. Others have distinguished between late onset and early onset alcoholism and between subjects with or without concurrent personality disorder or other psychopathology. Research has over recent years not given much support to the Type 1/Type 2 dichotomy (Koeter et al., 1995; Rubin et al., 1998; Sannibale and Hall, 1998), whereas the Type A/Type B distinction fares better (Schuckit et al., 1995). The overall conclusion to be drawn from this research is probably that statistical techniques have not as yet pointed to any consistent sub-species of dependence rooted in clinical reality (Peters, 1997).

Why an understanding of dependence matters

Having outlined the diagnosis of dependence, the manner in which degrees of the syndrome's development are to be identified, and the way in which personality and environment may shape the presentations, the question then arises: what is the practical purpose of such diagnostic work, the gain from developing this kind of diagnostic skill? The answers are both general and specific.

The dependence concept and the brokerage of understanding

The realization that there exists such a condition as alcohol dependence, and an understanding of the personal implications of this diagnosis, may often assist in the relief of the patient's sense of muddle and bafflement. It can contribute to a helpful framework for personal understanding, and enable patients to come to terms with a condition to which they had previously only reacted with confusion. The fact that alcohol is a drug which can produce dependence – 'a drug of addiction' – often comes as a surprise to a patient's family as much as to the patients themselves. The diagnosis, if sensitively explained, can, for the family too, mean a way of restructuring a reaction to a situation which previously engendered confusion, fear or anger. The spouse begins to realize that there is more than 'weakness of the will' that has to be understood, that expecting their partner 'to drink like other people' is unrealistic.

For the therapist, what flows from understanding the nature of dependence lies partly in accurate empathy for that person's experience. Baldly to impart no more than the diagnostic label – a sort of magisterial sentencing – is not what is meant by building up understanding.

Furthermore, it would be useful health education if the public in general was aware that alcohol has dependence potential. The public needs to know more of the dangers and the danger signals, what dependence can mean for themselves or someone in their family, for someone at work or someone they meet in the bar. Understanding of alcohol dependence should become part of ordinary social awareness, but it is equally important that society understands that alcohol problems also commonly occur without dependence.

The relevance of an understanding of dependence to the specifics of treatment

The ability to diagnose dependence and recognize its degrees is vital to setting the treatment goal (see Chapters 17 and 20). A severely dependent drinker is unlikely to be able to return to normal drinking (Edwards et al., 1986) and the clinician's ability accurately to recognize the degree of dependence is vital to this important aspect of care. Assessment of the patient's degree of dependence is also relevant to the choice of withdrawal regime and forewarning as to the risk of delirium tremens or withdrawal fits (see Chapter 16). Understanding of the severity of relapse requires an ability to recognize whether dependence has been reinstated. The monitoring of progress or regression of dependence intensity over time is relevant to the understanding of drinking career and drinking within the life course (Chapter 13).

There is also the question of whether intensity of dependence should be seen as indicating the intensity of the required treatment – a variant of the matching hypothesis (Glaser, 1980). There is common-sense appeal in the postulate that more heavily dependent drinkers should, say, be given more therapeutic time, be more readily admitted to in-patient care, and be provided with more intensive follow-up. However, some research does not support that proposition (Edwards and Taylor, 1994).

REFERENCES

American Psychiatric Association (1994) *Diagnostic and Statistical Manual of Mental Disorders,* 4th edn (DSM-IV). Washington, DC: American Psychiatric Association.

Babor, T.F., Del Boca, F.K., Hesselbrock, V., Meyer, R.E., Dolinsky, Z.S. and Rounsaville, B. (1992a) Types of alcoholics 1: evidence for an empirically derived typology based on indicators of vulnerability and severity. *Archives of General Psychiatry* 49, 599–608.

Babor, T.F., Dolinsky, Z.S., Meyer, R.E., Hesselbrook, M., Hoffman, M. and Tennen, H. (1992b) Types of alcoholics: concurrent and predictive validity of some common classification schemes. *British Journal of Addiction* 87, 1415–31.

Babor, T.F., Hesselbrock, V., Meyer, R.E. and Shoemaker, W. (1994) *Types of Alcoholics: Evidence from Clinical, Experimental and Genetic Research. Annals of the New York Academy of Sciences* Vol. 708. New York: The New York Academy of Sciences.

Ball, D.M. and Murray R.M. (1994) Genetics of alcohol misuse. In *Alcohol and Alcohol Problems,* ed. Edwards, G. and Peters, T.J. British Medical Bulletin No. 50. Edinburgh: Churchill Livingstone, 18–35.

Caetano, R. (1993) The association between severity of DSM-III-R alcohol dependence and medical and social consequences. *Addiction* 88, 631–42.

Carroll, K.M., Rounsaville, B.J. and Bryant, K.H. (1994) Should tolerance and withdrawal be required for substance dependence disorders? *Drug and Alcohol Dependence* 36, 15–22.

Chick, J. (1980) Alcohol dependence: methodological issues in its measurement: reliability of the criteria. *British Journal of Addiction* 75, 175–86.

Cloninger, C.R. (1987) Neurogenetic adaptive mechanisms in alcoholism. *Science* 236, 410–16.

Cloninger, C.R., Bohman, M. and Sigvardsson, S. (1981) Inheritance of alcohol abuse. *Archives of General Psychiatry* 38, 861–8.

Cottler, L.B. (1993) Comparing DSM-III-R and ICD10 substance use disorders. *Addiction* 88, 689–96.

Cottler, L.B., Phelps, D.L. and Compton, W.M. (1995) Narrowing of the drinking repertoire criterion: should it have been dropped from ICD10? *Journal of Studies on Alcohol* 56, 173–6.

Drummond, D.C., Lowman, C., Litten, R.Z. and Hunt, W.A. (eds) (2000) Research perspectives on alcohol craving. *Addiction* 95 (Suppl. 2).

Edwards, G. (1986) The alcohol dependence syndrome: a concept as stimulus to enquiry. *British Journal of Addiction* 81, 171–83.

Edwards, G. (1990) Withdrawal symptoms and alcohol dependence: fruitful mysteries. *British Journal of Addiction* 85, 447–61.

Edwards, G. (1994) Addiction, reductionism and Aaron's rod. *Addiction* 89, 9–12.

Edwards, G., Arif, A. and Hodgson, R. (1981) Nomenclature and classification of drug- and alcohol-related problems: a WHO memorandum. *Bulletin of the World Health Organization* 50, 225–42.

Edwards, G., Brown, D., Duckitt, A., Oppenheimer, E., Sheehan, M. and Taylor, C. (1986) Normal drinking in a recovering alcohol addict. *British Journal of Addiction* 81, 127–37.

Edwards, G. and Gross, M.M. (1976) Alcohol dependence: provisional description of a clinical syndrome. *British Medical Journal* 1, 1058–61.

Edwards, G., Gross, M.M., Keller, M., Moser, J. and Room, R. (1977) *Alcohol-related Disabilities.* WHO Offset Publication No. 32. Geneva: WHO.

Edwards, G. and Lader, M. (eds) (1990) *The Nature of Drug Dependence.* Society for the Study of Addiction Monograph No. 1. Oxford: Oxford University Press.

Edwards, G. and Taylor, C. (1994) A test of the matching hypothesis: alcohol dependence, intensity of treatment and 12 month outcome. *Addiction* 89, 553–61.

Feingold, A. and Rounsaville, B. (1995) Construct validity of the dependence syndrome as measured by DSM-IV for different psycho-active substances. *Addiction* 90, 1661–9.

Glaser, F. (1980) Anybody got a match? Treatment research and the matching hypothesis. In *Alcoholism Treatment in Transition,* ed. Edwards, G. and Grant, M. London: Croom Helm, 178–96.

Glautier, S. and Drummond, D.C. (1992) Alcohol dependence and cue reactivity. *Journal of Studies on Alcohol* 55, 224–9.

Glautier, S. and Drummond, C. (1994) Conditioning approaches: the analysis and treatment of drinking problems. In *Alcohol and Alcohol Problems,* ed. Edwards, G. and Peters, T.J. British Medical Bulletin No. 50. Edinburgh: Churchill Livingstone, 186–99.

Glue, P.W. and Nutt, D. (1990) Overexcitement and disinhibition. Dynamic neurotransmitter interactions in alcohol withdrawal. *British Journal of Psychiatry* 157, 491–9.

Grant, B.F., Harford, T.C., Chou, P. and Pickering, R. (1992) DSM-111-R and the proposed DSM-IV alcohol use disorders, United States 1988. A methodological comparison. *Alcoholism: Clinical and Experimental Research* 16, 215–21.

Greeley, J.D., Swift, W., Prescott, J. and Heather, N. (1993) Reactivity to alcohol-related cues in heavy and light drinkers. *Journal of Studies on Alcohol* 54, 359–68.

Hasin, D. and Paykin, A. (1999) Alcohol dependence and abuse diagnosis: concurrent validity in a nationally representative sample. *Alcoholism: Clinical and Experimental Research* 23, 144–50.

Hasin, D., Paykin, A., Meydan, J. and Grant, B. (2000) Withdrawal and tolerance: prognostic significance in DSM-IV alcohol dependence. *Journal of Studies on Alcohol* 61, 431–8.

Heather, N., Rollnick, S. and Winston, M. (1983) A comparison of objective and subjective measures of alcohol dependence as predictors of relapse following treatment. *British Journal of Clinical Psychiatry* 22, 11–17.

Hodgson, R., Rankin, H.J. and Stockwell, T. (1979) Alcohol dependence and the priming effect. *Behaviour Research and Therapy* 17, 379–87.

Jellinek, E.M. (1960) *The Disease Concept of Alcoholism.* New Brunswick, NJ: Hillhouse Press.

Johnson, A.L., Thevos, A.K. Randall, C.L. and Anton, R.F. (1991) Increased severity of alcohol withdrawal in in-patient alcoholics with a co-existing anxiety diagnosis. *British Journal of Addiction* 86, 719–25.

Johnson, E.O., Van den Bree, M.B.M., Gupman, A.E. and Pickens, R.W. (1998) Alcoholism: extension of a typology of alcohol dependence based on relative genetic and environmental loading. *Alcoholism: Clinical and Experimental Research* 22, 1421–9.

Jones, B.T., Corbin, W. and Fromme, K. (2001) A review of expectancy theory and alcohol consumption. *Addiction* 96, 57–72.

Jones, B.T. and McMahon, J. (1996) A comparison of positive and negative alcohol expectancy and value and their multiplicative composite as predictors of post-abstinence survivorship. *Addiction* 91, 89–99.

Kachler, C.W., Epstein, E.E. and McCrady, B.S. (1995) Loss of control and inability to abstain: the measurement of and relationship between two constructs in male alcoholics. *Addiction* 90, 1025–36.

Kalant, H. (1996) Current state of knowledge about the mechanisms of alcohol tolerance. *Addiction Biology* 1, 133–41.

Kerr, N. (1888) *Inebriety, its Etiology, Pathology, Treatment and Jurisprudence.* Edinburgh: H.K. Lewis.

Kivlahan, D., Sher, K.J. and Donovan, D.M. (1989) The Alcohol Dependence Scale: a validation study among in-patient alcoholics. *Journal of Studies on Alcohol* 50, 170–5.

Koeter, M.W.J., Van den Brink, W. and Hartgers, C. (1995) Cloninger's type I and type II alcoholics among treated alcoholics: prevalence and validity of the construct. *European Addiction Research* 1, 187–93.

Littleton, J. (2001) Receptor regulation as a unitary mechanism for drug tolerance and physical dependence – not quite as simple as it seemed. *Addiction* 96, 87–102.

Meehan, J.P., Webb, M.G.T. and Unwin, A.R. (1985) The Severity of Alcohol Dependence Questionnaire (SADQ) in a sample of Irish problem drinkers. *British Journal of Addiction* 80, 57–63.

Mundt, J.C., Searles, J.S., Peerrine, M.W. and Helzer, J.E. (1995) Cycles of alcohol dependence: frequency-domain analysis of daily drinking logs for matched alcohol-dependent and non-dependent subjects. *Journal of Studies on Alcohol* 56, 491–9.

Nutt, D.J. (1999) Alcohol and the brain. Pharmacological insights for psychiatrists. *British Journal of Psychiatry* 175, 114–19.

Peters, D. (1997) A natural classification of alcoholics by means of statistical grouping methods. *Addiction* 92, 1649–61.

Rankin, H., Stockwell, T. and Hodgson, R. (1982) Cues for drinking and degrees of alcohol dependence. *British Journal of Addiction* 77, 287–96.

Rapaport, M.H., Tipp, J.E. and Schuckit, M.A. (1993) A comparison of ICD10 and DSM-III-R criteria for substance abuse and dependence. *American Journal of Drug and Alcohol Abuse* 19, 143–51.

Rounsaville, B.J., Bryant, K., Babor, T., Kranzler, H. and Kadden, R. (1993) Cross system agreement for substance use disorders: DSM-III-R, DSM-IV and ICD10. *Addiction* 88, 337–48.

Rubin, G., Leon, G., Pascual, F.F.J. and Santo-Domingo, J. (1998) Clinical significance of Cloninger's classification in a sample of alcoholic Spanish men. *Addiction* 93, 93–101.

Sannibale, C. and Hall, W. (1998) An evaluation of Cloninger's typology of alcohol abuse. *Addiction* 93, 1241–9.

Schuckit, M.A. (1985) The clinical implications of primary diagnostic groups among alcoholics. *Archives of General Psychiatry* 41, 1043–9.

Schuckit, M.A., Smith, T.L., Daeppen, J-B. et al. (1998) Clinical relevance of the distinction between alcohol dependence with and without a physiological component. *American Journal of Psychiatry* 55, 733–40.

Schuckit, M.A., Tipp, J.E., Smith, T.L. et al. (1995) An evaluation of Type A and B alcoholics. *Addiction* 90, 1189–203.

Schuckit, M.A., Tipp, J.E., Smith, T.L. and Bucholz, K.K. (1997) Periods of abstinence following the onset of alcohol dependence in 1853 men and women. *Journal of Studies on Alcohol* 58, 581–9.

Stockwell, T., Hodgson, R., Edwards, G., Taylor, C. and Rankin, H. (1979) The development of a questionnaire to measure alcohol dependence. *British Journal of Addiction* 74, 145–55.

Stockwell, T., Murphy, D. and Hodgson, R. (1983) The severity of alcohol dependence questionnaire: its use, reliability and validity. *British Journal of Addiction* 78, 145–55.

Trotter, T. (1804) *An Essay on Drunkenness and its Effects on the Human Body.* London: Longman, Hurst, Rees and Orvine.

Vaillant, G.E. (1994) Evidence that the Type 1/Type 2 dichotomy in alcoholism must be re-examined. *Addiction* 89, 1049–57.

West, R. (2001a) *Addiction:* Special Issue on Theories of Addiction. *Addiction* 96, 1–192.

West, R. (2001b) Theories of addiction. *Addiction* 96, 3–13.

White, N.M. (1996) Addictive drugs as reinforcers: multiple partial action on memory systems. *Addiction* 91, 921–49.

Williams, R.J. and Ricciardelli, A. (1996) Expectancies related to symptoms of alcohol dependence in young adults. *Addiction* 91, 1031–9.

World Health Organization (1992) *The ICD-10 Classification of Mental and Behavioural Disorders.* Geneva: World Health Organization.

5

Drinking problems and the family

Drinking problems generally have a profound effect upon the family of the drinker. The spouse or partner and the children are the people commonly drawn into the drama, but parents, brothers, sisters, uncles or aunts or grandparents may in some way be involved. The nature of the involvement can be in terms of another person experiencing the adverse impact of the drinker's behaviour, the family's interaction in the genesis of the drinking problem, the family members' unhelpful connivance with or encouragement of the drinking problem, or, most positively, in terms of someone other than the drinker being able to aid the process of recovery.

A person with a drinking problem may appear to have lost all links with their family. Even so, they may harbour strong emotions in respect of those relationships which have been severed by death, dysharmony or neglect and it is likely that similar feelings are experienced by the estranged relatives. Where these relatives are alive, and if they can be traced, the question of renewing contact may arise. This can present a major challenge, both to the coping skills of the client and to the professional skills of the therapist.

The present chapter describes certain important aspects of family interaction, while full discussion of therapeutic implications is postponed to Chapters 17 and 19 of this book. Readers seeking a more detailed review of the impact of drinking problems upon children and spouses/partners should refer to Sher (1991), Velleman and Orford (1999) and Hurcom et al. (2000). Those seeking a more practical account, focused on the needs of the relative or friend of the problem drinker, should refer to Marshall (2001).

The spouse or partner

At the outset, it is necessary to emphasize that the spouse may be the husband of the woman with a drinking problem, or the wife of the man who is drinking. Although the initial discussion is largely in terms of the wife of the problem drinker – for this is the commoner situation – many of the considerations would apply equally to the reverse circumstances (a later section focuses on the husband of the woman with alcohol-related problems). Comments made here concerning spouses generally also apply to partners who are not legally married.

A history from the spouse in her own right

The assumption is too often made that the purpose of taking a history from the spouse is solely that of obtaining 'independent information'. What is frequently forgotten is the need to take a history from the spouse as a person in her own right. The result is that, after months have gone by, it is suddenly realized that treatment is proceeding on the basis of much being known about the patient while the wife remains a cipher, and their interaction is hence inexplicable. No one has bothered to see this woman in terms of her own being, and her own needs and expectations. Treatment of the patient is handicapped, and the fact that the wife herself needs help is overlooked.

What has to be overcome is a subconscious social constraint – the feeling that it is embarrassing to ask a woman whose role is presumed to be that of someone coming to the clinic to talk about her husband, then within that definition to talk about herself. Indeed, the interview may soon reveal that the wife has a great pressure of need to talk about herself. How the initial history is to be taken from the spouse in terms that honour her in her own right is fully discussed in Chapter 15.

Theories of the 'alcoholic marriage'

A number of different theories have been put forward to explain what may happen in a marriage in which one partner is an alcoholic. The term 'alcoholic' will be retained here, as it has been employed by most of the proponents of these theories. Each of these approaches can at times give useful understanding, but stereotyped descriptions of the alcoholic's wife have no general validity (Hurcom et al., 2000).

One of these theories is that the wife actually wishes her husband to be an alcoholic. The fact is noted that a proportion of wives had a father who was an alcoholic, and it is argued that the wife then marries an alcoholic with whom she can continue to enact her unresolved dynamic problems. She will subtly or overtly hamper treatment, persuade her husband to discharge himself prematurely from hospital, and tell him that a few drinks will not do him any harm. She will even buy the drink for him and bring it back to the house, and she will indicate to him that 'he's horrid now he's sober'. If the husband persists in his recovery, the wife herself may, in terms of this theory, then decompensate and develop a depressive illness.

There can be no doubt that marriages are occasionally encountered which astonishingly resemble such a bizarre picture as that just given, and where it is a reasonable supposition that the wife is subconsciously willing the husband's drinking. She married him knowing he was an alcoholic, she gains from seeing him as weak and despicable, has enjoyed taking over the management of home and finance, and wishes to have her expectations confirmed that men are dirt. She likes to show how badly she is used, enjoys mothering or dominating, and so on. But cruel mistakes result if the assumption is made that this is the common picture of *the* alcoholic marriage, and from forcing all such marriages into interpretations in these terms. For instance, the truth of the matter may be that when the husband began to drink excessively the wife inevitably had to make the choice between letting the home go to rack and ruin or taking much of its running into her own hands; her seeming 'dominance' is merely adjustive.

Some research has suggested that the wife's and family's reactions go through a predictable sequence of stages (Jackson, 1954). The evidence does not in fact support the notion that all wives follow exactly the same pathway, but certain phases can sometimes be recognized. At the beginning there is the reluctant admission that drinking is indeed a problem, and then the first attempts to control or prevent the problem behaviour. The family begins to be socially isolated, partly as a protective strategy; invitations are refused, people are not encouraged to call, relatives are not visited. Later, the wife may go into a phase in which she begins to realize her strategies are not working, that things are getting worse rather than better, that her reserves are being worn down. She may start to fear for her own sanity, and a feeling of hopelessness sets in. Sexual contact is diminished or ceases, and there is a general and continuing sense of estrangement, fear or anger. At this stage or earlier, the wife may begin to feel that 'something must be done'; she tries to persuade her husband to look for help. If no improvement follows, the marriage may either break up or continue for years in a phase characterized by strategies which might be called *circumvention*:

It's terrible really, but I suppose we've all got used to it. We'll all go to bed before he comes in at night and I'll pretend to be asleep when he comes into the room. I tell the kids to keep out of his way. Sometimes he gets back early but if we're in the sitting room watching the television, more often than not he just goes out to the kitchen. I take the children on holiday, he doesn't come, and frankly we don't ask him.

Coping styles

Past perspectives on the alcoholic marriage (not to mention some which are still current) have often been rather negative in outlook. A recognition of this bias has given rise to a shift in emphasis, away from that of the pathology of the spouse and their status as victim, towards an attempt to understand their ability to cope with the stresses presented by an intimate relationship with an alcoholic.

It is useful to try to make an assessment of the *coping style* that the wife is employing at any stage (Orford and Edwards, 1977). This knowledge can be useful in therapy, although there is some disagreement as to which coping styles are most effective and should therefore be encouraged. Furthermore, a wide range of different styles has been identified, and different approaches to classification are suggested. However, research suggests that they may all eventually be reduced to three main options: engagement, tolerance and withdrawal (Orford et al., 1998; Hurcom et al., 2000). A few suggestions are made here as to the kind of behaviours that might be found under each of these headings.

Engagement employs strategies which involve assertiveness, taking control, emotional responses or offering of support. For example, the wife may resort to *attack*, trying to control her husband's behaviour by scolding, shouting, threatening to leave him, or on occasions even by physical assault. She lets him know that she is contacting a solicitor. Drink is poured down the sink. *Manipulation* embraces a number of behaviours, such as seeking to shame the drinker, with the woman showing her own distress or emphasizing the children's suffering, while the wife herself may get purposely drunk 'to show him what it's like'. *Constructive help seeking* is a pattern characterized by behaviour such as the wife going to see the family doctor and asking him to speak to the husband, she finds out about Alcoholics Anonymous (AA) and leaves some pamphlets around for the husband to come upon, or goes to the public library and reads books on alcoholism, so as to help her own understanding.

Tolerance includes self-sacrifice, acceptance and inactivity. *Spoiling* may be a more active example of this approach: the spouse nurses her husband through his hangovers, and keeps the dinner warm for him whether he is drunk or sober. However, spoiling may also involve the promise of treats if he will ameliorate his behaviour, and in such circumstances might be better considered as a form of engagement. By contrast, *inaction* provides a more passive form of tolerance which simply accepts the *status quo*.

Withdrawal is illustrated by the case example of *circumvention* provided above. Contact is minimized as far as possible and there is emotional as well as physical avoidance. This might involve quite independent behaviours. For example, the wife might adopt an approach of *constructive management*: she retains her own sense of worth and protects and looks after the family by making sure that finances are in as good order as possible while she goes out to work. She makes sure that the children go short of nothing, and herself paints the house and cares for the front garden.

These various styles (summarized in Box 5.1) seldom exist in pure form, and there are other examples of coping behaviour which might be given. The choice of style may be influenced by the way in which the woman generally copes with life, by class expectations, by the type of behaviour which the husband is manifesting and by the duration of the problem. The coping style employed at a particular time may be a response in a sequence of experiments in which the wife is searching around, trying first one tack and then another.

BOX 5.1 Examples of each of three main options for action open to partners of problem drinkers

Engagement
- Attack
- Manipulation
- Spoiling (where used to attempt to induce change)
- Constructive help seeking

Tolerance
- Spoiling
- Inaction

Withdrawal
- Circumvention
- Constructive management

What is the wife having to cope with?

The particular stress of a situation in which there may often be social isolation rather than social support, and where there are no guidelines, has already been noted. A frequent additional feature is the stress imposed by the unpredictability of what is going to happen; the wife does not know whether, when the husband gets back from the pub, he will be in a sentimental or maudlin mood, or whether he will be in a raging temper and attack her with his fists. The exhaustion which can be engendered by the experience of dealing with continuing distress and peaks of crisis over a period of years can be the wife's dominant complaint.

Fundamentally, the wife is having to cope with the problems at both the emotional and the reality levels. The emotional problems include anxiety, fearfulness and misery. Often there is an element of self-doubt or self-blame: she wonders whether the problem has arisen because she is a bad wife and has sexually or in some other way failed her husband. She may also be perplexed by the acute conflict in the feelings which she develops towards her husband: she married this man because she loved him and yet now she at times feels almost murderous towards him. There is often also a sense of emotional deprivation and of loss: the man she married has disappeared. She herself begins to feel in some way diminished in her worth, or disgraced.

At the reality level, the problems can be tangibly threatening: there is the risk of eviction if the rent is not paid, or his violence may result in serious personal damage. More commonly it is the host of minor reality problems which have to be coped with: no housekeeping money this week, no money to pay the electricity, the neighbours complaining about the doors being slammed when he got home last night, constant rowing, his jealousy, his dirtiness or his wetting the bed.

It would, however, be a mistake always to picture such marriages only in extreme terms. Extremes of suffering certainly occur with unfortunate frequency, but there are all gradations. Sometimes the husband's deportment when drunk causes little distress; he is a bit silly and argumentative, tends to fall asleep in the chair after supper and can be difficult to get to bed, but in a drunken sort of way he remains polite and is never violent. He regularly hands over the housekeeping money and, if there are the finances to cushion the effects of his drinking and a job which is secure, some of the more distressing reality problems will not be so evident.

The types of hardship which the wife may encounter are discussed in more detail in relation to taking the 'independent history' from the spouse (Chapter 15).

Co-dependency

A popular concept which has emerged from AA and the Twelve Step movement (see Chapter 18) is the diagnosis of 'co-dependency'. According to this understanding of the alcoholic marriage and family, the spouse of the alcoholic becomes 'other orientated', excessively reliant on others for approval, low in self-esteem and unceasing in attempts to rescue their spouse, because they have an addictive disorder which renders them dependent upon relationships and caretaking. This concept is susceptible to criticism for being so broad as to defy objective definition, and because it has been used as a means of pathologizing, and thus blaming, the predominantly female spouses and partners of alcoholics (Hurcom et al., 2000). However, it has become enormously popular within the Twelve Step self-help movement.

Marriages in which the wife is the problem drinker

As was stated at the beginning of this chapter, most of the principles which apply to understanding the situation in which the husband has the drinking problem apply equally well when it is the wife who is the patient or client. There are, however, certain additional aspects to the marriage problem which may then develop, many of which relate to the generally punitive attitudes towards the female heavy drinker which many cultures display, and which are more fully discussed in Chapter 11. The husband's reaction may be coloured by a primitive disgust at his wife's behaviour, or by fear of social disapprobation and of the family being disgraced by a drunken woman. His feelings can lead to violence. To work through these feelings so that the husband is less frightened of what is happening and less blindly condemnatory may be the necessary prelude to any constructive changes.

If the husband is employed and the woman is the housewife and mother, he may find himself drawn into a managing role within the family to compensate for the wife's impaired competence. If he is also trying to keep going in a demanding job, he may find the double demands difficult to cope with, and the welfare of the children may be a particular worry. Failure of the woman to fulfil her expected roles sets neither greater nor lesser problems (though they are in some ways different) than a man's role failures. Sometimes the husband will seek to solve the family's plight by purposely promoting an elder daughter to the central female role within the household.

Another difference relates to the fact that, even in an era of greater equality between the sexes, economically it is often easier for a man to leave a drinking wife than for a wife to leave her drinking husband. Despite continued suffering, she may hold back from separation because she does not see an alternative way of providing a roof to shelter herself and the children. The husband can more readily see separation from his wife as an option, either taking the children with him or surrendering his responsibilities.

Marriages in which both partners have a drinking problem

This extraordinarily difficult situation is sometimes encountered. The story is usually that of a person with a drinking problem marrying someone else with an established and evident drinking problem. For one or both partners it may be a second marriage. They met, perhaps, in a bar or even in a hospital ward, and it is a marriage of convenience between drinkers. Their only shared interest is drinking, they have no knowledge of each other's sober beings and are, sadly, likely to drag each other down further. Alcohol-related problems do sometimes develop in both partners in an already established marriage. Quite often the development is not simultaneous, but the wife seems to follow in the husband's footsteps, her drinking being in part, perhaps, a reaction to the stress of the husband's behaviour. Another type of marriage involves partners who have met at AA, are both committed to 'recovery' and are able to give each other much support.

In general, where both husband and wife have a serious problem, it can be difficult to reach them with effective help. If they met in a pub and each purposefully married a drinking partner, the therapist may encounter a baffling pack of pathological motivations. In such instances all that may be possible is to make the offer of help, try to maintain some sort of monitoring contact, and wait for the event which can provide the therapeutic opening – one partner going into hospital with a physical illness, for example. Where the heavy drinking has developed during the marriage, rather than being the foundation of the marriage, the possibilities for therapy are usually more hopeful. Both partners may then simultaneously be able to seek help, or it may be necessary to start with the partner who is more motivated. If therapy can capture the potential for mutual understanding which can exist between partners who have shared the same problem, an initially difficult situation can be turned to special advantage.

Gay and lesbian couples

Problems similar to those which occur in a heterosexual marriage are encountered when one partner in a homosexual liaison has a drinking problem. A rather common story seems to be of the partner who is more emotionally dependent and more insecure beginning to drink heavily at a period when they fear that the relationship is going to break up:

I'd get home from work, and after I'd had a drink I'd start doing the cooking. All the time I was cooking the dinner I'd be wondering – is he coming home tonight? Who is he with? What lies is he going to tell? Not like the old days! So while I was cooking I'd have a few more drinks. By the time he came in I'd be all ready for a row.

Therapists may find that they are helping such people through the dissolution of their relationship or assisting in the exploration of basic and previously unresolved issues relating to sexuality and identity.

Children

For the children of the problem drinker to be entirely forgotten by the therapeutic team is sadly all too easy. Their names and ages are noted in the initial history taking, out of the corner of an eye there is the awareness of their continued existence, but the parents are the focus of attention and are taking up all the therapeutic time. There is the vague feeling that 'more ought to be done about the children', but the intention is all too seldom honoured.

Experiences to which children are exposed

The experiences of the child of an alcohol parent are varied, depending upon the degree of emotional support provided by either parent, the variety of other social and emotional supports which may be available, and the age of the child when the parent developed the drinking problem. Of great importance is the actual behaviour of the parent when intoxicated: if there is continued rowdiness, arguments or violence, the impact will be far more adverse than in those instances where drunkenness is not associated with verbal or physical aggression.

A drinking problem of whatever degree or nature, which as its end-result produces what can in summary be described as a bad home atmosphere, is attacking the centre of what family life should be able to give to a child. This is the kind of family about which the social worker will report that 'you know there is something wrong as soon as you go in at the door'. Whether it is more damaging for the mother rather than the father to be the person with the drinking problem is uncertain, and there may be a different impact on the boys and the girls in the family. If a parent when drunk continuously picks on a particular child, scolding them, finding fault, demeaning or hitting, then that child is immensely at risk.

In some families, the drinking of a parent will lead to separation and divorce, hospitalization of a parent, or even to death of a parent. Children may have to suffer criticism of their parents by family, neighbours or friends, and the behaviour of their parents may lead to embarrassment or shame. The behaviour of the drinking parent is likely to be unpredictable, and the behaviour of the sober parent may also be adversely affected as far as the child is concerned – even to the point where the child views this parent less favourably (Velleman and Orford, 1999).

Problems which children develop

At the psychological level, one effect may be a general and non-specific raising of the anxiety level in that child. In girls especially, there is also a higher incidence of depression, and in both sexes self-esteem is likely to be low (Zeitlin, 1994). But as well as this general impact on psychological health, a variety of important dynamic processes related to psychological growth can be affected. The child may, for instance, be very basically deprived of a satisfactory role model when the same-sex parent is the drinker, and a disturbed or ambivalent relationship with the parent of the opposite sex may result in feelings which are later going to be acted out in other relationships.

The psychological damages and the social disabilities which can result will inter-act. In the school setting, anxiety may lead to social disability, poor academic performance and other problems. Boys are especially likely to display antisocial behaviour. Children of both sexes may display temper tantrums or get involved in problems which come to the attention of the police (Zeitlin, 1994).

There is, however, little that is absolutely specific to the damaging psychological experience of this kind of home, and much the same types of disturbance must often result in homes where, for instance, one parent is chronically or repeatedly psychiatrically ill. What may be more specific is that the experience of intense family conflict centred on alcohol leaves children with conflicting attitudes towards drinking and drunkenness which are built into their psychological being as highly charged determinants of later feelings and behaviours. Part of the emotional damage is latently the risk of drinking problems in later life.

The absence of emotional regard within the home can mean that a child will, as an adolescent, develop particularly rejecting attitudes towards the parents, and enter precipitously into identification with an adolescent peer group. Such an extreme version of a normal process is not necessarily harmful, but the children from a disturbed home can be vulnerable to involvement with groups which are themselves disturbed and engaging in drug taking or delinquency. These associations may in part represent a revenge on the parents, or substitute comfort or excitement to replace the good inner feelings which are so lacking. There can, however, be no fixed predictions as to how a child from a drinking home will meet adolescence. Another outcome may be that the child is clinging, desperately and anxiously involved in the home, tied to protecting the non-drinking parent, and unable to make any identification with other young people.

At any stage of childhood, the possibility of actual physical damage must be considered. There is an association between drinking problems and baby battering, and in childhood and adolescence the risk of physical assault may continue; the damage is often no more than bruising, but the risk of more serious injury is not to be discounted. Accidental injury may occur due to inadequate supervision. Sexual abuse of children is more likely, and there is evidence that this is likely to increase the risk of alcohol or drug misuse in later life (Velleman and Orford, 1999; Bear et al., 2000). Help for the child is discussed in Chapter 17.

In adult life, children of parents with drinking problems are more likely to display low self-esteem, depression, anxiety, antisocial behaviour, marital dysharmony and generally poor strategies for coping with life (Box 5.2). There is evidence that women may be especially prone to depression, eating disorders, personality disorder and marriage to another problem drinker. However, for some there may even be a positive outcome, with increased achievement or autonomy (Velleman and Orford, 1999).

BOX 5.2 **Problems experienced by children of problem drinkers**
- Anxiety
- Depression
- Low self-esteem
- Relationship difficulties
- Poor school performance
- Antisocial behaviour
- Physical and sexual abuse
- Accidental injury
- Risk of alcohol-related problems in later life
- Other problems in later life (depression, marital dysharmony, etc.)

The concept of 'resilience' has been proposed in order to explain why some children who are brought up by an alcoholic parent fare better than others. It is not at all clear as to whether this concept explains variations in outcome, or whether it simply reflects varying levels of adversity to which such children are exposed (Sher, 2000). However, as with the move away from an emphasis on pathology towards a focus on the coping styles of the spouse or partner (see above), this would appear to emphasize a more constructive perspective upon the traumatic experience of being a child within an alcoholic family (Velleman and Orford, 1999).

Drinking problems and the family

Whether discussing the marriage or the children, what has essentially been argued in this chapter is that drinking problems will inevitably be embedded in a network of family interactions. Those interactions are in terms of both overt communications and direct impacts, and dynamic processes of great subtlety. Heavy and problematic drinking influences the spouse's behaviour, which in turn influences the drinker's behaviour, so that a sort of resonance is set up. Also, the children are not just passive recipients of what is done to them, but themselves actively participate. Not only are parents and children and other family members involved, but so also perhaps is the wife's friend 'who is always dropping in'. To become focused only on a single actor is to lose sight of the play.

However, a play comprises a stage set and script, as well as the actors. So in family life, the 'script' that the actors learn is a vital ingredient of the success of the play. A couple who come together in marriage, or in a partnership outside of marriage, bring with them all kinds of expectations based upon their different experiences of family life. In each area of family life, some of these scripts will come from one side of the family and some from the other partner. If one family of origin was adversely affected by the drinking of one or more of its members, then this may significantly influence the script that conveys the identity of the new family.

An established family is likely to display a range of behaviours which regulate daily life. Family therapists recognize these behaviours as including problem-solving strategies, routines and rituals (Steinglass et al., 1987). In 'alcoholic families', these processes may become unduly concerned with the need to accommodate the adverse consequences of chronic drinking. There is evidence that the extent to which family rituals become influenced by alcohol is important in determining not only the successful adjustment of that family in the face of chronic drinking, but also the risk of drinking problems occurring in the next generation. Where rituals are not sacrificed to the salient priority of heavy drinking, or where a new family makes a conscious decision not to perpetuate these kinds of unhelpful behaviour, the family identity is less likely to suffer, and drinking problems are less likely to be continued through into the next generation (Steinglass et al., 1987).

Christmas celebrations were frequently spoiled during Kate's childhood, as a result of her father's invariable drunkenness. Similarly, her memories of family holidays were dominated by alcohol, and most birthdays or anniversaries were associated with anxiety about her father's drunkenness. Even the normal routine of daily life had accommodated his unpredictable behaviour after 'a drink with colleagues' on the way home from work. When Kate married and started a family of her own, she and her husband determined that they would never let drinking spoil their family life, and they translated this into agreed family expectations on what would constitute acceptable drinking and the occasions when drinking might be done.

REFERENCES

Bear, Z., Griffiths, R. and Pearson, B. (2000) Childhood sexual abuse and substance abuse. *Executive Summary* 67, 1–4.

Hurcom, C., Copello, A. and Orford, J. (2000) The family and alcohol: effects of excessive drinking and conceptualizations of spouses over recent decades. *Substance Use and Misuse* 35, 473–502.

Jackson, J.K. (1954) The adjustment of the family to the crisis of alcoholism. *Quarterly Journal of Studies on Alcohol* 4, 562–86.

Marshall, E.J. (2001) Drinking problems. In *Mental Illness: A Handbook for Carers*, ed. Ramsay, R., Gerada, C., Mars, S. and Szmukler, G. London: Jessica Kingsley, 108–20.

Orford, J. and Edwards, G. (1977) *Alcoholism: a Comparison of Treatment and Advice, with a Study of the Influence of Marriage.* Maudsley Monograph, 26. Oxford: Oxford University Press.

Orford, J., Natera, G., Davies, J. et al. (1998) Tolerate, engage or withdraw: a study of the structure of families coping with alcohol and drug problems in South West England and Mexico City. *Addiction* 93, 1799–813.

Sher, K.J. (1991) *Children of Alcoholics.* Chicago: University of Chicago Press.

Sher, K. (2000) Risk and resilience: adults who were the children of problem drinkers – book review. *Addiction* 95, 631–3.

Steinglass, P., Bennett, L.A., Wolin, S.J. and Reiss, D. (1987) *The Alcoholic Family.* London: Hutchinson.

Velleman, R. and Orford, R. (1999) *Risk and resilience: Adults who were the Children of Problem Drinkers.* Amsterdam: Harwood.

Zeitlin, H. (1994) Children with alcohol misusing parents. *British Medical Bulletin* 50, 139–51.

6

Social complications of drinking

In this chapter, what is meant by social complications of drinking is explored (Klingemann and Gmel, 2001) and specific types of complication are then considered. Complications which occur within the family – an important type of social problem – are discussed in Chapter 5.

Convenient though it is to think in terms of three classical problem dimensions – physical, mental and social – this must not be allowed to obscure the fact that in the real lives of patients the dimensions are not separate at all. Problems in any one area lead to, and are exacerbated by, problems in the other areas. By and large, the more severe the dependence, the greater the likelihood of alcohol-related problems of all three kinds (Caetano, 1993). The clinical skill lies not only in making the detailed, one-dimensional assessment, but also in putting the dimensions together.

Even as the person from a helping profession other than medicine may be tempted, by training or habit of mind, to neglect the importance of the physical considerations in the equation, so may the physician be guilty of too narrow a concern with the patient's physical well-being at the cost of a proper awareness of the other issues. This chapter seeks to provide a checklist of what should be borne in mind in the social sphere, whatever one's professional affiliation.

The concept of 'social complication'

The idea of social complication often implies a failure adequately to fulfil an expected social role. The failure may be in meeting expectations as family member, employer or employee, good neighbour or law-abiding citizen. The result may be detrimental to both the individual and those around them. A social complication may also mean tangible alcohol-related loss or damage in the social dimension – the driving licence forfeited, for instance, or the doctor's loss of right to practise, the house gone, and so on.

As for the alcohol-mediated processes which lead to functional impairments, several factors usually interact. Excessive drinking can at an early stage result in a hangover which makes it difficult to get to work, while intoxication may impair the ability to manage the complexities of the job, and physical and mental impairment later make work impossible. Intoxication is, for many types of alcohol-related social problem, a prime mediating factor between the fact of drinking and the fact of harm, and frequent intoxication will carry heightened risk of harm (Midanik et al., 1996). More subtly, the drink centredness of the individual and the salience which dependent drinking begins to acquire over other demands can mean that work ceases to matter, and this person moves into an 'alcoholic role' which competes with any pre-existing roles.

A secondary process is likely to arise in terms of loss of reputation and the way that others now think about and react to the drinker and confirm them in the alcoholic role. These reactions will be influenced by the background of social attitudes towards drinking and drunkenness and public perspectives on possibilities for recovery. A series of self-fulfilling prophecies may be set up, with a process of amplification getting under way.

I wrote 30 job applications to various firms and told them I had been treated for a drink problem, was now sober and wanted to find my way back with everything in the open. Didn't get a single interview. So next time I kept quiet about my drinking, spun a yarn about that year off work, handed in two out-of-date references, lied on the medical form, and got the job. And then? They checked things out, I was fired on Friday, and yes, it's stupid, but I've been drinking. Just what they expected.

Social complications will almost inevitably spread to involve the *family and other people*, rather than affecting only the one individual. Such impacts on other people are referred to in the economist's language as *externalities*. In the USA for the year 1988, the total financial cost of alcohol-related problems was estimated at $85.8 billion (Rice et al., 1991), and social cost estimates are also available for a number of other countries (Gutjahr and Gmel, 2001).

So much for general principles. The headings which follow delineate major areas of social problem experience and a summary is given in Box 6.1. The ordering does not indicate precedence of importance and the list is not exhaustive. Social complications range from the trivial and the ephemeral to the major, and are widely distributed in the drinking population (Clark and Hilton, 1991; Edwards et al., 1994).

Problems at work

The difficulty that a person with a drinking problem may encounter when seeking employment has just been instanced, and the example shows how stigmatization

---

> **BOX 6.1 Social complications of excessive drinking**
> - Family and relationships
> - Problems at work
> - Housing
> - Financial difficulties
> - Homelessness and vagrancy
> - Alcohol and violence
> - Drink driving
> - Victimization
> - Impact on education and training

may compound the objective difficulties. The varieties of adverse influence that excessive drinking may have on work performance are many and costly (Jones et al., 1995; Romelsjö, 1995; Upmark et al., 1999). The impact is not limited to any one level of seniority in the employment hierarchy, and drinking problems are as likely to be found in the boardroom as on the shop floor.

The drinking doctor (Brooke, 1996) provides an instance of a profession in which alcohol-induced impairment can set special kinds of problem, but occupations and alcohol can interact in many different ways and, whatever the job, result in impaired efficiency or cause inconvenience, loss or danger to other people. In senior positions in industry or the armed services, in the diplomatic service or in the legal profession (Goodliffe, 1994), drunken indiscretion, irascibility or bad judgement at a crucial meeting may be the major problems. For the bus or train driver, the aeroplane pilot (Holdener, 1993), the ship's officer drunk on the bridge, intoxication carries enormous dangers for the public. In professions such as the church or teaching, the hint of scandal may be specially damaging, although it is surprising how tolerant or blind-eyed those in the individual's environment often appear to be. The seriousness with which excessive drinking is officially viewed by the medical profession is evidenced by the disciplinary procedures which in many countries are called into action if a doctor's drinking comes to official notice, although the story is again often one of complicity and cover-up. The conclusion to be drawn from this paragraph must therefore be that, whoever the individuals we are trying to assess and help, the analysis of their alcohol-related social problems requires a job-specific enquiry.

Housing

Urban housing problems and urban drinking problems often go together (each exacerbating the other). Where there are great concentrations of substandard housing and social deprivation, drinking is one of many endemic disorders contributing to, and deriving from, the totality of social disorganization.

However, cases are frequently encountered in which drinking is leading directly to a housing problem. In this type of instance, the patients' claim that they are 'drinking because of their unsatisfactory surroundings' has a hollow ring – theirs is the only house in the street which is shabby and unpainted and with an old sofa lying in the front garden. Housing problems of this kind will be more acute the more marginal the family's income. Bad relationships with neighbours, gross evidence of poor house maintenance, failure to meet the rent, services cut off, eviction, the sojourn in 'temporary accommodation' and multiple changes of address are familiar elements in the housing history as the drinking problem becomes more extreme.

Financial problems

An awareness of the possible financial complications of drinking problems and of the family's financial position is necessary for any complete case assessment. To maintain a major drinking habit is expensive and large additional sums are often spent without the drinker knowing how the money has gone – drinks for friends or drinks grandly offered to strangers, meals out and taxis home, a massive cigarette consumption, gambling, and so on. As with housing problems and many other social complications, the well-moneyed will be better protected for a longer time.

The financial balance is determined not only by the cost of the drinking and associated spendings, but also by the inflow of cash. Demotion, sickness and unemployment add to the stringencies. Complicated and devious stratagems may be engaged in to maintain the cash flow. 'Moonlighting' or a second job is common (often in a bar so as further to aid the drinking), loans are negotiated on preposterous terms, possessions are pawned, houses re-mortgaged. The employee 'works a bit of a racket' and a load of bricks disappears from the builder's yard. It becomes vital to evade income tax and to defraud Social Security. The rent is not paid and hire purchase payments fall behind.

The family may have reached the stage at which financial chaos has become the central and pressing pain. From the social work angle, sorting out that chaos may be the necessary first-aid, but it will be very temporary aid if the drinking problem is not radically met.

Homelessness and vagrancy

The vagrant way of life offers many pressures towards drinking, and at the same time the man or woman with a serious drinking problem may move towards vagrancy (Braumohl, 1989; Fischer, 1991). Drinking may mix with drug taking as a problem affecting runaway and vagrant young people (Kipke et al., 1997). Professionals with a special interest in alcohol do well also to remember that 'the homeless single person' may be homeless for many reasons other than drinking, but when a drinking problem exists it will add to the individual's vulnerabilities (Sosin and Bruni, 1997). Economic hardship and unemployment vary in the contribution they make to vagrancy from decade to decade, while mental illness, physical incapacity, epilepsy and personality disorders contribute continually to the genesis of a city problem which in many countries still seems intractable, come boom or slump.

With those other possible background factors noted, it is still true that the vagrant who is sleeping under the railway arch will often be someone who is manifesting the end-result of a drinking career – a 'social complication' of highly visible and dramatic nature, and the concern of the social reformer from the nineteenth century onwards (McDermott, 1994). The elements of this 'complication' constitute a complex system of related problems: the homelessness itself, the difficulty in getting a wash, the lack of clothes, the lack of fixed employment, the breakdown in family contacts and lack of any kinship or friendship supports, the petty criminal involvement, the poor nutrition and the risks of illness and accident. Drinking is what particularly contributes to the ultimate core characteristic of this situation – its seeming inevitability, the sense of the treadmill. It is easier to find a way into that degradation than a way out. On leaving hospital or the detoxification centre, the only friendship or support readily available may be that offered by a return to the company of the drinkers in the park.

What is the likely background of the man or woman who is begging at the street corner and hoping to raise funds for the next bottle of cheap wine? There are many routes into that situation, but with the need to avoid constructing a picture in terms of any stereotype again noted, the average story is as follows. That individual is more frequently a man than a woman, although women do reach this plight. The parents were often themselves holding onto socio-economic survival tenuously – the father an unskilled worker living in poor urban conditions or rural poverty, and the childhood family often large and lacking in care. Gross disruption of the childhood home is a frequent finding; education is likely to have been meagre and job training nil. The picture is therefore typically of someone who has started with few advantages and many handicaps. The vagrant drinker is, with overwhelming frequency, a casualty with origins in the underprivileged working class, and the shopkeeper or skilled tradesman who becomes involved in drink and falls on hard times seldom goes in that direction. The geographical origins may be well known and typical in a particular country: in London, the casualties will usually not be London born, but come from Scotland or Ireland.

After leaving school, the story tends to be of a few short-term jobs in the home town, a period perhaps in the armed forces or the merchant navy, a short-lived marriage and an unsuccessful attempt to settle down. Then the story will probably have been of the mobility and rootlessness of the casual labourer who moves from town to town and who follows the construction work and the big wages. Contacts with family and friends are lost. As the drinking becomes more incapacitating, there is a drift towards low-grade work such as kitchen portering, with periods of unemployment, spells in prison and psychiatric hospitals, and the final arrival at that disorganized way of life which is often referred to as Skid Row. That term was originally used in America to indicate the downtown tract of rooming houses, cheap hotels, blood banks, rescue missions, winos and bottle-gangs found in many North American cities. In the UK and other European countries, clearly segmented patches of social dizorganization generally do not exist. Skid Row refers more to a way of life than to particular streets.

As for the involvement of drinking in this unfolding story, excessive drinking has often started at an early age and then followed an accelerated course. Soon after the age of 30, drink has become a dominantly destructive influence. This man now begins to stand apart even from other heavy-drinking members of the casual workforce, is beginning to be picked up for drunkenness with alarming frequency, is violently shaky every morning, and is finally drawn into companionship with the bottle-gang and to sharing their cider, wine or industrial spirits. The Skid Row way of life may appear to be chaos and disorder, but it has its own social organization and sub-culture; it becomes the individual's only support system and gives them values and expectations as well as drink. The pathways through which women move towards a life of alcohol and vagrancy may overlap with the typical male routing, but can often involve evident negative life experience, with a history of spousal violence a not uncommon feature.

Accurate and sympathetic understanding of this extreme social complication of drinking is needed if we are to cope with such problems. Too often the person in this condition tends to be even further alienated and his or her pessimism further reinforced by responses which indicate that we do indeed regard them as alien, hopeless, beyond the pale. One of the lessons of close experience is, in fact, that this condition is recoverable and that there are pathways off Skid Row, however difficult to find (Cook, 1975).

Crime

Multiple relationships

The relationship between crime and drinking is as complex as with any other social complications of alcohol. Simple, direct and one-way causality is seldom a sufficient analysis, and various models of understanding have been proposed (Zhang et al., 1997; Graham et al., 1998; Graham and West, 2001). Personality, background and social circumstances which predispose to crime may as much and independently predispose to drinking. Genetic influences may need to be considered. A drinking problem may also in passing affect a dedicated and professional criminal, perhaps at a later stage of their career. Alternatively, one may see the person who is alcohol dependent and who, at a much later age than the usual 'first offender', falls foul of the law or is caught up in a flurry of recidivism. Sometimes the person is seen who suddenly shifts from a circulation around the prisons to a hospital and voluntary agency circuit: their drinking remains much the same, but they have learnt to present themselves and their problems differently. The offence may by definition involve the actual intoxication itself: for instance, 'the drunkenness offender' (Greenfield and Weisner, 1995) and 'the drink driver' (National Institute on Alcohol Abuse and Alcoholism, 1996). The drunkenness offender overlaps with the vagrant drinking population. Social context may be very important in determining whether a drunken assault will occur or a drunken driver take off in their car, and certain kinds of poorly ordered public drinking place may engender particularly high risk (Stockwell et al., 1992)

The variations on the alcohol–crime connection are legion. There is no type of offence which will not sometimes be related to drinking, and many types of offence which will often be so related. The problems load at the petty end of the spectrum: petty theft, minor assault, travelling on public transport without a ticket, failing to pay for the meal in the cheap café, urinating in the subway, begging. The person with a drinking problem may know that when they are drunk (and only when they are drunk), they are apt to engage in their own particular offence, for example taking cars and driving them away, 'going burgling' in a clumsy sort of fashion, or passing dud cheques. Drinking may be the story behind an embezzlement.

Alcohol and violence

To the judge or the magistrate, the relationship between drinking and violence may appear to be evident and to make a repeated contribution to the offences coming before the courts. Often drinking seems to be responsible for disinhibition and release of violent or sexually violent behaviour. A Skid Row drinker hits a fellow member of a bottle-gang on the head with an iron bar; a man comes out of a pub and follows a woman down an alleyway and rapes and murders her; three drunken youths brutally assault and rob the owner of a liquor store.

Although to the courts and the ordinary citizen it may appear evident that alcohol causes or considerably contributes to the genesis of these kinds of serious crime, researchers have repeatedly pointed out the dangers in assuming an identity between correlation and causality in this arena (Shepherd, 1994; Graham and West, 2001). Many case series have shown a high frequency of intoxication among violent offenders at the time of the criminal act (Roslund and Larson, 1979), but that does not prove that the drinking *caused* the crime. People bent on violence may coincidentally choose to drink, drinking can be a mere adjunct to intrinsically dangerous situations and confrontations, and alcohol may be used for excuse.

Several different research approaches have been used to examine the validity of the assumption that alcohol can contribute to the genesis of these types of offence, and the inherent difficulties in the interpretation of simple, cross-sectional studies have been referred to above. One approach has come from anthropological research, which has suggested that the degree to which people behave violently or sexually when drunk is not so much determined by their drinking, but by the way in which society and culture believe or propose that people will behave when intoxicated (MacAndrew and Edgerton, 1969). Psychologists have explored the influence of alcohol on aggression within experimental paradigms (Gustafson, 1993; Hoaken and Pihl, 2000). Population surveys (Rossow, 1996; Fergusson and Horwood, 2000), including surveys of young people (Rossow et al., 1999), have explored the relationship between intoxication and violence. From the various lines of work mentioned in this paragraph, it is reasonable to infer that culture and set, and setting, will influence the individual's response to alcohol, but these studies still leave unanswered the question of whether alcohol is likely to contribute significantly and directly to violent crime in an industrial society.

Further light has, however, been thrown on an issue for which everyday experience and rational analysis have previously sometimes seemed to be at odds, by research which explores the correlation over time in national per-capita alcohol consumption and rates for assault or homicide (Lenke, 1990; Edwards et al., 1994). For some but not all countries, the correlations are positive. Other research has looked specifically at the relationship between drinking and offending among juveniles and has shown that, with correction for shared risk factors, there is in this age group a significant association between drinking and violent offending (Fergusson et al., 1996).

A similar literature has been developing on the relationship amongst drinking, self-harm and suicide (Murphy and Wetzel, 1990; Rossow, 1996). That a true causal link of some significance exists here is becoming increasingly evident.

Drink driving offenders

The bulk of drink driving offences are committed by the generality of the drinking population and it is to that broad target that counter-measures should predominantly be directed (Edwards et al., 1994). The factors which predict involvement in this kind of offence include not only drinking behaviour (quantity and frequency of drinking), but also other groups of variables such as socio-demographic factors, drinking behaviour and psychological characteristics (National Institute on Alcohol Abuse and Alcoholism, 1996).

Estimates of the proportion of subjects among drink driving offenders variously defined as 'alcoholics' or 'problem drinkers' have varied from 4% to 87% across samples and jurisdictions, with prevalence rates influenced by operational definition and tending to be lower when definitions are more tightly drawn. Alcohol dependence is likely to have a stronger association with drink driving the higher the blood alcohol concentration at the time of offence and among repeat offenders, and a research literature attempts to identify the differential characteristics of drinkers in treatment who are likely to offend (MacDonald and Pederson, 1990). Multiple offenders are not only likely to be more alcohol involved but also to show wider personality and background disturbance.

From the clinical angle, the conclusion must be that enquiry into driving behaviour and drink driving offences should be an integral part of any assessment. By no means everyone who has been convicted of driving while intoxicated will have an otherwise manifest drinking problem (Gruenewald et al., 1990), but among clinical populations there will be a significant proportion of individuals whose driving poses a threat to themselves and other people, with that fact putting distinct responsibility on the clinician.

The individual's drinking and the risk of being a victim of crime

There is a positive relationship in the general population between the quantity an individual drinks and the likelihood of being assaulted (Room, 1983; Edwards et al., 1994). A grossly intoxicated person will easily fall prey to having their pockets turned out or be deprived of the capacity to resist violence or rape. Thus, victimization is a common social complication of heavy drinking. Intoxication among young people may be associated with early or unwanted sexual experience (Traeen and Kvalem, 1996).

Impact on education and training

A social complication of drinking which deserves greater note is the long-term handicap which results when an educational or training opportunity is partly wasted or totally lost. Being sent down from university, failing to complete a post-graduate degree, the abandonment of an apprenticeship because of a drinking problem may all have serious long-term consequences.

The essential themes

Having started this chapter with a general discussion of the nature and genesis of social complications and having then worked through a listing of specific problem areas, it is useful finally to emphasize again certain essential themes. Drinking, and in particular drinking to intoxication, can impair many aspects of social adjustment and lead to many types of social loss or damage, but is usually an element which *contributes* to causality. The social impact of excessive drinking can seldom be understood in uni-causal and single-directional terms. Impairment of social well-being is as real and important as the physical and mental impairments with which it may interact, and concern for this dimension is therefore fundamental, both to the initial assessment and to the work of recovery.

Awareness of the social dimension to alcohol-related harm is essential to professional responses both to the drinker and to the family of the drinker. Besides the relevance of such insights for competence and roundedness at the individual level of care, there are implications for public health. Research indicates that community initiatives can help reduce the prevalence of the adverse social consequences of drinking (Holmila, 1997; Holder, 1998). Furthermore, enlightened self-interest should lead society to provide help for people with drinking problems, because so much of the burden of costs generated by drinking fall on society. Treatment will often reduce the cost of those social externalities. For instance, treatment of the husband's drinking problem has been shown over 2-year follow-up to produce sustained reduction in domestic violence (O'Farrell et al., 1999).

In short, the essential themes of this chapter are that drinking problems have social consequences, and that informed alertness to these problems is of fundamental importance to effective treatment and community responses.

REFERENCES

Braumohl, J. (ed.) (1989) Alcohol, homelessness and public policy. *Contemporary Drug Problems* 16(3), Special Issue.

Brooke, D. (1996) Why do some doctors become addicted? *Addiction* 91, 317–19.

Caetano, R. (1993) The association between severity of DSM-III-R alcohol dependence and medical and social consequences. *Addiction* 88, 631–42.

Clark, W.B. and Hilton, M.F. (eds) (1991) *Alcohol in America: drinking practises and problems.* Albany, NY: State University of New York Press.

Cook, T. (1975) *Vagrant Alcoholics.* Boston: Routledge and Kegan Paul.

Edwards, G., Anderson, P., Babor, T.F. et al. (1994) *Alcohol Policy and the Public Good.* Oxford: Oxford University Press.

Fergusson, D.M. and Horwood, J. (2000) Alcohol abuse and crime: a fixed effects regression analysis. *Addiction* 95, 1525–36.

Fergusson, D.M., Lynskey, M.T. and Horwood, L.J. (1996) Alcohol misuse and juvenile offending in adolescence. *Addiction* 91, 483–4.

Fischer, P. (1991) *Alcohol, Drug Abuse and Mental Health Problems among Homeless Persons: a Review of the Literature 1980–1990.* Rockville, MD, National Institute on Alcohol Abuse and Alcoholism.

Goodliffe, J. (1994) Alcohol and depression in England and American lawyer disciplinary proceedings. *Addiction* 89, 1237–44.

Graham, K., Leonard, K.E., Room, R. et al. (1998) Current directions in research in understanding and preventing intoxicated aggression. *Addiction* 93, 659–76.

Graham, P. and West, P. (2001) Alcohol and crime: examining the link. In *International Handbook of Alcohol Dependence and Problems*, ed. Heather, N., Peters, T.J. and Stockwell, T. Chichester: John Wiley and Sons, 439–70.

Greenfield, T.K. and Weisner, C. (1995) Drinking problems and self-reported criminal behavior, arrests, and convictions: 1990 US national and 1989 county surveys. *Addiction* 90, 361–74.

Gruenewald, P.J., Stewart, K. and Klitzner, M. (1990) Alcohol use and the appearance of alcohol problems among first offender drunk drivers. *British Journal of Addiction* 85, 107–17.

Gustafson, R. (1993) What do experimental paradigms tell us about alcohol-related aggressive responses? *Journal of Studies on Alcohol* (Suppl. 11), 20–9.

Gutjahr, E. and Gmel, G. (2001) The social costs of alcohol consumption. In *Mapping the Social Consequences of Alcohol Consumption*, ed. Klingemann, H. and Gmel, G. Dordrecht: Kluwer Academic Publishers, 133–43.

Hoaken, P.N.S. and Pihl, R.O. (2000) The effects of alcohol intoxication on aggression responses in men and women. *Alcohol and Alcoholism* 35, 471–7.

Holdener, F.O. (1993) Alcohol and civil aviation. *Addiction* 88 (Suppl.), 953–8.

Holder, H.D. (1998) *Alcohol and the Community: a Systems Approach to Prevention*. International Research Monographs in the Addictions 1. Cambridge: Cambridge University Press.

Holmila, M. (ed.) (1997) *Community Prevention of Alcohol Problems*. London: Macmillan.

Jones, S., Casswell, S. and Zhang, J-F. (1995) The economic costs of alcohol-related absenteeism and reduced productivity in the working population of New Zealand. *Addiction* 90, 1453–62.

Kipke, M.D., Montgomery, S.B., Simon, T.R. and Iverson, E.F. (1997) 'Substance abuse' disorders among runaway and homeless youth. *Substance Use and Misuse* 32, 969–86.

Klingemann, H. and Gmel, G. (eds) (2001) *Mapping the Social Consequences of Alcohol Consumption*. Dordrecht: Kluwer Academic Publishers.

Lenke, L. (1990) *Alcohol and Criminal Violence – Time Series Analyses in a Comparative Perspective*. Stockholm: Almqvist and Wiksell.

MacAndrew, C. and Edgerton, R.B. (1969) *Drunken Comportment*. Chicago: Aldine.

MacDonald, S and Pederson, L.L. (1990) The characteristics of alcoholics in treatment arrested for driving while impaired. *British Journal of Addiction* 85, 97–105.

McDermott, I. (1994) Journal interview 34. Conversation with Monsignor Ignatius McDermott. *Addiction* 89, 791–8.

Midanik, L.T., Tam, T.W., Greenfield, T.K. and Caetano, R. (1996) Risk functions of alcohol-related problems in a 1988 US national sample. *Addiction* 91, 1427–37.

Murphy, G.E. and Wetzel, R.D. (1990) The lifetime risk of suicide in alcoholism. *Archives of General Psychiatry* 47, 383–92.

National Institute on Alcohol Abuse and Alcoholism (1996) Drinking and driving. *Alcohol Alert* 31, 1–3.

O'Farrell, T.J., Van Hutton, V. and Murphy, C.M. (1999). Domestic violence before and after alcoholism treatment: a two-year longitudinal study. *Journal of Studies on Alcohol* 60, 317–21.

Rice, D.P., Kelman, S. and Miller, L.S. (1991) The economic cost of alcohol abuse. *Alcohol Health and Research World* 15, 307–16.

Romelsjö, A. (1995) Alcohol consumption and unintentional injury, suicide, violence, work performance and intergenerational effects. In *Alcohol and Public Policy: Evidence and Issues*, ed. Holder, H.D. and Edwards, G. Oxford: Oxford University Press, 114–42.

Room, R. (1983) Alcohol and crime, behavioral aspects. In *Encyclopedia of Crime and Justice, Vol. 1*, ed. Kadish, S. New York: The Free Press, 35–44.

Roslund, B. and Larson, C.A. (1979) Crimes of violence and alcohol abuse in Sweden. *International Journal of the Addictions* 14, 1103–15.

Rossow, I. (1996) Alcohol and suicide. Beyond the link at the individual level *Addiction* 91, 1413–16.

Rossow I., Pape H. and Witchstrøm L. (1999) Young, wet and wild? Association between alcohol intoxication and violent behaviour in adolescence. *Addiction* 94, 1017–31.

Shepherd, J. (1994) Violent crime: the role of alcohol and new approaches to the prevention of injury. *Alcohol and Alcoholism* 29, 5–10.

Sosin, M.R. and Bruni, M. (1997) Homelessness and vulnerability among adults with and without alcohol problems. *Substance Use and Misuse* 32, 939–68.

Stockwell, T., Somerford, P. and Lang, E. (1992) The relationship between license type and alcohol-related problems attributed to licensed premises in Perth, Western Australia. *Journal of Studies on Alcohol* 53, 495–8.

Traeen, B. and Kvalem, I.L. (1996) Sex under the influence of alcohol among Norwegian adolescents. *Addiction* 91, 995–1006.

Upmark, M., Möller, J. and Romelsjö, A. (1999) Longitudinal, population-based study of self-reported alcohol habits, high levels of sickness absence, and disability pensions. *Journal of Epidemiology and Community Heath* 53, 223–9.

Zhang, L., Wieczoreix, W.F. and Welte, J.W. (1997) The nexus between alcohol and violent crime. *Alcoholism: Clinical and Experimental Research* 21, 1264–71.

7

Drinking problems as cause of neuropsychiatric disorders

In some instances heavy drinking actually causes mental illness. This usually indicates that the drinking problem is serious and of relatively long duration, and that a degree of neuroadaptation is already present (see Chapter 3). This chapter deals with the neuropsychiatric complications seen in individuals with drinking problems. It looks firstly at alcohol-related hallucinatory states as exemplifying conditions for which drinking or withdrawal of alcohol is of undoubted and central causality. Delirium tremens, alcohol hallucinosis and alcohol-induced psychotic disorder with delusions are considered, followed by a review of pathological intoxication and alcoholic blackouts. Finally, the Wernicke–Korsakoff syndrome, alcoholic pellagra encephalopathy and alcohol-related brain damage are discussed.

Transient hallucinatory experience

Transient hallucinatory experience deserves note for two reasons. First, it may herald the onset of delirium tremens or alcoholic hallucinosis, and can often give early warning of the likelihood of these much more serious illnesses. It may therefore be viewed as continuous with these states, rather than as an altogether discrete clinical entity. Second, it is important to be aware that transient hallucinations may occur without the illness progressing to either of the major presentations. The diagnostician who is unfamiliar with these transient phenomena may be tempted to record incorrectly that the patient has 'suffered from DTs', when this was not the case.

The essence of this condition is that the patient fleetingly and suddenly experiences any one of a variety of perceptual disturbances, often very much to their surprise and consternation, and with the episode then immediately over. These occurrences may be experienced during periods of continued, heavy and chaotic dependent drinking or during withdrawal. There is no delirium or evidence of severe physiological disturbance as seen in delirium tremens. Here are some examples of how patients described such experiences.

I would be driving along the road and suddenly something would run across in front of the car – a dog, a cat, I couldn't be sure – and I would slam on the brakes. A real fright. And then I'd realise there was nothing there.

I would be walking down the road and, ZOOM, a car would come up behind me and I'd jump on the pavement. Frightened out of my life. But it was all imagination.

What used to happen was that I would turn around thinking someone had called my name.

The degree of insight is often characteristic; the patient immediately disconfirms the reality of the hallucination. A relatively stereotyped and limited kind of hallucinatory experience is also typical; for one patient it is nearly always the car coming up from behind, for another a pigeon flying into the room. It is important to realize that some patients can experience such discomforting happenings for many months without progressing to a major disturbance. The meaning and significance of 'continuity' will immediately become clear as we go on below to discuss delirium tremens and alcoholic hallucinosis.

Delirium tremens

The clinical picture

Delirium tremens is a short-lived, toxic, confusional state which usually occurs as a result of reduced alcohol intake in alcohol dependent individuals with a long history of use (World Health Organization, 1992).

Delirium tremens can produce a variety of clinical pictures, but it is best viewed as a unitary syndrome with a continuum of severities and a variation in symptom clustering. The disturbance is often fluctuating, with the patient's condition worsening in the evening or when the room is unlit and shadowy. The classical triad of symptoms includes clouding of consciousness and confusion, vivid hallucinations affecting any sensory modality and marked tremor. Delusions, agitation, sleeplessness and autonomic arousal are frequently also present.

Symptoms of delirium usually occur from about 24 hours to 150 hours after the last drink (within this band earlier rather than later onset is more typical), peaking between 72 and 96 hours (Naranjo and Sellers, 1986). Prodromal symptoms are usually evident, but may be overlooked. The onset is often at night, with restlessness, insomnia and fear (Lishman, 1998).

Delirium

The patient is more or less out of contact with reality and potentially disorientated as to person, place and time. For instance, they may believe that they are cruising on a liner, mistake the nurse for a steward and order a drink, but 5 minutes later know that they are in hospital and correctly identify the people around them.

Hallucinations and illusions

Hallucinations and illusions are characteristically vivid, chaotic and bizarre and occur in any sensory modality: the patient may see visions, hear things, smell gases or feel animals crawling over them. The classical visual hallucinations are vivid and horrifying and typically include snakes and rats and other small animals which may appear to attack the patient as they lie in bed. They may also take a 'microscopic' form (small, furry men dancing on the floor), but any type of visual hallucination can occur. These visions are often brightly coloured and have been described by Hemmingsen and Kramp (1988) as 'kaleidoscopic with a niavistic, animated, cartoon-like flavour'. One patient in their series had visual hallucinations of soldiers outside the window, Marilyn Monroe on the roof, policemen selling flowers, and insects. Patients often become completely preoccupied by, and interact with, the hallucinated objects. Thus, they feed the dogs or argue with the little men.

Hallucinatory voices or bursts of music may be heard, or the threatening screams of animals. Hallucinations are often based on a ready tendency to illusional misrepresentation: the wrinkles in the bedclothes become snakes, patterns in the wallpaper become faces.

Tremor

As the illness develops, the patient become anxious and more fearful and develops tremor. At worst, they may be shaking so severely that the bed is rattling, but, as with other symptoms, there can be a continuum of severity and the tremor may not be very noticeable unless the patient is asked to stretch out their hands.

Fear

The patient may be experiencing extremes of horror in reaction for instance to the snakes which writhe all over their bed, but on other occasions the hallucinations appear to be enjoyable or entertaining, and the patient is perhaps happily watching a private cinema show.

Paranoid delusions

The illness often has a degree of paranoid flavouring: enemies are blowing poisonous gas into the room, assassins lurk at the window and there is a nameless conspiracy afoot. The mood can, in fact, be paranoid, with every happening and stimulus being misrepresented as it comes along, but the patient's mental state is too muddled for the delusional ideas to become systematized.

Occupational delusions or hallucinations

The barman, for instance, may believe that he is serving in his cocktail bar and pour out imaginary drinks, or the bricklayer may be building an imaginary wall.

Restlessness and agitation

Partly as a consequence of the fearfulness of the hallucinatory experiences, the patient is often highly restless, clutching and pulling at the bed clothes, starting at any sound, or attempting to jump out of bed and run down the ward. This over-activity, when combined with a degree of weakness and unsteadiness, can put the patient seriously at risk of falls and other accidents.

Heightened suggestibility

The patient who is suffering from delirium tremens can show a heightened susceptibility to suggestion, which occasionally becomes evident spontaneously but may only come out on testing. The older text books often mention such stories as the patient agreeing to deal from an imaginery pack of cards or 'drinking' from a proffered but empty glass.

Physical disturbances

Heavy sweating is typical, with the consequent risk of dehydration. Appetite is usually lacking, the pulse is rapid and the blood pressure is likely to be raised and the patient feverish. If the illness continues over many days, the picture gradually becomes that of dehydration, exhaustion and collapse, with the possibility of a sudden and disastrously steep rise in temperature.

Aetiology and course

Delirium tremens is today generally viewed as essentially an alcohol withdrawal state, although it is conceded that other factors such as infection or trauma sometimes play an ancillary part. The withdrawal which precipitates the attack may have been occasioned by admission to hospital, arrest and incarceration, or a self-determined effort to give up drinking. Often, though, there is no history of abrupt withdrawal and the illness starts while the patient is still drinking, but there has probably been at least partial withdrawal. In some instances the patient seems to have hovered on the brink of delirium tremens for many preceding weeks, with much evidence of transient hallucinatory experience, whereas in other instances the illness has a more explosive onset. It is unusual for a patient to experience

delirium tremens without a history of at least several years of severe alcohol dependence and many years of excessive drinking, but an attack may occur even after 1 or
2 weeks if a previously abstinent patient rapidly reinstates dependence. Recurrent
attacks are common once a patient has had one such episode.

The condition usually lasts for 3–5 days, with gradual resolution. On rare occasions, the illness drags on for some weeks, fluctuating between recovery and relapse.
The possibility of severe physical complications has been mentioned and, before
the advent of antibiotics, intercurrent chest infection or pneumonia constituted a
serious risk. Reported mortality rates have varied from centre to centre and even
with skilled care a degree of risk remains, with death occurring in about 5% of
admissions (Chick, 1989; Cushman, 1987). Death is typically due to cardiovascular
collapse, hypothermia or intercurrent infection.

Possibilities of diagnostic confusion

It might be supposed that delirium tremens would give a picture so vivid and distinct
as to make diagnostic mistakes unlikely. There is always the possibility that an
underlying condition which is contributing to the picture is being overlooked. Liver
failure, pneumonia and head injury should always be borne in mind. Confusion may
also occur when the possibility of delirium tremens is entirely overlooked, although
in retrospect the diagnosis was plainly evident. This is often the case in the setting of
a general hospital ward, where the patient is noted to be suffering from 'confusion',
to be 'rambling a bit', or to be trying to get out of bed at night. In this situation
the condition may be put down to the non-specific effects of infection, trauma or
operation. The diagnosis is at times overlooked in the psychiatric hospital setting,
when it may be misdiagnosed as an 'acute schizophrenic reaction', for instance
when the acutely disturbed person with delirium tremens has florid paranoid ideas
and is found running up the street with a knife in their hand and presents as an
emergency admission from the police.

The treatment of delirium tremens is outlined on page 272.

A 65-year-old widower was admitted to a general hospital via ambulance following a period
of heavy drinking. On admission he was written up for one dose of chlordiazepoxide (25 mg
orally). An adequate dosage regime was not commenced, even though nursing and medical
staff were aware that he had an alcohol problem. During the first two days of admission he
was 'pleasantly confused'. On the third day he went into the nursing office, where he saw
a nurse 'organizing patients into groups'. He suddenly realized that this meant everyone
had to be evacuated because of a bomb scare. He left the ward in his pyjamas and bare
feet, walked out of the hospital into a busy street, 'shouting vividly' that the hospital was in
danger. He was duly found, returned by porters and reassured by nursing staff. Ten days later
he had a hazy recall of the event: 'I knew it wasn't true, and yet I experienced a mounting

and inexplicable fear and I knew that I had to escape.' Since then nothing extraordinary has happened.

Alcoholic hallucinosis

The term alcoholic hallucinosis is used to describe auditory or visual hallucinations that occur either during or after a period of heavy alcohol consumption (Glass-Crome, 1989a, 1989b; Tsuang et al., 1994). The hallucinations are vivid, of acute onset and typically occur in the setting of clear consciousness (World Health Organization, 1992). They may be accompanied by misidentifications, delusions, ideas of reference and an abnormal affect. Alcoholic hallucinosis typically resolves over a period of weeks, but can occasionally persist for months. Delirium tremens and psychotic disorders must be ruled out before a diagnosis of alcoholic hallucinosis can be made.

In alcoholic hallucinosis the auditory hallucinations may consist of unformed noises or snatches of music, but usually take the form of voices. These voices may be talking to the patient directly, but more often take the form of a running commentary about them. Sometimes there is only one voice, but often several engage in discussion, and the same voice may come back again on different occasions. The commentary may be favourable and friendly, or accusatory and threatening. Sometimes the voices command the patient to do things against their will and this may result in acting-out behaviour or a suicide attempt. There is a lack of insight and the voices are considered as real, but the patient will seldom elaborate any complex explanation as to the supposed mechanism by which the voices are reaching them. The voices may come and go or haunt the patient more or less incessantly.

The majority of studies of alcoholic hallucinosis were carried out before the widespread use of operational criteria and standardized assessment, and were therefore based on mixed samples of patients having hallucinations associated with alcohol withdrawal, schizophrenia, major depression and psychostimulant use such as amphetamines or cocaine. Tsuang et al. (1994) have shown that the prevalence of 'alcoholic hallucinosis' varies according to the diagnostic criteria used.

There is little evidence to support the view that alcoholic hallucinosis is a form of latent schizophrenia. Nevertheless, it may superficially resemble acute paranoid schizophrenia and the differential diagnosis may be difficult. The delusions associated with alcoholic hallucinosis are usually attempts to explain the hallucinations. There is no evidence of a complicated delusional system, schizophrenic thought disorder or incongruity of affect, and insight is regained as the voices diminish (Lishman, 1998). While these guidelines provide useful indications, it can still in practice be difficult to make the distinction, and in such circumstances the sensible course of action is to admit the patient to hospital, withdraw them from alcohol and observe what happens. Recovery may take place abruptly, but more often there is a slow fading of the symptoms. The voices become less persistent, do not make such an urgent demand on attention and their reality begins to be doubted.

The possibility that the illness will finally declare itself to be schizophrenia has, of course, to be borne in mind, and if symptoms have not ceased within a couple of months, the latter diagnosis becomes more likely, although it has been reported that alcoholic hallucinosis may sometimes require even 6 months for complete recovery. Some drug intoxications, including most notably amphetamine psychosis, can also result in a picture mimicking alcoholic hallucinosis and with a presentation of this sort it is always wise to carry out urine testing for drugs.

When a patient has experienced one attack of alcoholic hallucinosis, they are at risk of recurrence of this condition if they drink again, although such reinstatement is not inevitable.

The possible pathophysiological mechanisms underlying alcoholic hallucinosis are described by Soyka (1995). The acute onset of hallucinations during alcohol withdrawal may reflect increased dopamine activity and decreased serotonin (5-HT) in the brain (see Chapter 3). More recent work points to the role of beta-carbolines and essential fatty acids.

Alcohol-induced psychotic disorder with delusions

The category alcohol-induced psychotic disorders with delusions has been included in DSM-IV (American Psychiatric Association, 1994) and deserves mention here. Although few studies have systematically focused on this clinical condition, it has been reported in the literature for at least 150 years. Such patients typically develop paranoid or grandiose delusions in the context of heavy drinking, but remain alert and do not display any confusion or clouding of consciousness. Although psychiatric hospitalization may be required, the prognosis is generally good and the delusional syndrome clears within days to weeks of abstinence. As with alcoholic hallucinosis, there appears to be no association with schizophrenia.

'Pathological intoxication'

Pathological intoxication, sometimes referred to as mania à potu, is a term used to describe a sudden onset of aggressive and often violent behaviour, not typical of the individual when sober, and occurring soon after drinking small amounts of alcohol that would not produce intoxication in most people (Coid, 1979). There is classically an amnesia for the event and it is alleged that the aggressor was in a trance state or displaying automatism. The episode is usually followed by a long sleep. There may be an association with EEG abnormalities and other signs of brain damage, particularly frontal lobe dysfunction.

Pathological intoxication is an ill-defined entity (Coid, 1979) and it is doubtful whether such a distinct entity deserves recognition. Clearly, a relationship between drinking and aggression does exist (see page 88), and the aggressor in such circumstances often manifests an alcohol-induced amnesia if there has been a high blood-alcohol level at the time of the offence. Careful questioning will usually reveal that the amount of alcohol ingested was more than a 'small amount' and that there has been previous evidence of propensity to violence. This is borne out by Maletzky's (1976) work, which demonstrated that large amounts of alcohol were required before disturbed behaviour was evident. Other instances of supposed pathological intoxication may be attributable to alcohol-induced hypoglycaemia, organic brain damage or personality disorder.

Here is an account of the type of case which frequently comes before the courts.

A young man aged 23 had a pattern of frequent but intermittent heavy drinking. At his brother's wedding he became very drunk and argumentative. The best man tried to quieten him down but a quarrel ensued, and without warning this young drinker picked up a knife and stabbed a bystander, narrowly missing the victim's heart. The assailant said that he had 'only taken a drink or two', but this was clearly untrue. He displayed a patchy amnesia for the surrounding events. Enquiry revealed that he had on several previous occasions been involved in dangerous fights, both when drunk and when sober.

It can hardly be doubted that this young man's intoxication contributed to his loss of impulse control, and it was probably the crucial additional factor which sparked off his violence, given also the background importance of predisposition and circumstance. The position taken here is not that intoxication is irrelevant to understanding such events, but rather that it is unproductive to segment cases into those due to 'intoxication', as opposed to instances in which 'pathological intoxication' is deemed to be the cause. This distinction is encouraged by legal systems, which give simple drunkeness no standing, and which therefore lead defence lawyers to search for a medical basis on which to argue that their client's intoxication was a disease manifestation. From the strictly medical point of view, 'pathological drunkeness' is a very uncertain concept.

Alcoholic blackouts (alcohol-induced amnesic episodes)

The widely used but somewhat confusing lay term 'alcoholic blackout' refers to transient memory loss which may be induced by intoxication. There is no associated loss of consciousness. Clinicians should not enquire simply whether the patient has had a blackout and leave it at that. It is preferable to ask: 'Have you ever forgotten things you did while drinking?' Although such occurrences are reported in some two-thirds or more of alcohol dependent individuals (Schuckit et al., 1993; Goodwin et al., 1969a, 1969b), alcoholic memory blackouts are also relatively common in social drinkers after incidents of heavy indulgence. Approximately one-third of young men in the general population are likely to have experienced memory blackouts (Goodwin et al., 1969a). Thus, while they are an important warning sign of problem drinking, they are not pathognomonic of alcohol dependence.

Blackouts have been described as being of two types (Goodwin et al., 1969a, 1969b). The 'en bloc' variety is characterized by a dense and total amnesia with abrupt points of onset and recovery, and with no subsequent recall of events for the amnesic period, either spontaneously or with prompting. This period may extend from 30 to 60 minutes up to as long as 2 or 3 days. In contrast, 'fragmentary' blackouts or 'greyouts' are patchy episodes of amnesia, with indistinct boundaries and islands of memory within these boundaries. They are often characterized by partial or complete subsequent recall, and usually extend over a shorter period than the 'en bloc' variety. In reality, alcoholic memory blackouts can occur with every degree of gradation and, although it is useful to recognize the two types, the experience of each patient has to be described separately.

Blackouts may begin to occur at a late stage in a career of excessive drinking or never at all. Once they start to be experienced with any frequency, they tend to recur, and often patients may be able to identify the phase at which they 'began to get bad blackouts'. The reason for such varied susceptibility to the disorder is unknown, but blackouts are associated with an early onset of drinking, high peak levels of alcohol and a past history of head injury (Kopelman, 1991). Concurrent use of sedatives and hypnotics may increase the likelihood of amnesia. Blackouts are not predictive of long-term cognitive impairment.

During an alcoholic blackout, the individual can engage in any type of activity. To the observer, the drinker will not obviously be in an abnormal state of mind (other than being intoxicated), although a spouse or someone else who knows them well may claim to recognize subtle changes – for instance, 'they get that glazed look'.

The journey syndrome

Patients sometimes report that during an alcohol blackout period they wandered away from home, later 'waking up' in a strange place, an event which is described as a 'fugue state' in psychiatric terms. Here is an example.

When I came round I was sitting in a barber's chair having a shave. Hadn't a clue where I'd got to this time, terribly embarrassed, didn't like to ask. I had to go outside and look at the shop signs until I found the answer, and then to my amazement I discovered I was in this town 150 miles from home. To this day I don't know how I got there. That was the worst experience of this kind, but time after time I woke up in strange places or found myself sitting on a train going to the coast.

Blackouts and their significance to the patient

One patient may mention their blackouts only on direct questioning and appear not to be at all worried about such experiences, while another patient may be very worried about these experiences and see them as a leading reason for seeking help. Blackouts for the latter type of patient are often a matter of dread, with, for instance, recurrent, anguished fear that they may have hurt or killed someone while driving home; they do not remember getting their car into the garage the previous night, and they go out in the morning fearfully to check the paint work.

Wernicke–Korsakoff syndrome

Although Wernicke's encephalopathy and Korsakoff's psychosis were originally described as different entities (in 1881 and 1887, respectively), both are caused by thiamine (vitamin B_1) deficiency and show the same underlying pathological lesions in the periventricular and periaqueductal grey matter (Victor et al., 1971). Cortical abnormalities have also been reported in a proportion of cases. Prevalence rates of the Wernicke–Korsakoff syndrome vary, with autopsy studies reporting rates of about 1.5% (Cook et al., 1998). The condition is commoner in autopsy studies of 'alcoholics'. Incidence rates are reported to have increased in Scotland over recent years (Ramayya and Jauhar, 1997). Wernicke's encephalopathy is the acute or sub-acute manifestation of the syndrome and Korsakoff's psychosis the chronic form.

Wernicke's encephalopathy

Wernicke's encephalopathy occurs in alcohol misuse and dependence and in a variety of other disorders associated with a poor intake or absorption of thiamine. These other disorders include gastric carcinoma, other malignancy, hyperemesis in pregnancy, anorexia nervosa and haemodialysis. In alcohol dependent individuals, Wernicke's encephalopathy is often precipitated by alcohol withdrawal or the stress of an intercurrent illness. Some individuals may have a particular susceptibility to developing the condition.

The encephalopathy usually has an abrupt onset, although it may take a few days for the full picture to develop (Lishman, 1998). Mental confusion or staggering or unsteady gait is often the first feature to be seen. The patient may be aware of ocular abnormalities – they complain of wavering vision or double vision on looking to the side. The classic triad of confusion, ataxia and ocular abnormalities (nystagmus, an oscillatory movement of the eyeballs; and ophthalmoplegia, a paralysis of the eye muscles that might cause a squint) is diagnostic. However, these symptoms and signs may only be present in part, or not at all, and the diagnosis is often missed in life. There must always, therefore, be a high index of suspicion, particularly in cases of unexplained confusion. Other common features include anorexia, nausea and vomiting (Lishman, 1998). There is usually a degree of memory disorder. Lethargy and hypotension have also been described. Rarely, the disorder presents with hypothermia, stupor or coma. About 17–20% of patients die in the acute stage (Cook et al., 1998).

Given the difficulties in making a definitive diagnosis, there should be a low threshold for making a presumptive diagnosis (see Box 7.1).

BOX 7.1 Wernicke's encephalopathy

A presumptive diagnosis of Wernicke's encephalopathy should be made in heavy-drinking and alcohol dependent individuals who develop one or more of the following unexplained symptoms:

- Confusion/apathy
- Drowsiness
- Coma/unconsciousness
- Abnormal eye movements that might seem like a squint
- Double vision
- Poor balance

Patients with a presumptive diagnosis of Wernicke's encephalopathy should be treated promptly with high-dose parenteral B-complex vitamins.

Wernicke's encephalopathy is a medical emergency. Treatment with high-dose parenteral thiamine should be given promptly to offset the risk of death or irreversible brain damage. Parenteral thiamine is itself associated with a small risk of anaphylactic reactions and should only be given when appropriate resuscitation facilities are available. Up to 1 g of thiamine may be needed initially to achieve a clinical response. Thereafter, 500 mg thiamine should be given once or twice daily for 3–5 days (Cook and Thomson, 1998).

Hypomagnesaemia may impair the clinical response to treatment and it is therefore worth checking serum magnesium levels. Electrolyte imbalance and dehydration must be avoided, and any intercurrent infection treated. Oral B vitamins are usually continued for several weeks.

Ocular abnormalities usually recover quite quickly (within days or weeks) and the ataxia usually responds within the first week, but takes about 1–2 months to resolve (Lishman, 1998). Some patients are left with a residual nystagmus and ataxia. Improvements in acute confusion or delirium usually occur within 1–2 days. Global confusion begins to improve after 2–3 weeks, but may take 1–2 months to clear. As it improves, so the amnesic (memory) defects become more obvious.

A milder, sub-clinical form of Wernicke's encephalopathy exists in which patients do not manifest the clinical signs and symptoms outlined above. Undiagnosed and untreated episodes are experienced, resulting in chronic pathological changes at autopsy. The existence of sub-clinical Wernicke's encephalopathy has important implications for the prophylactic use of high-dose parenteral vitamin B therapy (Cook and Thomson, 1998).

In Wernicke's encephalopathy, pathological changes are symmetrical and occur in the walls of the third ventricle, the periaqueductal region, the floor of the fourth ventricle, certain thalamic nuclei, the maxillary bodies, the terminal portions of the fornices, the brainstem and the anterior lobe and superior vermis of the cerebellum (Lishman, 1998).

Korsakoff's syndrome

Korsakoff's syndrome often emerges as a chronic disorder following an episode of Wernicke's encephalopathy. It can, however, develop insidiously, with no clear prior history of a Wernicke episode. The main defect in Korsakoff's syndrome is in recent memory (Lishman, 1998). New learning is impaired. In some instances there is no new learning and an anterograde amnesia is evident (this is an inability to lay down new memories). However, the immediate memory span is unimpaired, so performance on a test of digit span (ability to repeat a list of numbers) is usually normal. Some retrograde amnesia (loss of memory for events occurring before the onset of the syndrome) is usually evident and this may be of long duration. Individuals with Korsakoff's syndrome also manifest a disturbance in time sense, for instance some recent memory is allocated to the past, or a past event is brought up as a recent happening. Remote memory for matters beyond the retrograde gap is better preserved, but may also be impaired. Confabulation (the fabrication of ready answers and fluent descriptions of fictitious experiences compensating for gaps in memory) has been described. However, it is more likely that patients produce false memories without realizing this (Knight, 2001). Confabulation may come and go and seems to be commoner in the early stages (Lishman, 1998).

Other cognitive functions may appear to be superficially intact, but are often found to be impaired when examined carefully. These individuals therefore find it difficult to sustain mental activity, have an inflexible set and reduced capacity to shift attention from one task to another. Their thinking is often stereotyped, perseverative and facile (Lishman, 1998). There are marked disturbances in personality, with a degree of apathy and self-neglect. Some patients are chatty, but the content of the conversation is superficial and repetitive. They often lack interest in their surroundings and may show little interest in alcohol. They show a remarkable lack of insight, with few realizing that they have memory deficits.

In Korsakoff's syndrome, the pathology at the base of the brain is usually associated with cortical shrinkage and ventricular dilatation. It is likely that Korsakoff's syndrome is misdiagnosed in clinical practice and that there is some overlap between it and 'alcoholic dementia' (Lishman, 1998). Neuroimaging studies report a range of subcortical lesions and cortical atrophy. Functional imaging studies report impaired frontal cortical blood flow (Joyce, 1994). Neuropsychological studies also reveal frontal lobe deficits, which could explain aspects of the syndrome such as lack of insight and apathy.

The amnesia of Korsakoff's syndrome does not generally respond to treatment with thiamine. This raises the possibility that thiamine deficiency may not be the sole factor contributing to the development of the disorder. Alcohol neurotoxicity must also be considered, either alone or in association with thiamine deficiency.

These rather strange-sounding eponyms should not deflect the non-specialist from trying to understand what is being talked about, and the following case abstract illustrates both how the acute element can present very suddenly and the type of chronic disorder which may occur when the Wernicke–Korsakoff syndrome supervenes.

A woman aged 48, who had been drinking a bottle of whisky each day for 10 or more years, was admitted to a psychiatric hospital for detoxification. It was noted that she was suffering from severe peripheral neuropathy (weakness, tingling, and pain in the legs). On the evening of admission, she was found to be rather confused, to be complaining of double vision, and to be staggering. By the next evening, she was stuporose, and her eye movements were unco-ordinated (external ocular palsies). At this stage, and much too late, she was started on massive doses of thiamine – the classical picture of confusion, staggering gait and ocular palsies should have alerted the staff to the dangerous onset of Wernicke's encephalopathy. After 5 days of the acute illness, the confusion cleared and the patient was then found to have a grossly impaired memory for recent events, a tendency to make things up to fill her gaps in memory (confabulation) and very little ability to remember new information, as witnessed by her difficulty in finding her way around the ward. This amnesic syndrome (Korsakoff syndrome) showed little recovery over the ensuing months, and arrangements had to be made for the patient's transfer to long-term residential care.

This is a story of a tragedy which might have been averted, and there is a good argument for giving thiamine prophylactically to any patient who is in danger of this sort of complication.

Alcoholic pellagra encephalopathy

This is caused by a deficiency of nicotinic acid and its precursor tryptophan in association with chronic alcohol misuse. It is rarely reported in the British and American literature, perhaps because of the routine use of parenteral multi-vitamin therapy (Lishman, 1981). However, this may be due to under-diagnosis because it is still evident in other countries, such as Japan. Clinical features include a fluctuating confusional state with global memory loss, visual hallucinations, restlessness alternating with apathy and other neurological signs, including myoclonic jerks and hyper-reflexia. Differential diagnosis can be difficult and it can be misdiagnosed as delirium tremens. Treatment with thiamine and pyridoxine can aggravate the condition, which responds to treatment with nicotinic acid.

Alcoholic 'dementia'

Many individuals with a history of chronic alcohol misuse have mild to moderate impairment in short-term and long-term memory, learning, visuo-spatial organization, visuo-perceptual abstraction, maintenance of cognitive set and impulse control (Oscar-Berman, 1990). Neuropsychological tests improve with abstinence, but some impairments may still be evident even 5 years later. With the advent of computerized tomographic (CT) scanning, cortical shrinkage (particularly in the frontal area) and ventricular enlargement were confirmed in about two-thirds of 'alcoholics', compared with age-matched controls (Lishman, 1998). Abstinence was shown to lead to reversal of brain shrinkage, particular in younger individuals and in women. Neuropathological studies have shown that, in comparison with controls, brain weight is significantly reduced in heavy drinkers at autopsy with selective neuronal loss.

Magnetic resonance imaging (MRI) confirms cortical atrophy and mild ventricular enlargement, as well as volume reductions in various parts of the brain (Jernigan et al., 1991; Pfefferbaum et al., 1992, 1997, 1998; Agartz et al., 1999). Functional imaging studies suggest a reduced cerebral blood flow within the medial frontal cortex. Implications of alcohol-related brain damage for the treatment of alcohol dependence are discussed on page 126.

It is likely that cognitive deficits represent one possible factor contributing to poor treatment outcome. Therapeutic programmes may be too complex for these individuals to grasp. Clinicians should therefore be familiar with the risk factors and early signs of cognitive impairment in their patients. Simple objective feedback about neuropsychological test results and brain scans may help to motivate the patient to abstinence. Patients with moderate to severe brain damage who appear cognitively intact may not be able to understand the principles of motivational interviewing, cognitive–behavioural therapy and relapse prevention (see Chapter 18). Their initial needs are more basic and likely to include good nutrition, treatment with parenteral and oral thiamine and residential placement in a supervised setting. The repetitive structure and routine of Alcoholics Anonymous (AA) are well suited to those with mild–moderate brain damage. AA, of course, also has within it much complexity, but the cognitively handicapped patient will perhaps be able to focus on the simpler aspects of the AA programme.

Neuropsychiatric disorders: the broad implications

The types of problem discussed in this chapter are of varying degrees of potential clinical threat, but some may be dangerous or life threatening for the patient. These syndrome profiles are in principle recognizable, but the clinician must be sensitive to their degrees and varieties of presentation – a failure to make the diagnosis or respond appropriately can, at the worst, have tragic consequences. Everyone working in this field needs therefore to be alert to the reality of these conditions, which may be met with any day.

REFERENCES

Agartz, I., Momenan, R., Rawlings, M.S., Kerrich, M.J., and Hommer, D.W. (1999) Hippocampal volume in patients with alcohol dependence. *Archives of General Psychiatry* 56, 356–63.

American Psychiatric Association (1994) *Diagnostic and Statistical Manual of Mental Disorders*, 4th edn. Washington, DC: American Psychiatric Association.

Coid, J. (1979) 'Mania a potu': a critical review of pathological intoxication. *Psychological Medicine* 9, 709–19.

Chick, J. (1989) Delirium tremens. *British Medical Journal* 298, 3–4.

Cook, C.C.H. and Hallwood, P.M. and Thomson, A.D. (1998) B vitamin deficiency and neuro-psychiatric syndromes in alcohol misuse. *Alcohol and Alcoholism* 33, 317–36.

Cook, C.C.H. and Thomson, A.D. (1998) B-complex vitamins in the prophylaxis and treatment of Wernicke–Korsakoff syndrome. *British Journal of Hospital Medicine* 57, 461–5.

Cushman, P. (1987) Delirium tremens – update on an old disorder. *Postgraduate Medicine* 82, 117–22.

Glass-Crome, I.B. (1989a) Alcoholic hallucinosis: a psychiatric enigma – I. The development of an idea. *British Journal of Addiction* 84, 29–41.

Glass-Crome, I.B. (1989b) Alcoholic hallucinosis: a psychiatric enigma – 2. Follow-up studies. *British Journal of Addiction* 84, 151–64.

Goodwin, D.W., Crane, B.J. and Guze, S.B. (1969a) Phenomenological aspects of the alcoholic 'blackout'. *British Journal of Psychiatry* 115, 1033–8.

Goodwin, D.W., Crane, B.J. and Guze, S.B. (1969b) Alcoholic 'blackouts': a review and clinical study of 100 alcoholics. *American Journal of Psychiatry* 126, 191–8.

Hemmingsen, R. and Kramp, P. (1988) Delirium tremens and related clinical states. *Acta Psychiatrica Scandinavica* 345 (Suppl.), 94–107.

Jernigan, T.L., Butters, N., Di Traglia, G. et al. (1991) Reduced cerebral gray matter observed in alcoholics using magnetic resonance imaging. *Alcoholism: Clinical and Experimental Research* 15, 418–27.

Joyce, E.M. (1994) Aetiology of alcoholic brain damage: alcoholic neurotoxicity or thiamine malnutrition? In *Alcohol and alcohol problems*, ed. Edwards, G. and Peters, T.J. *British Medical Bulletin* 50, 99–114. London: Churchill Livingstone.

Knight, R.G. (2001) Neurological consequences of alcohol use. In *International Handbook of Alcohol Dependence and Problems*, ed. Heather, N., Peters, T.J. and Stockwell, T. Chichester: John Wiley and Sons, 129–48.

Kopelman, M. (1991) Alcoholic brain damage. In *The International Handbook of Addictive Behaviour*, ed. Glass, I.B. London: Routledge, 141–51.

Lishman, W.A. (1981) Cerebral disorders in alcoholism. *Brain* 104, 1–20.

Lishman, W.A. (1998) *Organic Psychiatry*, 3rd edn. Oxford: Blackwell Scientific Publications.

Maletzky, B.M. (1976) The diagnosis of pathological intoxication. *Journal of Studies on Alcohol* 37, 1215–28.

Naranjo, C.A. and Sellers, E.M. (1986) Clinical assessment and pharmacotherapy of the alcohol withdrawal syndrome. In *Recent Developments in Alcoholism*, Vol. 4, ed. Galanter, M. New York: Plenum Press, 265–81.

Oscar-Berman, M. (1990) Learning and memory deficits in detoxified alcoholics. *NIDA Research Monograph* 101, 136–55.

Pfefferbaum, A., Lim, K.O., Zipursky, R.B. et al. (1992) Brain gray and white matter volume loss accelerates with aging in chronic alcoholics: a quantitative MRI study. *Alcoholism: Clinical and Experimental Research* 16, 1078–89.

Pfefferbaum, A., Sullivan, E.V., Mathalon, H.M. and Lim, K.O. (1997) Frontal lobe volume loss observed with magnetic resonance imaging in older chronic alcoholics. *Alcoholism: Clinical and Experimental Research* 21, No. 3, 521–9.

Pfefferbaum, A., Sullivan, E.V., Rosenbloom, M.H. and Mathalon. D.H. (1998) A controlled study of cortical gray matter and ventricular changes in alcoholic men over a 5-year interval. *Archives of General Psychiatry* 55, 903–12.

Ramayya, A. and Jauhar, P. (1997) Increasing incidence of Korsakoff's psychosis in the East End of Glasgow. *Alcohol and Alcoholism* 32, 281–5.

Schuckit, M.A., Smith, T.L., Anthenelli, R.M. and Irwin, M. (1993) The clinical course of alcoholism in 636 male inpatients. *American Journal of Psychiatry* 150, 786–92.

Soyka, M. (1995) Pathophysiological mechanisms possibly involved in the development of alcohol hallucinosis. *Addiction* 90, 289–94.

Tsuang, J.W., Irwin, M.R., Smith, T.L. and Schuckit, M.A. (1994) Characteristics of men with alcoholic hallucinosis. *Addiction* 89, 73–8.

Victor, M., Adams, R.D. and Collins, G.H. (1971) *The Wernicke–Korsakoff Syndrome*. Oxford: Blackwell Scientific Publications.

World Health Organization (1992) *The ICD-10 Classification of Mental and Behavioural Disorders*. Geneva: World Health Organization.

8

Alcohol problems and psychiatric co-morbidity

Anyone working in the field of drinking problems must cultivate an awareness of the range of mental illnesses that may result from, or lie behind, the drinking. Very serious issues will otherwise be overlooked. Alcohol problems and psychiatric disorders are both common and some degree of overlap should be expected in any population. More importantly, alcohol is a readily available medication for many types of mental distress, and in these cases drinking is a complication of the underlying and primary pathology. Some aspects of the relationship between personality, mental illness and alcohol problems have already been touched on briefly in Chapter 2 when discussing the causes of excessive drinking.

In the Epidemiologic Catchment Area (ECA) study, 37% of individuals in the general population with an alcohol disorder also experienced another psychiatric disorder (Regier et al., 1990). The most common co-morbid disorders were anxiety disorders (19%), antisocial personality disorders (14%), affective disorders (13%) and schizophrenia (4%) (Helzer and Pryzbeck, 1988; Table 8.1).

Another American survey, the National Co-Morbidity Survey (NCS), reported a slightly higher level of co-morbidity (Kessler et al., 1994, 1997). The evidence for lifetime co-morbidity was stronger for alcohol dependence than for alcohol 'abuse', and co-morbidity was more likely to occur in women than in men. Anxiety and affective disorders were the main contributors to co-morbidity in women. The predominant co-morbid disorders among men were substance use disorders, conduct disorder and antisocial personality disorder (ASPD).

The British Psychiatric Morbidity Survey (Farrell et al., 1998) was a national survey of three populations: a household population, a population of long-term residents in psychiatric institutions and a homeless population. Rates of current and 12-month alcohol dependence were 5% in the household sample, 7% in the institutional sample and 21% in the homeless sample. Heavy drinking and alcohol dependence were associated with higher rates of psychological morbidity.

Table 8.1 Life-time prevalence and odds ratios (ORs) of various mental disorders among persons with any alcohol disorder diagnosis[a]

Co-morbid disorder	Any alcohol disorder	
	% (SE)	OR
Any mental	36.6[b] (1.4)	2.3
Any anxiety	19.4[b] (1.0)	1.5
Antisocial personality disorder	14.3[b] (1.1)	21.0
Any affective (mood)	13.4[b] (0.9)	1.9
Schizophrenia	3.8[b] (0.6)	3.3

[a] Five-site ECA combined community and institutional sample standardized to the US population.
[b] $p < 0.001$ prevalence in exposed versus non-exposed group.
From Regier et al. (1990).

There is a great deal of clinical heterogeneity in the co-morbid disorders experienced by individuals with drinking problems. The causes of co-morbidity are of theoretical and clinical importance, because co-morbidity complicates treatment and prognosis. Psychiatric disorders often pre-date the alcohol problem and are clinically significant independent disorders. As mentioned above, another explanation for co-morbidity is the 'self-medication hypothesis', which proposes that alcohol is used to alleviate psychiatric symptoms. A genetic linkage between alcohol dependence and some psychiatric disorders such as bipolar affective disorder and ASPD has also been proposed (Winokur et al., 1995). Clinical samples have higher prevalence rates of co-morbidity than community samples, because the presence of the co-morbid disorder increases the likelihood that people will seek help (Hall and Farrell, 1997). It is also possible that the psychiatric symptoms experienced by alcohol dependent individuals are related to the experience of intoxication and withdrawal and are substance induced. Many studies exploring co-morbidity have assessed clinical samples during the first few weeks of abstinence, and this does not give an overview of how the various syndromes wax and wane over time.

A number of themes are explored in this chapter. Co-morbid depressive illness, suicide, bipolar disorder, anxiety disorder, post-traumatic stress disorder (PTSD), personality disorder, eating disorders and psychosis are reviewed. This is followed by a discussion of so-called dual diagnosis issues and consideration of service models.

Depression

Depression is common amongst individuals with drinking problems and may be the decisive factor in seeking treatment. However, the nature of the relationship between the two is still poorly understood. What seems, on the surface, to be a simple association is in fact extremely complex. Part of the problem is a lack of clarity in terminology. The word 'depression' has a variety of meanings and a distinction has to be made between the experience of being depressed and depressive illness.

The experience of being depressed
The ordinary range of experience

Feelings of sadness and unhappiness can occur as a normal reaction to adversity. Individuals vary greatly in temperament and response to psychological stress.

Persistent mood disorder

Some individuals experience persistent but fluctuating depression of mood which is not severe enough to merit a diagnosis of depressive illness. This usually begins in early and adult life and lasts for several years, sometimes for the greater part of the individual's adult life, causing considerable distress.

Depression associated with other psychiatric syndromes

Depressive symptoms are often evident in other psychiatric syndromes, for instance schizophrenia, obsessional illness or dementia.

Depressive illness

Depression as a psychiatric illness must be distinguished from feelings of depression which have been described above. The essential feature of a depressive episode is a period of at least 2 weeks during which there is depressed mood and loss of interest or pleasure in nearly all activities. The mood disturbance is often worse at a particular time of day, usually the morning. Loss of energy, fatigue and diminished activity are common, as is marked tiredness after slight effort. Other symptoms include reduced concentration and attention, reduced self-esteem and self-confidence, ideas of guilt and unworthiness, bleak and pessimistic views of the future, disturbed sleep and early morning wakening, diminished appetite and weight loss, and ideas of self-harm and suicide (World Health Organization, 1992). Sexual interest is lost. Somatic complaints, rather than feelings of sadness, may be emphasized and the patient thinks that they are physically ill. There is often increased irritability, an impaired ability to think or make decisions and poor concentration. The patient may be agitated or slowed down. Psychotic symptoms such as delusions, hallucinations or depressive stupour can occur in a severe depressive episode.

Depressive illness exists in degrees, and there are many variations in which symptoms cluster and present. No one description can do justice to the true variety of presentations. The picture will be influenced by culture and the patient's age and personality. There have been many attempts to typologize this disorder – endogenous versus reactive, 'neurotic depression' versus true depressive illness, and so on. The most up-to-date classification can be found in ICD-10 (World Health Organization, 1992) and DSM-IV (American Psychiatric Association, 1994). A distinction is made between unipolar affective disorder and bipolar affective disorder, the latter characterized by repeated episodes in which the patient's mood and activity levels are significantly disturbed, sometimes in terms of elevation of mood (elation), increased energy and activity (mania or hypomania), and at other times by episodes of depression.

So much for the basic concepts. Deciding whether a person is just miserable or, on the contrary, ill with depression can, however, be extraordinarily difficult when they are drinking, and there is the ever-looming possibility of suicide as the price of a mistake. Depressive illness is often over-diagnosed in problem drinkers, with consequent needless prescribing of drugs or pointless administration of electroconvulsive therapy (ECT), whereas on other occasions the diagnosis may be overlooked. This is an instance in which correct diagnosis will speak very importantly to correct management. If the patient is suffering from non-specific unhappiness rather than a depressive illness, that aspect of their situation may require skilled help, but not the same type of help as would be indicated for the undoubted illness. A picture of drinking problems together with a complaint of depression is illustrated by the following case abstract.

A married woman aged 35 had been drinking excessively for 3 or 4 years. Visited at home by a social worker, the house was in a terrible state and the children much neglected. The patient herself was dishevelled, obviously rather drunk and declaring in a maudlin fashion that she was no good and that the family might as well be rid of her.

How should the social worker respond to this situation? Quite certainly, an entirely inadequate course of action would be simply to arrange for a prescription of antidepressant drugs and let the patient mix these drugs with the drinking. Treatment cannot be intelligently and usefully started until it is known what there is to treat. The obverse approach, and one as misguided as the ill-thought-out use of drugs, is to assume that all problem drinkers can be a bit maudlin at times, and to dismiss this woman's complaint as 'just the alcoholic miseries' – later, perhaps, to hear that she killed herself.

How is the question as to whether such a patient as this is suffering from a depressive illness in practice to be decided? Assessment of the history is very important: a previous history of depressive illness, an event such as childbirth or bereavement which might have precipitated the illness, a sense of some more or less demarcated point at which 'things changed' and the patient knew that whatever the previous ups and downs of mood, something was now being experienced which was fixed and of different degree. A family history of depression can also be an important indicator. With the history has to be integrated what details can be observed of present behaviour and mental state. But it is also true that many problem drinkers will, when drinking, show emotional lability, will cry easily, will talk of the hopelessness of their lives. Immediately in all such instances to leap to a diagnosis of depressive illness would result in a great deal of over-diagnosis. The dilemma can be very real, and even experienced clinical judgement may be unable to resolve this diagnostic question while that patient is intoxicated. The patient's account may be inconstant, it may seem to be over-dramatized, the immediate life situation may be distressingly fraught and chaotic, but it is still unclear whether or not behind this drinking lies a depressive illness.

In such circumstances the sensible rule is to admit that diagnosis cannot be made in the presence of drinking, and to see the patient's stopping drinking as the prerequisite to a resolution of the diagnostic difficulty. After a week of sobriety, it may be obvious that the misery has almost miraculously faded away – this often happens. Alternatively, it may become very apparent that a classical depressive illness now stands out as certainly as a rock left by the tide. Sometimes, however, even after a few weeks of in-patient observation and continued sobriety, it may be difficult to know whether what is emerging is a depressive illness or a personality chronically prone to unhappy feelings and explosive declarations of misery. The ultimate resolution of the diagnostic problem might, for instance, be that the woman described above had always been a rather unhappy and insecure person, that in this setting and to relieve these feelings she had gradually started to drink and had been drinking heavily for 5 or more years, but that against all this background she had undoubtedly a year previously and following childbirth developed a true and severe depressive illness which had been untreated. The unravelling of such a story may require a lot of time, but arriving at a proper understanding is no optional extra if the depressed drinker is effectively to be helped.

Drinking problems and depression – their relationship

In most cases depression is secondary to the alcohol problem. However, a proportion of problem drinkers have primary depression, which may predispose them to the direct development of an alcohol problem, or exacerbate it once it has developed. It is worth noting that depression pre-dated alcohol abuse or dependence in 66% of women in the ECA study (Helzer and Pryzbeck, 1988).

Depression is commoner in women drinkers and in problem drinkers who have a family history of alcohol problems, an earlier onset of heavy drinking, are divorced and of lower social status (O'Sullivan et al., 1983). Other predisposing factors include a history of anxiety, other drug misuse and previous suicide attempts (Roy et al., 1991). A history of recent, particularly 'negative', life events and a family history of depression appeared to be risk factors for secondary depression in male 'alcoholics' (Roy, 1996).

Depressive symptoms are common during alcohol withdrawal, particularly following a period of heavy consumption. Clinically significant levels of depression are found among in-patients with drinking problems during the early stages of admission (Brown and Schuckit, 1988; Davidson, 1995), but typically improve after 2–3 weeks of abstinence. However, depressive symptoms may persist or even emerge during abstinence and the astute clinician should always be on the look-out for this. Long-term follow-up studies suggest that depressive experience declines with continued abstinence.

The frequent co-occurrence of depression and alcohol dependence has raised the question of whether these two disorders might be genetically linked. Current research suggests that, although both disorders are to an extent familial, they are transmitted independently in families (Merikangas et al., 1985: Maier et al., 1994). A recent population-based study of a sample of US twins (3755 twin pairs) has shown that familial transmission of lifetime major depression and alcohol dependence was largely disorder specific (Prescott et al., 2000). Co-morbidity appears to be due to sex-specific genetic and environmental factors.

In the clinical situation, it may be helpful to differentiate between alcohol-induced depressive syndromes (concurrent depression) and independent depressive episodes (Schuckit et al., 1997). Major depressive episodes occurring during a period of active alcohol dependence are considered to be alcohol-induced. Independent major depression is defined as an episode that occurred either before the onset of alcohol dependence or during a period of 3 or more months of abstinence.

Depression and drinking problems: the practical importance of the diagnostic question

The reasons for it being of practical importance to determine whether a patient with drinking problems is suffering from a depressive illness are several (see Box 8.1). If such an illness exists, it of course deserves treatment as well as whatever psychological or social help may be necessary – the illness may respond to an antidepressant drug, or ECT may still sometimes be indicated if the patient does not respond to drug treatment. The second important reason for believing that every effort must be made not to miss this diagnosis is that if depression is untreated, any attempts

---

BOX 8.1 **Drinking problems and depression**
- Drinking problems are a major cause of depression
- Abstinence from alcohol alleviates depression
- A small proportion of problem drinkers will benefit from antidepressants but the alcohol problem must be tackled first

to treat the drinking problem will be grossly handicapped (Mueller et al., 1994). A depressed patient may find it extremely difficult to stop drinking, and untreated depression can, on occasion, run on for 2 or 3 years, or even longer, perhaps then with partial remissions and further relapses making the time course even more blurred and extended. Another important reason for taking the diagnostic question extremely seriously is the influence which the answer must have on the assessment of suicidal risk (see below). Problem drinkers who are not suffering from depressive illness may kill themselves, but the risk is certainly enhanced if this illness is present.

For the long-term management, knowledge that there has been a depressive illness has a bearing which must be openly discussed with the patient. Once someone has suffered from one such illness they are at some risk of later again developing depression after a shorter or longer interval, and if they can recognize early signs and seek appropriate help, a lot of trouble may be averted. A depression is not an uncommon cause of relapse into drinking after a longish period of sobriety. Paradoxically, the development of an underlying depression may be the reason after many years for drinkers eventually seeking help. It may be an expression of their depressive illness when they say they 'can't carry on any more', start to blame themselves rather than others for their drinking, or make the suicidal gesture which gets them into hospital.

Summing the matter up, it can fairly be said that an awareness of the significance of depressive illness is so essential to working with problem drinkers that anyone who is going to take a close interest in drinking problems will also need to develop a good understanding of depression. If in relation to this question there exists a golden rule, it is that when a drinker is suffering from depressive illness, the therapeutic priority is to aid and persuade that patient first to stop drinking (offering perhaps immediate admission to achieve this purpose). Treating the depression is then the second phase of help and the immediate follow-through. It is generally messy and ineffective to try to treat a depressive illness when the patient is still drinking.

Suicide

The lifetime risk of death by suicide in alcohol dependent individuals is between 60 and 100 times that of the general population (Murphy and Wetzel, 1990). Alcohol dependence is also associated with a higher lifetime risk of suicide (7%) than either affective disorders (6%) or schizophrenia (4%) (Harris and Barraclough, 1997; Inskip et al., 1998). This has implications for clinicians. It is important to identify psychiatric co-morbidity in these individuals (Driessen et al., 1998). Depressive disorders are not the only disorders closely associated with suicidal behaviour in alcohol dependence. Anxiety disorders and the combination of anxiety and depressive disorders are also associated with a high risk of suicidal behaviour. Co-morbid personality disorders confer moderate risk. Multiple co-morbid disorders (depression and anxiety and personality disorders) appear to be associated with the greatest risk of suicidal behaviour (Driessen et al., 1998). Hazardous and harmful alcohol use are also implicated in suicidal behaviour, and a number of studies have helped to characterize risk groups, particularly male adolescents and young men (Vassilas and Morgan, 1997; Fombonne, 1998: Pirkola et al., 1999).

A 25-year follow-up study of almost 50 000 Swedish male conscripts born in 1950 and 1951 has explored the association between alcohol abuse and suicidal behaviour in young and middle-aged men (Rossow et al., 1999). Men abusing alcohol had an elevated risk of attempted suicide (odds ratio 27.1), as well as completed suicide (odds ratio 4.7). This stronger association between alcohol abuse and parasuicide persisted even after controlling for psychiatric morbidity and can probably be attributed to impulsive acts carried out in a state of intoxication.

Bipolar disorder

Hypomania

Pathological elevation of mood is not as common a condition as pathological depression, and when it occurs does not carry a particularly high risk of being associated with drinking. Occasionally, hypomanic patients may, however, find that alcohol relieves unpleasant elements in their feelings: accompanying the basic elevation of mood, the hypomanic state may be characterized by considerable admixture of anxiety, irritability and suspiciousness. Mixed affective illnesses exist in which the patient is both excited and tearful, with a confusing presentation that moves within minutes from elation to depression. A patient with repeated hypomanic bouts may give the appearance of 'bout drinking'. In an attack these patients are likely to lose their social judgement, and to spend large sums of money and live things up, and this general disinhibition, as well as the more specific seeking of relief from unpleasant feelings, may contribute to the drinking. The treatment is primarily that of the underlying illness.

A more difficult diagnostic problem arises when there is a suspicion that the patient's mood may phasically become slightly elevated but with the condition not approaching a hypomanic illness in severity. This slight elevation and disinhibition may appear to be sufficient to spark off some weeks of drinking, and on occasion this is a plausible explanation of 'periodic drinking', although there are many other explanations for such a drinking pattern (see page 63). What is being discussed here is a mood disturbance which would usually be seen as a character trait (cyclothymic personality) rather than as an illness, but there is no absolute demarcation between this sort of state and hypomania. In turn, hypomania merges with mania, with the latter term indicating a state of appalling over-excitement, or the traditional picture of 'raving madness'. A patient with fully developed mania is far too disordered to be other than rapidly admitted to hospital, and drinking as a complication of this illness is not a question which arises other than in the very short term.

Anxiety

The relationship between alcohol problems and anxiety disorders is complex. Clinical studies consistently report an association and it is estimated that about one-third of problem drinkers may have significant anxiety experience (Mullaney and Trippett, 1979; Kushner et al., 1990; Allan, 1995). Alcohol problems can sometimes develop as a result of agoraphobia and social phobia, and may reflect attempts at self-medication (Mullaney and Trippett, 1979; Stockwell et al., 1984). The association with panic disorder is less clear cut (Ross et al., 1988). Individuals with alcohol dependence appear to have higher lifetime rates of panic disorders, generalized anxiety disorders and social phobias than the general population. Rates of agoraphobia and obsessive–compulsive disorder are similar (Schuckit and Hesselbrock, 1994).

Symptoms of anxiety are particularly prominent after a bout of heavy drinking and during alcohol withdrawal (Schuckit et al., 1990; Brown et al., 1991). Alcohol withdrawal symptoms can mimic anxiety and panic disorder, and it is possible that a common neurochemical process underlies both (George et al., 1990). Individuals with alcohol dependence and anxiety disorder have been found to experience more severe alcohol withdrawal symptoms than a non-anxious control group, even though the two groups had similar drinking histories (Johnston et al., 1991). Anxiety symptoms diminish in the early stages of abstinence and continue to improve with prolonged abstinence.

Here is a case example which illustrates one kind of possible clinical relationship between alcohol and anxiety.

A woman aged 50 was admitted to hospital with a long history of drinking. Her immediate presentation was that of a working woman who earned her living by getting up early and going out to do office cleaning. She would have a drink at 6.00 a.m. before leaving the house, and then put a couple of bottles of wine into her bag. What was to be found in the old notes was that many years previously her first presentation to the hospital was as someone with a phobic state who found great difficulty in leaving her house. Careful questioning revealed that phobic anxiety symptoms still very much persisted, although alcohol dependence had now been contracted as a problem in its own right.

The practical clinical approach when a problem drinker appears to be suffering from a phobic anxiety state is usually to arrange hospital admission, for the purposes of both diagnosis and treatment. It is difficult to assess the true severity or fixedness of the phobic symptoms until the patient has been completely off alcohol for some weeks, and sometimes a longer period of observation is required. What may then happen is that seemingly rather severe phobic symptoms fade away, and in the event there is no phobic anxiety to be treated. The symptoms were part of general 'bad nerves' related to alcohol dependence.

If, however, phobic symptoms persist in severe degree, an effort then has to be made to treat them, with treatment started while the patient is in hospital. Treatment of the underlying condition requires sobriety, and an attempt to treat these symptoms when the patient is still drinking is a hopeless undertaking. Treatment will today usually involve the planned application of cognitive–behaviour therapy, and the response is often excellent provided that the patient can co-operate, that there is not a too high background level of anxiety, and that the phobic situations are not too universal. It would, however, be optimistic to suppose that behaviour therapy is a panacea and those favourable conditions are not always fulfilled. The use of minor tranquillizers or hypnotics with such patients has to be approached with extreme caution. To treat phobic, alcohol dependent patients while they are still drinking, by giving them a minor tranquillizer, is likely to be both dangerous and ineffective. Drugs and alcohol will be haphazardly mixed, with the risk of super-added drug dependence. Indeed, by the time severely phobic problem drinkers present for treatment, it is not uncommon to find that they have a medically induced drug problem, as well as their alcohol dependence.

Post-traumatic stress disorder

Post-traumatic stress disorder is an anxiety disorder which develops following exposure to an extremely traumatic stressor considered to be exceptionally threatening or catastrophic in nature (American Psychiatric Association, 1994). Characteristic symptoms include persistent re-experiencing of the traumatic event, persistent avoidance of stimuli associated with the trauma, numbing of general responsiveness and persistent symptoms of hyper-arousal. PTSD may exist with major depressive disorder, may present as a combination of the above symptoms and typical grief, and often leads to drug and alcohol misuse.

Several hypotheses have been proposed to explain the link between PTSD and alcohol misuse, including the self-medication hypothesis (Khantzian, 1990). However, other studies have shown that alcohol misuse may precede the onset of PTSD symptoms (Cottler et al., 1992). It may be that early substance misuse occurs in the context of other 'high-risk' behaviours which increase the likelihood of exposure to potentially traumatizing events and hence the likelihood of developing PTSD. Additionally, individuals who begin using alcohol at an early stage may also be susceptible to the development of PTSD following traumatic exposure, because they have historically relied on alcohol as a way of combating stress and have failed to develop more effective stress reduction strategies.

The association between PTSD and alcohol misuse or dependence is particularly strong for women, and this is associated with the higher incidence of childhood physical and sexual abuse in women. A history of childhood sexual abuse has been shown to increase the risk of later alcohol problems by a factor of 3 (Winfield et al., 1990). Early experiences of physical and sexual abuse put individuals at a greater risk of developing PTSD symptoms following traumatic events in adulthood (Breslau et al., 1999).

In an ideal world, individuals with alcohol dependence and PTSD should tackle both problems simultaneously. Therapeutic strategies help them to cope with the trauma and situations that remind them of the event or events. They learn how to control or avoid such situations. However, this is not always possible, and 'therapy' may, in some individuals, be so traumatic as to cause relapse to heavy drinking, as is illustrated in the following case example.

A 36-year-old man was referred to a specialist PTSD clinic. He had a long history of alcohol dependence and PTSD, secondary to childhood sexual abuse. Now abstinent for 1 year, he was motivated for treatment. Unfortunately, he relapsed to dependent drinking after only four treatment sessions, during which he was 'exposed' to the traumatic memories and encouraged to re-live them as vividly as possible. His wife left him because he was repeatedly violent to her while intoxicated. She was also worried that he might repeat the pattern of sexual abuse with their two children. There followed a number of admissions to an alcohol unit but no substantial period of abstinence over the next 5 years, despite in-patient and out-patient treatment, cognitive–behavioural therapy and pharmacotherapy for alcohol dependence and depressive illness. He now lives on his own, continues to drink and has lost custody of his children, whom he rarely sees. He is 'obsessed' with the man who sexually abused him as a child.

Schizophrenia

Since the early 1980s, a population of 'difficult to treat' patients with severe mental illness (mainly psychosis) and substance misuse (Bachrach, 1982) has emerged. The term 'dual diagnosis' is now regularly used to describe these individuals with co-existent severe mental illness and substance abuse disorders. The ECA study reported a 3.8% prevalence of schizophrenia in individuals with any alcohol disorder (Regier et al., 1990). With schizophrenics, the odds of having an alcohol disorder were three times as high as for the general population, and the odds of having another drug disorder six times as high. Rates of substance misuse in schizophrenic patients have been increasing over time (Cuffel, 1992). This might reflect a real increase in alcohol and drug use amongst this group, but could also be explained by improved methods of detection. Several factors may have contributed to the increased use of drugs and alcohol by schizophrenics. Drugs are readily available in the community, and are popular and socially acceptable. Schizophrenics may use substances to facilitate social interaction and to cope with stress, depression, anxiety or boredom.

A number of studies have compared psychotic patients who misuse substances with psychotic patients who do not. Findings suggest that the psychotic substance users have a better premorbid personality, and are more likely to develop psychosis at an earlier age, to have a family history of mental illness and to be male. From the symptom viewpoint, these patients are more likely to show hostility, disordered speech and suicidal behaviour. They are also more likely to be admitted to hospital, to be violent and to be non-compliant with medication (see Marshall, 1997, for references).

Alcohol misuse and drug misuse usually precede the onset of psychosis (Soyka et al., 1993). This is not fully understood but has been explained in a number of ways. Firstly, substance misuse may play a role in the development of a severe psychiatric disorder such as schizophrenia. It may even precipitate or cause mental illness in more vulnerable patients (Andreasson et al., 1987). Alternatively, individuals in the prodromal or early stages of a psychotic disorder may use alcohol or drugs to self-medicate unpleasant symptoms.

Alcohol, cannabis, psychostimulants (amphetamines and cocaine) and hallucinogens are the main substances used by individuals with severe mental illness. Opioids and sedatives are used less frequently. The drugs used are likely to reflect drug exposure and the pattern and degree of drug misuse within the general population. In the USA, drug use currently appears to be more prevalent amongst these patients, whereas alcohol problems are commoner in the UK and Germany (Soyka et al., 1993; Duke et al., 1994; Menezes et al., 1996). Alcohol disorders in this group are as severe as in individuals presenting to services with a primary alcohol problem (Lehman et al., 1994). Cannabis also appeared to antedate other drug use in a fashion reminiscent of substance use in non-psychotic adolescents.

Alcohol consumption is a risk factor for violence in individuals with schizophrenia (Lindquist and Allebeck, 1989). Violence may be associated with intoxication or withdrawal effects and their impact in mentally ill individuals, or with personality changes associated with prolonged use of substances. Antisocial and personality traits and brain damage are also important risk factors for violence.

The relationship between schizophrenia and alcohol problems is an important one. High rates of alcohol problems have been reported in individuals with schizophrenia (22.1%; Duke et al., 1994) and psychosis (31.6%; Menezes et al., 1996).

Alcohol use may be an added risk factor for the development of tardive dyskinesia in some schizophrenics (Duke et al., 1994).

Personality disorder

The relationship between alcohol problems and personality factors is complex and still poorly understood. It is impossible to work with drinking problems without becoming aware of the relevance of personality to an understanding of the genesis of drinking and the treatment of excessive drinking and dependence. Personality has multiple dimensions and is influenced by genetic, environmental and cultural factors. Cross-sectional studies of male 'alcoholics' in treatment have suggested that they are 'anti-social, rebellious and impulsive individuals who have difficulty delaying gratification' (Bates, 1993). However, these studies are flawed, because such characteristics may either pre-date or follow the development of excessive alcohol use, and are not unique to it.

More recent behavioural genetic research suggests that certain personality sub-types and temperaments may increase the risk for developing alcohol problems in adulthood. Tarter (1991) proposed that there are heritable dimensions of temperament which make individuals vulnerable to the development of alcohol problems in adulthood. Zuckerman (1991) postulated a sensation-seeking trait based on inherited, biological traits of reactivity to stimulation. Cloninger (1987) hypothesized a typological classification. His theory postulates inheritance of a predisposing personality type manifesting high levels of impulsivity and novelty seeking and low harm avoidance. This personality type in turn predisposes to type II 'alcoholism', which occurs exclusively in men, has an early age of onset (under 25 years) and is associated with childhood antisocial behaviour and criminality in the father. Although this typology has been validated empirically in some studies (Babor et al., 1992), and the traits of impulsivity and novelty seeking are closely related to Zuckerman's sensation-seeking traits, this concept remains controversial. The question of typologies has also been discussed earlier in this book (see page 62). Recent work suggests that men and women who score highly on two broad dimensions of personality, negative emotionality and behavioural disinhibition, have especially high rates of 'alcoholism'. It is uncertain whether these personality characteristics pre-date the onset of alcoholism (McGue et al., 1997).

Although the association between ASPD and alcohol problems has gained acceptance in the USA, it has not been taken up with as much enthusiasm in Britain, largely, perhaps, because it is seen as potentially unhelpful in working with individuals troubled by their drinking. Studies suggest poor outcomes for individuals with antisocial personality and alcohol problems, but do not take into account the heterogeneity within this population. The consequence of a rigid categorical approach may be therapeutic nihilism.

As far as this chapter is concerned, there is common ground between the two seemingly divergent schools of thought in that both parties would agree that patients with drinking problems are sometimes, and to various degrees, angry, unhappy, non-conformist, rule-breaking, aggressive and handicapped in their ability to deal with social demands and expectations. It would also be common ground that when a patient is first met it can be difficult to determine how much such seeming disturbances are cause, and how much are the consequence of excessive drinking. Furthermore, it would be widely agreed that personality disturbance can make treatment difficult and has to be dealt with therapeutically as a significant issue.

Eating disorders

The most common disorders of body weight which result from excessive drinking are obesity, due to the high calorie content of the alcohol which is being consumed, and, paradoxically, the loss of weight and general malnutrition which are consequent on the dietary neglect which frequently accompanies heavy drinking.

It is these two common types of disorder to which the diagnostician is likely to be very properly alert. There is, however, increasing evidence that certain eating disorders, which were until recently considered to be only rare accompaniments of alcohol problems, are not, in fact, uncommon. These conditions are anorexia nervosa and bulimia nervosa.

Eckert et al. (1979) reported a 6.7% lifetime prevalence of 'alcohol problems' among patients with anorexia nervosa. However, a controlled 10-year follow-up study of women with anorexia nervosa found no significant relationship with drinking problems (Halmi et al., 1991). Higher rates of 'alcoholism' were found in the first-degree relatives of patients with anorexia nervosa, compared with relatives of the controls. Prevalence rates of alcohol misuse in bulimic subjects vary from 9% to 49% (Goldbloom, 1993).

Fewer studies have explored the prevalence of eating disorders in patients referred for treatment of drinking problems (Lacey and Moureli, 1986; Peveler and Fairburn, 1990). Depending on sampling and the criteria employed, it seems possible that up to about 30% of women with drinking problems may at some time experience a significant eating disorder. The prevalence of eating disorders in Japan are lower than those reported in Western countries, and yet 11% of an in-patient sample of women 'alcoholics' fulfilled DSM-III-R criteria for eating disorders, especially bulimia nervosa (Higuchi et al., 1993). Clinical research suggests that eating disorders complicated by drinking problems respond as well to treatment as those in which alcohol is not a problem (Goldbloom, 1993). However, individuals with eating and drinking problems may also have a predisposition towards other 'impulse' disorders such as self-mutilation, parasuicide, misuse of illicit or prescribed drugs, and shoplifting (Lacey, 1993).

Pathological jealousy

Jealousy is a normal human emotion, and it is not easy to set a cut-off point between the normal and the pathological. At one end of the spectrum there is, however, a group of people whose lives are plagued and corrupted by their jealous feelings, and who make life miserable for the objects of their jealousy. For reasons which are discussed below, this condition is likely to be met quite frequently in the treatment of drinking problems, and one should know how to recognize its features.

A 34-year-old garage owner said that he had been painfully jealous ever since his adolescence. His jealousy was now threatening to break up his marriage. He would repeatedly charge his wife with infidelity, taunting her and threatening her, as well as accusing her. There would then be explosive rows, and sometimes violence resulted. Later he would be desperately sorry, and transiently realize the falseness and cruelty of his accusations. But very shortly worrying doubts would again return. He would come home secretly and keep watch on the house, and sometimes he would follow his wife down the road. His wife's handbag was regularly searched, and he checked on her underclothes for seminal stains. Recently he had thought of hiring a detective. He remained sexually potent, and wanted to keep his wife pregnant so as to make her uninteresting to other men. His drinking appeared to be inextricably mixed with the jealousy story, but his jealousy only came to light when his wife was interviewed.

The essential characteristics of this syndrome suggest that it may sometimes parallel an obsessional disorder, although this is not a view of the condition which finds approval in the standard psychiatric texts. The constant rumination, the fact that there is frequent (if only short-lived and partial) realization of the falseness of the belief, the unpleasantness of the associated feelings, the compulsive need to check, and the transient relief from the active checking are features very reminiscent of obsession. But it seems certain that pathological jealousy cannot be related to any one all-embracing psychiatric diagnosis, and underlying the common presenting features may be any one of several psychiatric disorders, including paranoid schizophrenia.

The usual view is that alcohol dependence is a cause of jealousy, rather than jealousy a cause of alcohol dependence. The psychodynamic explanations offered for this chain of events are complex, but can be sketched out in very abbreviated terms as the individual doubting his own masculinity and therefore drinking, drinking leading to impotence, and the reaction to impotence being jealousy. Impotence and pathological jealousy are thus alleged frequently to co-exist. Pathological jealousy is also sometimes vaguely subsumed (if not explained) under the general heading of 'alcoholic paranoia'. There is much still to be found out about this condition, but it may be questioned whether the conventional view that alcohol dependence causes pathological jealousy is too simple. The story which the patient gives more often suggests that jealousy has been in some degree a life-long feature, perhaps even with manifestations in childhood, and very early family dynamics can be rather obviously related to the genesis of the problem. The distress which is associated with the experience of jealousy may be appalling, and the patient in adulthood discovers that this distress is at least temporarily relieved by drinking. This may therefore sometimes provide just another illustration of the fact that anyone for whom drink is available, and who suffers from any kind of chronic psychological distress, may be led into excessive drinking as a result of self-medication. The general level of heightened anxiety so often associated with alcohol dependence may then make the jealousy more intractable, and the situation becomes circular.

However, by the time the patient comes for help, both jealousy and drinking have probably been going on for many years, and it can be extremely difficult to untangle the true, historical relationship of the two elements. In the here-and-now, they are usually best seen as mutually interacting, as exacerbating each other, rather than as either taking precedence. The practical approach is to try somehow to persuade the patient to stop drinking, and then assess the severity of the jealousy. What happened to the garage owner is fairly typical, and shows that pessimism is by no means always well founded if drinking can be got out of the way.

He 'realized that something had to be done about it', and as an act of faith he stopped drinking. He immediately needed to talk about his jealousy, which was at first very painful for him. But the terrible scenes of destructive accusation forthwith ceased. He was able to realize that drinking had been making matters worse, and been leading to drunken acting-out of his anxieties. He and his wife were, for the first time, able safely to discuss his jealousy, both admitting its irrationality, but agreeing that his feelings were a serious and painful problem for both of them. As his mood lifted, the intensity of his jealously considerably faded, and to his surprise he and his wife settled on a rather joking way of dealing with the problem, and one which helped them both. 'Come on, love, I say to him, none of that old nonsense, you're my one and only and you know it'. Seen a year later, he still on occasion had a surge of jealous feelings (he would not take his wife to a party), but these feelings were less severe than they had been for many years and his wife could live with the situation.

The extracts from this case story illustrate an approach which focused initially on the drinking, in the hope that the jealousy would then become more manageable. This is almost inevitably the best approach, for unless one is dealing with an underlying psychotic illness (which is seldom the case), there is no specific treatment available for the jealousy. Drugs have no part to play, and behavioural treatments are largely untried. Talking the matter through in a sympathetic and common-sense fashion, bringing husband and wife together to work on the problem, encouraging a sense of optimism may, if the patient stays off alcohol, often bring good results. Sometimes, however, the condition is intractable. The patient simply cannot stop drinking, and the result is break-up of the marriage (with the husband still haunting the doorstep), or even a tragic drunken murder.

The reasons for giving this space to what has often been termed a rare syndrome are several. It may be doubted whether the condition is in fact all that rare; with an open eye and alert questioning, many more cases will come to light. Although the basic description of the syndrome is to be found in the textbooks, the clinical handling of this problem seldom receives due attention. It is a condition easily missed, but very real once recognized, and it needs to be given a definite place on the checklists of anyone working with alcohol problems.

Damage to the tissue of the brain

The question often arises as to whether the patient with a drinking problem is suffering from brain damage. If the damage is gross, there will be no diagnostic difficulty, but the diagnosis (and significance) of lesser degrees of damage commonly sets problems.

The most familiar picture is that of an associated alcoholic 'dementia', and this condition is discussed more fully on page 107 in relation to the physical damages which can result from drinking. Much the same sort of picture is to be seen when the patient is developing a dementia for any other reason (pre-senile dementia, for instance, or senile or multi-infarct dementia). The patient with alcoholic dementia will typically give a history of many years heavy drinking, with the ultimate development of brain damage. With non-alcoholic dementia, the sequence of events is the other way round: the patient develops dementia and, as a result of the ensuing disinhibition and personality deterioration, becomes involved in drinking.

The fact that brain damage can be cause as well as consequence of drinking needs to be written into any diagnostic checklist. Besides brain damage due to degenerative processes such as those already mentioned, the significance of a history of brain injury should be specially borne in mind. Instances occur in which personality change as a sequel to head injury is disproportionate to any fall-off in intellectual functioning, and this type of personality change may, for instance, result in drinking problems as a late sequel of a road accident. The following brief case extracts show some of the many possible organic relationships which should be on that checklist.

A woman civil servant, aged 50, of previously unblemished record, suffered a subarach-noid haemorrhage (a bleed into the space around the brain). The leaking blood vessel was operated on and she 'recovered completely' but she had, in fact, sustained a degree of brain damage. Work habits which had for a life time been almost over-meticulous now deteriorated, and she was found to be drinking secretly in the office.

A man, aged 40, suffered from crippling obsessional symptoms, and a leucotomy was per-formed. His obsessional symptoms were relieved, but although up to the time of his oper-ation he had been a very moderate drinker, he now rapidly developed alcohol dependence.

A woman of 60 presented with alcohol dependence, seemingly of recent onset. She was found to have a brain tumour.

Some of these case histories illustrate only rather rare associations, and the precise part that brain damage played in the aetiology of the drinking is in some instances difficult to establish. The general picture which is being built up by listing these diverse cases, however, is valid and important. Some associations between brain damage and alcohol dependence are relatively common (personality deterioration following head injury, for example), whereas others, such as tumour, are rare, but the general message that no diagnostic assessment is complete without thinking about the possible significance of brain involvement has to be stressed. Alcohol dependence can also supervene as a complication of learning disability of any origin.

Whatever the underlying brain syndrome associated with alcohol dependence, the clinical features can be grouped under a number of headings. There are, of course, firstly the primary symptoms of the brain damage itself. Features of the drinking problem will also stand in their own right, but it is the interaction of the underlying brain damage and the drinking which gives these cases their colouring. Personal and social deterioration may seem to be disproportionate to the drinking, or suddenly to have accelerated. Drunken behaviour where there is underlying brain damage often appears to be particularly heedless of consequences, or antisocial. There are increasing episodes of violence, or the patient sets their lodgings on fire. There is also an increased sensitivity to alcohol; the patient gets drunk on less drink, and with relatively little alcohol becomes disinhibited or begins to fall about.

Given proper alertness to the possibility of such underlying problems, what are then the practical implications? If brain involvement is in any way suspected, this usually constitutes an indication for hospital admission so that appropriate neuro-logical and psychological investigations can be carried out with a sober patient. The sad fact is that most of the possibly relevant brain conditions are going to prove more diagnosable than treatable, but even so an accurate diagnostic formulation is the necessary basis for working out what is best to be done. If, for instance, an individual with alcohol dependence is severely brain damaged, the only kind and safe policy may be to propose long-term hospital care, or care in a supportive residential community. If there is milder damage, the patient will be able to keep going outside an institution, but brain damage can adversely affect the course of alcohol problems, and relapse and further troubles are probably to be expected. The continuing treatment policy must be set up so as to be able to meet these sorts of eventuality, and be designed to support the family in what may well be a difficult situation. The emphasis may sometimes have to be on rather directive intervention such as ensuring that money is properly handled or that the local publicans will not serve drinks. But even here there is no cause for absolute pessimism, for sometimes a patient with brain damage will be able to stop drinking, the progression of such damage will be arrested and the patient's behaviour will improve. Treatment implications are discussed further on page 107.

Mental illness: the general implications

The account which has been given in this chapter of the many types of mental illness which can be associated with excessive drinking, and of the nature of those possible relationships, must not be interpreted as meaning that only the psychiatrist can treat the problem drinker. Neither does the fact that psychiatric treatment or admission to a psychiatric hospital may be indicated for some of these patients mean that the treatment of alcohol problems is a psychiatric preserve. However, what must be evident is that psychiatry may quite often have a part to play, and that a working liaison with psychiatric services should be available to anyone helping with drinking problems. Moreover, an awareness of this psychiatric dimension must be important, whatever the therapist's professional discipline.

REFERENCES

Allan, C.A. (1995) Alcohol problems and anxiety disorders – a critical review. *Alcohol and Alcoholism* 30, 145-51.

American Psychiatric Association (1994) *Diagnostic and Statistical Manual of Mental Disorders,* 4th edn. Washington, DC: American Psychiatric Association.

Andreasson, S., Allebeck, P. and Engstrom, A. (1987) Cannabis and schizophrenia: a longitudinal study of Swedish conscripts. *Lancet* 11: 1483–6.

Babor, T.F., Hofmann, M., Del Boca, F.K. et al. (1992) Types of alcoholics, I: Evidence for an empirically derived typology based on indicators of vulnerability and severity. *Archives of General Psychiatry* 49, 599–608.

Bachrach, L.L. (1982) Young adult chronic patients: an analytic review of the literature. *Hospital and Community Psychiatry* 33, 187–97.

Bates, M.E. (1993) Social and cultural perspectives: psychology. In *Recent Developments in Alcoholism*, ed. Galanter, M. Vol. 11, *Ten Years of Progress*, New York: Plenum Press, 45–72.

Breslau, N., Chilcoat, H.D., Kessler, R.C. and Davis, G.C. (1999) Previous exposure to trauma: results from the Detroit Area Survey of Trauma. *American Journal of Psychiatry* 156, 902–7.

Brown, S.A., Irwin, M. and Schukit, M.A. (1991) Changes in anxiety among abstinent male alcoholics. *Journal of Studies on Alcohol* 52, 55–61.

Brown, S.A. and Schuckit, M.A. (1988) Changes in depression amongst abstinent alcoholics. *Journal of Studies on Alcohol* 49, 412–17.

Cloninger, C.R. (1987) Neurogenetic adaptive mechanisms in alcoholism. *Science* 236, 410–16.

Cottler, L.B., Compton, W.M., Mager, D.E., Spitznagel, E.L. and Janca, A. (1992) Post-traumatic stress disorder among substance users from the general population. *American Journal of Psychiatry* 149, 664–70.

Cuffel, B. (1992) Prevalence estimates of substance abuse in schizophrenia and their correlates. *Journal of Nervous and Mental Disease* 180, 589–92.

Davidson, K.M. (1995) Diagnosis of depression in alcohol dependence: changes in prevalence with drinking status. *British Journal of Psychiatry* 166, 199–204.

Driessen, M., Veltrup, C., Weber, J., John, U., Wetterling, T. and Dilling, H. (1998) Psychiatric co-morbidity, suicidal behaviour and suicidal ideation in alcoholics seeking treatment. *Addiction* 93, 889–94.

Duke, P., Pantelis, C. and Barnes, T.R.E. (1994) South Westminster Schizophrenia Survey. Alcohol use and its relationship to symptoms, tardive dyskinesia and illness onset. *British Journal of Psychiatry* 164, 630–6.

Eckert, E.D., Goldberg, S.C., Halmi, K.A., Casper, R.C. and Davis, J.M. (1979) Alcoholism in anorexia nervosa. In *Psychiatric Factors in Drug Abuse*, ed. Pickens, R.W. and Heston, L.L. New York: Grieve and Stratton, 267–83.

Farrell, M., Howes, S., Taylor, C. et al. (1998) Substance misuse and psychiatric comorbidity: an overview of the OPCS National Psychiatric Morbidity Survey. *Addictive Behaviours* 23, 909–18.

Fombonne, E. (1998) Suicidal behaviours in vulnerable adolescents. *British Journal of Psychiatry* 173, 154–9.

George, G.T., Nutt, D.J. and Dwyer, B.A. (1990) Alcoholism and panic disorders: is the co-morbidity more than coincidence? *Acta Psychiatrica Scandinavica* 81, 97–107.

Goldbloom, D.S. (1993) Alcohol misuse and eating disorders: aspects of an association. *Alcohol and Alcoholism* 28, 375–81.

Hall, W. and Farrell, M. (1997) Comorbidity of mental disorders with substance abuse. *British Journal of Psychiatry* 171, 4–5.

Halmi, K.A., Eckert, E., Marchi, P., Sampugnaro, V., Apple, R. and Cohen, J. (1991) Comorbidity of psychiatric diagnosis in anorexia nervosa. *Archives of General Psychiatry* 48, 712–18.

Harris, E.C. and Barraclough, B.M. (1997) Suicide as an outcome for mental disorders. *British Journal of Psychiatry* 170, 205–28.

Helzer, J.E. and Pryzbeck, T.R. (1988) The co-occurrence of alcoholism with other psychiatric disorders in the general population and its impact on treatment. *Journal of Studies on Alcohol* 49, 219–24.

Higuchi, S., Suzuki, K., Yamada, K., Parrish, K. and Kono, H. (1993) Alcoholics with eating disorders: prevalence and clinical course. A study from Japan. *British Journal of Psychiatry* 162, 403–6.

Inskip, H.M., Harris, E.C. and Barraclough, B. (1998) Lifetime risk of suicide for affective disorder, alcoholism and schizophrenia. *British Journal of Psychiatry* 172, 35–7.

Johnston, A.L., Thevos, A.K., Randall, C.L. and Anton, R.F. (1991) Increased severity of alcohol withdrawal in in-patient alcoholics with a co-existing anxiety diagnosis. *British Journal of Addiction* 86, 719–25.

Kessler, R.C., Crum, R.M., Warner, L.A., Nelson, C.B., Schulenberg, J. and Anthony, J.C. (1997) Lifetime co-occurrence of DSM-III-R alcohol abuse and dependence with other psychiatric disorders in the National Comorbidity Survey. *Archives of General Psychiatry* 54, 313–21.

Kessler, R.C., McGonagle, K.A., Zhad, S. et al. (1994) Lifetime and 12-month prevalence of DSM-III psychiatric disorders in the United States: results from the National Comorbidity Survey. *Archives of General Psychiatry* 51, 8–19.

Khantzian, E.J. (1990) Self regulation and self medication factors in alcoholism and addictions: similarities and differences. In *Recent Developments in Alcoholism*, Vol. 8, ed. Galanter, M. New York: Plenum Press, 255–69.

Kushner, M.G., Sher, K.J. and Beitman, B. (1990) The relation between alcohol problems and anxiety disorders. *American Journal of Psychiatry* 147, 685–95.

Lacey, J.H. (1993) Self-damaging and addictive behaviour in bulimia nervosa. *British Journal of Psychiatry* 163, 190–4.

Lacey, J.H. and Moureli, E. (1986) Bulimic alcoholics: some features of a clinical sub-group. *British Journal of Addiction* 81, 389–93.

Lehman, A.F., Myers, C.P., Corty, E. and Thompson, J. (1994) Severity of substance use disorders among psychiatric in-patients. *Journal of Nervous and Mental Disease* 182, 164–7.

Lindquist, P. and Allebeck, P. (1989) Schizophrenia and assaultive behaviour: the role of alcohol and drug abuse. *Acta Psychiatrica Scandinavica* 82, 191–5.

McGue, M., Slutske, W., Taylor, J. and Iacono, W.G. (1997) Personality and substance use disorders: I. Effects of gender and alcoholism subtype. *Alcoholism: Clinical and Experimental Research* 21, 513–20.

Marshall, E.J. (1997) Dual diagnosis: comorbidity of severe mental illness and substance misuse. *Journal of Forensic Psychiatry* 9, 9–15.

Maier, W., Lichtermann, D. and Minges, J. (1994) The relationship between alcoholism and unipolar depression – a controlled family study. *Journal of Psychiatric Research* 3, 303–17.

Menezes, P., Johnson, S., Thornicroft, G. et al. (1996) Drug and alcohol problems among individuals with severe mental illness in South London. *British Journal of Psychiatry* 168, 612–19.

Merikangas, K.R., Leckman, J.F., Prusoff, B.A., Pauls, D.L. and Weissman, M.M. (1985) Familial transmission of depression and alcoholism. *Archives of General Psychiatry* 42, 367–71.

Mueller, T.I., Lavori, P.W., Keller, M.B. et al. (1994) Prognostic effect of the variable course of alcoholism on the 10-year course of depression. *American Journal of Psychiatry* 151, 701–6.

Mullaney, J.A. and Trippett, C.J. (1979) Alcohol dependence and phobias: a clinical description and relevance. *British Journal of Psychiatry* 135, 565–73.

Murphy, G.G. and Wetzel, R.D. (1990) The lifetime risk of suicide in alcoholism. *Archives of General Psychiatry* 47, 383–92.

O'Sullivan, K., Whillans, P., Daly, M., Carroll, B., Clare, A. and Cooney, J. (1983) A comparison of alcoholics with and without co-existing affective disorder. *British Journal of Psychiatry* 143, 133–8.

Peveler, R. and Fairburn, C. (1990) Eating disorders in women who abuse alcohol. *British Journal of Addiction* 85, 1633–8.

Pirkola, S., Marttunen, M.J., Henriksson, M.M., Isometsa, E.T., Heikkinen, M.E. and Lönnqvist, J.K. (1999) Alcohol-related problems among adolescent suicides in Finland. *Alcohol and Alcoholism* 34, 320–9.

Prescott, C.A., Aggen, S.H. and Kendler, K. (2000) Sex specific genetic influences on comorbidity of alcoholism and major depression in a population-based sample of US twins. *Archives of General Psychiatry* 57, 803–11.

Regier, D.A., Farmer, M.E., Rae, D.S. et al. (1990) Comorbidity of mental disorders with alcohol and other drug abuse. *Journal of the American Medical Association* 264, 2511–18.

Ross, H.E., Glaser, F.B. and Stiasny, S. (1988) Sex differences in the prevalence of psychiatric disorders in patients with alcohol and drug problems. *British Journal of Addiction* 83, 1179–92.

Rossow, I., Romelsjö, A. and Leifman, H. (1999) Alcohol abuse and suicidal behaviour in young and middle-aged men: differentiating between attempted and completed suicide. *Addiction* 94, 1199–207.

Roy, A. (1996) Aetiology of secondary depression in male alcoholics. *British Journal of Psychiatry* 169, 753–7.

Roy, A., DeJong, J., Lamparski, D., George, T. and Linnoila, M. (1991) Depression among alcoholics. *Archives of General Psychiatry* 48, 428–32.

Schuckit, M.A. and Hesselbrock, V. (1994) Alcohol dependence and anxiety disorders: what is the relationship. *American Journal of Psychiatry* 151, 1723–34.

Schuckit, M.A., Irwin, M. and Brown, S.A. (1990) The history of anxiety symptoms among 171 primary alcoholics. *Journal of Studies on Alcohol* 51, 34–41.

Schuckit, M.A., Tipp, J.E., Bereman, M., Reich, W., Hesselbrock, V.M. and Smith, T.L. (1997) Comparison of induced or independent major depressive disorder in 2,945 alcoholics. *American Journal of Psychiatry* 154, 948–57.

Soyka, M., Albus, M., Kathmann, N. et al. (1993) Prevalence of alcohol and drug abuse in schizophrenic in-patients. *European Archives of Psychiatry and Clinical Neuroscience* 242, 362–72.

Stockwell, T., Smail, P., Hodgson, R. et al. (1984) Alcohol dependence and phobic anxiety states. II: a retrospective study. *British Journal of Psychiatry* 144, 58–63.

Tarter, R.E. (1991) Developmental behavior – genetic perspective of alcoholism etiology. In *Recent Developments in Alcoholism*, Vol. 9, ed. Galanter, M. New York: Plenum Press, 69–85.

Vassilas, C.A. and Morgan, H.G. (1997) Suicide in Avon. Life stress, alcohol misuse and use of services. *British Journal of Psychiatry* 170, 453–5.

Winfield, I., George, L.K., Swartz, M. and Blazer, D.G. (1990) Sexual assault and psychiatric disorders among a community sample of women. *American Journal of Psychiatry* 147, 335–41.

Winokur, G., Coryell, W., Akiskal, H.S. et al. (1995) Alcoholism in manic–depressive (bipolar) illness: familial illness, course of illness, and the primary secondary distinction. *American Journal of Psychiatry* 152, 365–72.

World Health Organization (1992) *The ICD-10 Classification of Mental and Behavioural Disorders.* Geneva: World Health Organization.

Zuckerman, M. (1991) Sensation seeking: the balance between risk and reward. In *Self-Regulatory Behavior and Risk Taking*: *Causes and Consequences*, ed. Lipsitt, L.P. and Multnick, L.L. Norwood, NT: Ablex, 143–52.

9

Alcohol and other drug problems

'Chemical dependence'

In many countries the contemporary pattern of substance misuse, particularly in individuals under the age of 40, is of multiple substances. Drug and alcohol problems may occur either concurrently or as problems which develop in sequence. The patterns of relationship which can exist between the use of different types of mind-acting chemical are many and the following case extract illustrates one variation on this theme.

The patient was a successful and wealthy entrepreneur aged 35. His working day was lived at a great pitch of tension and every evening he would go out to restaurants and night clubs and get through a lot of alcohol. He would on average drink a couple of bottles of wine and up to a dozen double vodkas before becoming, in his terms, 'pretty incoherent'. He was beginning to feel 'dreadful, sick, sweaty' on most mornings and would often be unable to remember how he had reached his bed. Cocaine then began to be available in his social circle and before long he discovered that this drug appeared to provide an antidote to some of the unwanted effects of alcohol. For instance, if he snorted (sniffed) cocaine a few times during the evening, 'it lifted me up, I could go on drinking, it stopped me passing-out with the alcohol'. He also found that a snort or two of cocaine helped to alleviate the unpleasant early-morning symptoms caused by the previous night's drinking. Within a few months he progressed from snorting to free-basing (inhaling) cocaine, and his cocaine use rapidly and disastrously went out of control. His problem came to attention when a club was raided and he was arrested for possession of cocaine. Seen by a doctor at the request of the defence solicitor this man said, 'OK, I'm addicted to cocaine but let's not keep on about the alcohol'.

What this patient's history illustrates is that another type of chemical often lies behind the immediately presenting drug. It would be unprofitable in such circumstances to debate whether alcohol or cocaine was the 'real' problem. This man's problem was his tendency to misuse chemicals. Both the alcohol and cocaine aspects of his history have to be taken seriously, but what the patient himself and those who are seeking to help him need to realize is that dependence can often resemble the many-headed Hydra of mythology: one head can be lopped off and another grows. Unless with such a patient there is a focus on the central issue of his tendency to develop dependence on chemicals, the story will all too probably progress in terms of a further switching or mixing of different substances – in terms, perhaps, of tranquillizers or sleeping tablets then being added to alcohol. Nicotine is an almost inevitable part of the mix.

The most common reason for concurrent drug use is to enhance effects. For instance, alcohol can enhance the effects of stimulants such as cocaine and amphetamines, and also the effects of benzodiazepines and volatile solvents. Alcohol is commonly used to counteract the effects of other drugs. It reduces jittery feelings associated with stimulant use and may help in the withdrawal phase. A heroin user may substitute with alcohol, cannabis or benzodiazepines, either alone or in combination, to tide him or her over until heroin is again available. A further reason for multiple drug use is peer influence. The combined use of alcohol, cannabis and nicotine is commonplace.

This chapter describes some of the more commonly encountered connections between alcohol and other drug problems. The issue of multiple dependencies is then considered in some detail. Lastly, discussion turns to the general implications both for prevention and for clinical practice which stem from the realization that alcohol and other drug problems potentially constitute one continuous domain rather than two distinct problem areas. Box 9.1 summarizes some of the main points which this chapter emphasizes.

BOX 9.1 **Drug problems and alcohol problems: key issues**
- Multiple substance use is the contemporary pattern of substance misuse
- Alcohol is almost always implicated in multiple substance use
- Other drugs are not always implicated in alcohol misuse
- Multiple substance use is associated with significant physical and psychosocial morbidity
- Therapists and treatment services need the skills to meet mixed problems

---

Multiple substance use

Multiple substance use has become increasingly prevalent over recent decades and shows no sign of abating. It occurs in the general population and is not confined to individuals heavily involved in the 'drug scene' or in contact with treatment services. Nevertheless, the number of multiple substance users in contact with treatment services is increasing, and is a cause of serious concern.

The initiation of substance use in adolescents is largely determined by environmental rather than genetic factors (Han et al., 1999). These factors include availability, price, the social situation, peer group usage and fashion. Adolescent substance use is a powerful predictor of substance use disorders in adulthood (Grant and Dawson, 1997).

Over the past 10 years or so, increasing numbers of young people are using alcohol, tobacco and illicit drugs. This is a matter of concern worldwide. A number of studies have examined associations between different substances, and a clear relationship between alcohol, tobacco and drug use in adolescents has been shown. Young people using one or more of these substances, especially alcohol, are more likely to use the other substances subsequently. Teenagers with heavier drinking and smoking patterns are at greater risk of later drug use. Research from the USA suggests a protective effect of church affiliation or 'religiosity'. However, a UK study of church-affiliated young people found that illicit drug use was 50 times more likely amongst those who had ever smoked cigarettes (Cook et al., 1997).

Recent studies of English schoolchildren confirm that rates of cigarette smoking, alcohol and illicit drug use rise rapidly in the teenage years (Sutherland and Willner, 1998; Sutherland and Shepherd, 2001). Alcohol is the most heavily used substance, followed by cigarettes and then by illicit drugs. These findings suggest that there is a 'low threshold' for alcohol use among adolescents, and a higher threshold for cigarette and illicit drug use.

Initiation into the recreational drug scene is subtle. Young people think that drug use is 'cool – that everyone is doing it'. They take risks and some use a variety of drugs over a number of years without any 'overt' problems. Drug fashions come and go, but alcohol is almost always implicated in the shifting picture of multiple substance use.

Multiple substance use can develop in stages, with individuals moving from licit to illicit drugs, and from less to more serious drugs. Substances used at earlier stages in their career are often used at increasing levels of severity.

There is now evidence to suggest that, at least in men, the factors underlying vulnerability to the use or abuse of one drug also put individuals at risk of abusing every other class of drug (Tsuang et al., 2000). Thus, some characteristic of the individual seems to underlie vulnerability to the abuse of all categories of drugs. In the literature this characteristic is referred to as the 'shared' or 'common' vulnerability. This shared vulnerability is influenced by genetic factors, family environmental factors and non-family environmental factors. Not every drug is influenced to the same extent by the shared vulnerability factor. For instance, most of the genetic influence on heroin abuse is specific to heroin and not shared with other drugs, whereas most of the genetic influence on abuse of cannabis, stimulants and sedatives is shared across drugs, with a modest degree of genetic variance specific to each substance. There is something about the family environment that imparts a substantial risk for all categories of drug abuse. However, something else about the family environment imparts a specific risk for cannabis abuse.

History taking should incorporate a set of questions for each drug class, in order to define the sequencing and pattern of drug use and the combinations of drugs used (alcohol and cannabis; alcohol and cigarettes; alcohol and cocaine, and so on). It will be helpful to work out whether or not the problem amounts to dependence. Multiple substance users are often dependent on one or two drugs, but also use other drugs in a problematical way. It must be remembered that multiple substance use is associated with significant medical and psychosocial complications which must also be elicited. The interaction of alcohol with other drugs such as opioids and benzodiazepines is potentially dangerous (White and Irvine, 1999; Warner-Smith et al., 2001). Overdose death is an intrinsic hazard of multiple substance use.

Specific combinations

Alcohol and cocaine

The combination of alcohol and cocaine is an increasingly familiar pattern of multiple drug use and in the USA alcohol is more likely to be used in conjunction with cocaine than with any other type of drug (Regier et al., 1990; Carroll et al., 1993b). Alcohol is typically used during a cocaine binge in order to prolong the euphoriant effects of cocaine and, as already mentioned, to diminish unpleasant experiences associated with cocaine use, such as agitation and paranoia, and to ameliorate the dysphoria associated with acute abstinence from cocaine (the 'crash'). Once regular cocaine and alcohol use is established, it may be difficult to give up one substance without giving up the other. Alcohol can become a powerful conditioned cue for cocaine. Cocaethylene, a pharmacologically active metabolite of alcohol and cocaine, is thought to enhance and extend cocaine euphoria (McCance et al., 1995).

For many people, treatment of the cocaine problem may lead to an improvement in the alcohol problem (Kosten, 1989). However, the presence of alcohol problems and dependence in treated cocaine users is associated with more severe dependence, poorer retention in treatment and a poorer outcome compared with either disorder alone (Walsh et al., 1991; Carroll et al., 1993a, 1993b; Brady et al., 1995), and more needs to be learnt about how to treat this difficult combination (Brower et al., 1994). A recent report suggested that treatment with disulfiram for 12 weeks was associated with better treatment retention and abstinence, particularly when combined with 'active' out-patient psychotherapy (cognitive–behavioural coping skills and therapy) and Twelve-Step Facilitation (Carroll et al., 1998). The disulfiram effect persisted at 1-year follow-up (Carroll et al., 2000).

A 40-year-old lawyer was referred for a combined alcohol and cocaine problem. He first drank at 16 and soon alcohol became 'an all-embracing hobby'. His 20s were spent in an intoxicated haze. Already alcohol dependent at 35, he began to use cocaine, always in the context of alcohol use, and always in exactly the same way. Soon after commencing treatment he managed a 6-month period of abstinence from both drugs. On relapse to drinking, he started to use cocaine again, in exactly the same manner as before.

Alcohol and opioids

Problematic use of alcohol is a common problem in opioid users. Alcohol consumption typically precedes the first use of heroin in the early career of heroin addicts, but levels of alcohol use tend to drop off when regular opioid use is established (Rounsaville et al., 1982). However, the impact of treatment of opioid dependence on alcohol use is uncertain, some studies finding that rates of alcohol misuse remain constant or decline, and others reporting that treatment entry is associated with increased alcohol use. The theme that emerges from these studies is that alcohol problems frequently pre-date opioid use, and that when one dependence has developed, a variety of drugs will be misused.

Two general patterns of drinking have been recognized in heroin dependent subjects during and following treatment: *concurrent* use while on licit or illicit opioids and use of alcohol as *a substitute for* opioids. Methadone treatment, in particular, is associated with alcohol problems, because it blocks the intoxicating effect of opioids, thus causing addicts to look for another intoxicating substance. Prevalence rates of problem drinking in patients undergoing methadone treatment programmes have varied from 20% to 50% in the majority of (mainly American) studies (Liebson et al., 1973). A British study, of patients enrolled in a methadone treatment programme in a London teaching hospital, reported that 32% had actual or potential drinking problems (Stastny and Potter, 1991). Those with alcohol problems were also likely to use benzodiazepines.

Multiple substance use is widespread among heroin users and people on methadone maintenance treatment. Although a variety of drugs can be used, there are particular problems with alcohol and benzodiazepine dependence in this group. An Australian study found that 91% of 222 heroin injectors (mean age 29.8 years) had used benzodiazepines (35% had injected), and 67% were current users (Ross and Darke, 2000). Of the currently using group, 22% were benzodiazepine dependent. Those with a lifetime of benzodiazepine dependence were more likely to have a lifetime history of alcohol and cocaine dependence, as well as an anxiety and depressive disorder.

Alcohol problems may substitute for opioids when heroin users attempt to detoxify on their own, in a treatment programme or during prolonged periods of abstinence. A seemingly promising recovery from a drug problem is being brought down because the danger of contracting a later cross-dependence on alcohol was not foreseen. A long-term national study in the USA found that substitution of alcohol for heroin occurred in approximately 10% of the clients followed up, and was strongly associated with cannabis use (Sells and Simpson, 1987). Treated opioid addicts who go on to develop alcohol problems are more likely to have had disruptive childhoods, more legal problems and poly-drug use, more problems with social functioning and higher rates of psychiatric disorders than 'non-alcoholic addicts' (Rounsaville et al., 1982). Here is a typical story of early heavy drinking in a setting of poly-drug use; this youthful pattern of mixed use may lead to a dominant use of heroin, and recovery from heroin dependence being followed a few years later by a plunge into alcohol.

A 34-year-old unemployed man was referred for assessment of his heavy drinking and depression. He had experienced extreme emotional deprivation in childhood and had been in care. At 14 he began to drink beer and to smoke cannabis 'for comfort'. He soon began to use amphetamines and diazepam, and his daily alcohol consumption gradually increased to three to four cans of strong lager. He first smoked heroin in his early 20s and very soon switched to intravenous use, sharing needles. He also snorted cocaine on a regular basis, injecting it on occasion. Other drug use included LSD intermittently, 'mushrooms' and Ecstasy. When he was 30 he entered a residential rehabilitation unit and gave up all illicit drug use. However, his alcohol consumption escalated and 4 years later, at the time of referral, his drinking was out of control. He was also experiencing marked craving for heroin and cocaine and was worried that he would begin to use them again.

Alcohol and benzodiazepines

The risk of benzodiazepine abuse in the general population is very low, in the region of 1% (Posternak and Mueller, 2001). Benzodiazepine abuse is associated with illicit drug abuse, particularly opiate abuse. It occurs much less frequently in individuals with alcohol problems. There is evidence to suggest that 'alcoholics' who develop concurrent benzodiazepine abuse are also more likely to have an antisocial personality disorder (Sokolow et al., 1981; Ross, 1993). Benzodiazepine use does not appear to increase the risk of alcohol abuse or relapse.

Benzodiazepines were introduced to clinical practice in 1960 and soon became widely used in the treatment of anxiety and insomnia. They are also accepted as the treatment of choice for alcohol withdrawal symptoms. A wide variety of benzodiazepines has been marketed and Table 9.1 lists the commoner substances, giving both their official and trade names. In many countries, including the UK, prescriptions for benzodiazepines as anxiolytics have fallen over the past two decades, whereas prescriptions for their use as hypnotics are little changed (Lader, 1998).

Table 9.1 Some common benzodiazepines

Non-proprietary name	Proprietary name	Active metabolites	Approximate duration of action	Approximate equivalent dose (mg)
Diazepam	Valium	Several	2–4 days	5
Chlordiazepoxide	Librium	Several	2–4 days	15
Nitrazepam	Mogadon	None	12–24 hours	5
Clonazepam	Rivotril	Several	1–2 days	0.5
Lorazepam	Ativan	None	8–12 hours	0.5
Temazepam	Normison	None	8 hours	10
Oxazepam	Oxanid	None	8–12 hours	15

Source: British National Formulary (2002).

Drugs within the benzodiazepines group have many properties in common. Important differences exist, however, in relation to duration of action either of the drug itself or of its active metabolite. Lorazepam, oxazepam and temazepam are all relatively short acting; chlordiazepoxide and diazepam are long acting; and the other substances listed in the table produce an action of intermediate duration.

Most benzodiazepine prescribing is appropriate (Woods et al., 1988). Nevertheless, long-term, continuous use of benzodiazepines carries a risk of dependence. This is most evident for high doses, but dependence can develop in patients who take therapeutic doses for as little as 6 weeks (Mant et al., 1987). The relatively short-acting compounds may have a greater dependence potential than the long-acting compounds. The proportion of patients taking therapeutic doses of benzodiazepines at risk of developing dependence is not known. Neither is there enough information, other than in broad terms, to identify the level of exposure (dose and duration) associated with an increased risk of dependence. New prescriptions of benzodiazepines should be restricted to approximately 2 weeks, and certainly no longer than 4 weeks, and lorazepam should be avoided.

Patients with alcohol problems should not generally be given benzodiazepines, except for the treatment of acute alcohol withdrawal, and then only on a careful and time-limited basis. Patients with concurrent anxiety should be referred for cognitive–behavioural therapy. A selective serotonin reuptake inhibitor (SSRI) or antidepressant can be prescribed; there is evidence for their efficacy in anxiety disorders, social phobia and obsessive–compulsive disorder (Lader, 1998). However, there will still be patients who have taken benzodiazepines for many years, are dependent and prefer to stay on this medication.

The use of benzodiazepines as a hypnotic in alcohol dependent individuals should be avoided. There may well be problems with the newer non-benzodiazepine compounds, zopiclone and zolpidem, and these are detailed below.

Dependence is not the only potential problem encountered with benzodiazepine use. Ataxia, falls, confusion, depression and irritability are all significant sequelae of long-acting compounds, with the elderly being at particular risk (Lader, 1998). Short-acting benzodiazepines at high doses appear to be associated with amnesia.

Alcohol and zopiclone

Zopiclone is a cyclopyrrolone, licensed for the short-term treatment of insomnia. Although chemically unrelated to the benzodiazepines, it acts at the GABA-benzodiazepine receptor. Several instances of dependence have now been reported, and it is possible that individuals with alcohol dependence and multiple drug use are more at risk (Ayonrinde and Sampson, 1998; Jones and Sullivan, 1998). Withdrawal symptoms include severe anxiety and panic attacks, palpitations, tremor, sweating and rebound insomnia. In the instances of zopiclone dependence reported, individuals had increased the dose from the recommended amount of 7.5 mg nocte to between 15 and 30 mg nocte.

There have also been a number of reports of abuse. In a survey of 100 multiple drug users attending a methadone maintenance clinic, six subjects abusing zopiclone in doses of 90–380 mg daily were identified (Sikdar and Ruben, 1996). Abuse of intravenous zopiclone has also been reported (Clee et al., 1996).

Alcohol and nicotine

About 80% of alcohol dependent men and women smoke regularly (Hughes, 1996) and there may be a common genetic vulnerability (True et al., 1999). They are often heavy smokers, have difficulty quitting smoking and, when they stop drinking, may compensate by even heavier use of cigarettes (Hays et al., 1999). Nicotine dependence is associated with a greater severity of alcohol dependence and alcohol-related problems (Daeppen et al., 2000). 'Alcoholics' who smoke have high rates of tobacco-related disease, and are more likely to die from tobacco-related diseases than from their alcohol dependence (Rosengren et al., 1993; Hurt et al., 1994; Marshall et al., 1994). Both alcohol and nicotine dependence are associated with mood disorders. Individuals with concurrent alcohol and nicotine dependence have a substantially increased risk of bipolar disorder, use of illicit drugs and antisocial personality disorder (ASPD) (Helzer et al., 1991).

Several psychological and neuropharmacological models have been proposed to explain the association between alcohol use disorders and cigarette smoking. The overlap between the two substances suggests that there are many shared cues.

Theoretically, then, it might be more difficult to stop using either alcohol or nicotine than to quit both substances at the same time. Despite the fact that alcohol and nicotine are commonly used together, the feasibility of quitting smoking at the same time as drinking has largely been unexplored. Nevertheless, the implications for counselling problem drinkers to quit smoking are persuasive. Alcohol dependent individuals are open to advice on smoking (Harris et al., 2000). Counselling is safe, even in the early stages of recovery, and may have a positive effect on drinking outcome at 6-month and 12-month follow-up (Bobo et al., 1995, 1998; Martin et al., 1997). Smoking cessation programmes in residential alcohol treatment units have shown good outcomes for nicotine abstinence.

Bupropion, an atypical antidepressant recently licensed in the USA as an aid for smoking cessation, was shown to be effective in a sample of smokers with a former history of major depression and alcoholism (Hayford et al., 1999).

'A web of dependence'

Multiple substance use complicates our understanding of the concept of dependence and raises fundamental questions about the nature of dependence (Gossop, 2001; West, 2001). Should dependence be viewed as a condition that spans more than one substance, rather than multiple substance-specific conditions residing in the same person (West, 2001)? This has profound implications for treatment. For instance, should we routinely be trying to help alcohol dependent individuals in recovery to quit smoking too?

Behavioural pharmacology can provide insights into these questions (Stolerman, 2002). Animals and humans can be trained to discriminate between two drugs on the basis of their subjective effects (stimulus generalization). This type of work explores whether the effects of two substances are treated as similar under particular circumstances. A different approach, the self-administration paradigm, has been used to explore substitution of one drug for another. This work has been mostly carried out in animals. Self-administration tends to continue when the original substance is changed to a different drug of abuse, even when the second drug is pharmacologically very different, and is more pronounced if the substitute drug is similar to the original drug. In this paradigm, transfer from one drug to another indicates whether the substitute drug can act as a positive reinforcer. It does not mean that subjects cannot detect the difference between them (discrimination). The effects of drugs clearly depend on the circumstances in which they are assessed.

Alcohol and drug dependence disorders run in families. This suggests that they are, in part, caused by genetic factors. What is the nature of these underlying genetic factors? Is a general addictive risk factor transmitted or are there specific risk factors for particular drugs? This research is extremely complicated and still in progress. Although risk factors underlie substance disorders in general, the clustering of different substance use disorders within families seems to be substance specific (Bierut et al., 1998; Merikangas et al., 1998). This means that independent factors may be involved in the development of each type of substance dependence.

The behavioural economic perspective may provide a framework in which the demand for multiple commodities (multiple substances) can be conceptualized (Vuchinich and Tucker, 1998; Tucker, 2001). Choice behaviour is considered to be context-dependent. Thus, preference for a given commodity (e.g. drug) is thought to vary inversely with constraints or access to it and directly with constraints on access to alternatives. Essentially, a reduction in multiple substance use can be promoted by enriching the environment with attractive non-drug alternatives and reducing delays in their availability, and by reducing the availability of preferred 'substances' and other commodities that function as complements to their use (Tucker, 2001). Thus reducing drug availability has to be paired with increasing environment enrichment, a considerable challenge for the 'real world' drug clinic setting.

Alcohol and other drugs as one domain: the practical implications

Several of the most immediate implications of this perspective have already been discussed in earlier sections of this chapter. At this point it may, however, be useful to bring together the core implications, and in Box 9.2 we draw attention to some matters of special clinical relevance.

BOX 9.2 **Tips for therapists**
- Have a good working knowledge of alcohol *and* other substances
- Always take a complete alcohol *and* drug history
- Update the history regularly
- Organize spot urinary drug screens where indicated

Implications for training and service organization

Anyone taking professional responsibility for the treatment of alcohol problems should recognize that multiple substance use is pervasive and possess a good working knowledge of drug problems (and *vice versa*). There may be a continuing place for specialized drug or specialized alcohol treatment services, but the intensity of specialization must not be of such a degree as to be out of tune with clinical realities. The problems with which patients present often do not respect the specialists' demarcations. Inadequate training may mean that individuals with combined drug and alcohol problems find it difficult to obtain treatment, are incompletely evaluated and treated, and often rejected. If treatment services are to face the challenge of multiple substance use successfully, they must have a capacity to integrate alcohol and drug treatment.

A prime responsibility for prevention

Therapists who are treating patients with drinking problems have a special responsibility not to do their patients damage by careless prescription of sedatives and minor tranquillizers. It is similarly important that anyone who is treating opioid-dependent patients should offer counselling on the use of alcohol and the dangers of alcohol dependence.

Diagnosis and screening

With a patient whose presenting problem is with one type of substance, an open eye should be kept on the possible existence of problems with other types of chemical. It is, for instance, less than useful to concentrate exclusively on a patient's drinking while failing to detect the fact that massive quantities of benzodiazepines are being consumed. A complete alcohol and drug history should be obtained. This means charting as necessary the evolution of use and dependence for every drug taken, as well as for alcohol. In this way the sequence of drug use can be mapped out, for example solvents as a child, alcohol and later amphetamines in the teenage years, heroin as an adult. Many clients presenting to alcohol services may have a past history of intravenous drug use and will need assessment of risk behaviour and counselling with respect to testing for hepatitis and human immunodeficiency virus (HIV) status. Routine urine testing should be more widely employed. The history should be updated at regular intervals.

Treatment goals

Therapists working within treatment programmes which take the concept of chemical dependence as a central tenet would probably advise a patient who has encountered difficulties with either alcohol or other drugs to avoid all mood-altering chemicals for ever after. For many patients this is the best advice, although it is unlikely to be acceptable to all patients (some former heroin addicts may, for instance, later use alcohol moderately and safely). The insistence that patients should be made aware of the dangers of crossing over from one substance to another is very generally appropriate. Essentially, the needs of individuals with multiple substance use must be met. Services also need to cope with co-existing anxiety and depressive disorders.

A constant two-way vigilance

This heading cross-cuts with all the other entities in this section. When seeing a patient or client for the first time, when planning and carrying through a treatment programme and when assessing success, patient and therapist should be thinking in terms of drugs and alcohol and not just alcohol or just drugs. Also, to turn a blind eye to nicotine is not in the patient's best health interests.

REFERENCES

Ayonrinde, O. and Sampson, E. (1998) Physical dependence on zopiclone: risk of dependence may be greater in those with dependent personalities (letter). *British Medical Journal* 317, 146.

Bierut, L.J., Dinwiddie, S.H., Begleiter, H. et al. (1998) Familial transmission of substance dependence: alcohol, marijuana, cocaine, and habitual smoking. *Archives of General Psychiatry* 55, 982–8.

Brady, K.T., Sonne, E., Randall, C.L., Adinoff, B. and Malcolm, R. (1995) Features of cocaine dependence with concurrent alcohol use. *Drug and Alcohol Dependence* 39, 69–71.

Bobo, J.K., McIlvain, H.E., Lando, H.A., Walker, R.D. and Leed-Kelly, A. (1998) Effect of smoking cessation counseling on recovery from alcoholism: findings from a randomised community intervention trial. *Addiction* 93, 877–87.

Bobo, J.K., Slade, J. and Hoffman, A.L. (1995) Nicotine addiction counselling for chemically dependent patients. *Psychiatric Services* 46, 945–7.

British National Formulary (2002) London: British Medical Association and Royal Pharmaceutical Society of Great Britain.

Brower, K.J., Blow, F.C., Hill, E.M. and Mudd, S.A. (1994) Treatment outcome of alcoholics with and without cocaine disorders. *Alcoholism: Clinical and Experimental Research* 18, 734–9.

Carroll, K.M., Nich, C., Ball, S.A., McCance, E., Frankforter, T.L. and Rounsaville, B.J. (2000) One-year follow-up of disulfiram and psychotherapy for cocaine–alcohol users: sustained effects of treatment. *Addiction* 95, 1335–49.

Carroll, K.M., Nich, C., Ball, S.A., McCance, E. and Rounsaville, B.J. (1998) Treatment of cocaine and alcohol dependence with psychotherapy and disulfiram. *Addiction* 93, 713–28.

Carroll, K.M., Power, M.-E.D., Bryant, K. and Rounsaville, B.J. (1993a) One-year follow-up status of treatment-seeking cocaine abusers. *Journal of Nervous and Mental Disease* 181, 71–9.

Carroll, K.M., Rounsaville, B.J. and Bryant, K.J. (1993b) Alcoholism in treatment seeking cocaine abusers: clinical and prognostic significance. *Journal of Studies on Alcohol* 54, 199–208.

Clee, B.C., McBride, A.J. and Sullivan, G. (1996) Warning about zopiclone misuse (letter). *Addiction* 91, 1389–90.

Cook, C.C.H., Goddard, D. and Westall, R. (1997) Knowledge and experience of drug use among church affiliated young people. *Drug and Alcohol Dependence* 46, 9–17.

Daeppen, J.-B., Smith, T.L., Danko, G.P. et al. and the Collaborative Study Group on the Genetics of Alcoholism (2000) Clinical correlates of cigarette smoking and nicotine dependence in alcohol dependent men and women. *Alcohol and Alcoholism* 35, 171–5.

Gossop, M. (2001) A web of dependence. *Addiction* 96, 677–8.

Grant, B.F. and Dawson, D.A. (1997) Age at onset of alcohol use and its association with DSM-IV alcohol abuse and dependence: results from the National Longitudinal Alcohol Epidemiologic Survey. *Journal of Substance Abuse* 9, 103–10.

Han, C., McGue, M.K. and Iacono, W.G. (1999) Lifetime tobacco, alcohol and other substance use in adolescent Minnesota twins: univariate and multivariate behavioural genetic analyses. *Addiction* 94, 981–93.

Harris, J., Best, D., Man, L.-H., Welch, S., Gossop, M. and Strang, J. (2000) Change in cigarette smoking among alcohol and drug misusers during in-patient detoxification. *Addiction Biology* 5, 443–50.

Hayford, K.E., Patten, C.A., Rummans, T.A. et al. (1999) Efficacy of bupropion for smoking cessation in smokers with a former history of major depression or alcoholism. *British Journal of Psychiatry* 174, 173–8.

Hays, J.T., Schroeder, D.R., Offord, K.P. et al. (1999) Response to nicotine dependence treatment in smokers with current and past alcohol problems. *Annals of Behavioural Medicine* 21, 244–50.

Helzer, J.E., Burnam, A. and McEvoy, L.T. (1991) Alcohol abuse and dependence. In *Psychiatric Disorders in America*, ed. Robins, L. N. and Regier, D.A. New York: The Free Press, 81–115.

Hughes, J.R. (1996) Treating smokers with current or past alcohol dependence. *American Journal of Health Behavior* 20, 286–90.

Hurt, R.D., Eberman, K.M., Croghan, I.T. et al. (1994) Nicotine dependence treatment during inpatient treatment for other addictions: a prospective intervention trial. *Alcohol: Clinical and Experimental Research* 18, 867–72.

Jones, I.R. and Sullivan, G. (1998) Physical dependence on zopiclone: case reports. *British Medical Journal* 316, 117.

Kosten, T.R. (1989) Pharmacotherapeutic interventions for cocaine abuse. *Journal of Nervous and Mental Disease* 177, 379–89.

Lader, M. (1998) Iatrogenic sedative dependence and abuse – have doctors learnt caution? *Addiction* 93, 1133–5.

Liebson, I., Bieglow, G. and Flamer, R. (1973) Alcoholism amongst methadone patients. A special treatment method. *American Journal of Psychiatry* 130, 483–5.

McCance, E.F., Price, L.H., Kosten, T.R. and Jatlow, P.I. (1995) Cocaethylene: pharmacology, physiology and behavioural effects in humans. *Journal of Pharmacology and Experimental Therapeutics* 274, 215–23.

Mant, A., Wodak, A. and Day, R. (1987) Benzodiazepine dependence. Strategies for prevention and withdrawal. *Current Therapeutics* Feb., 59–79.

Marshall, E.J., Edwards, J.G. and Taylor, C. (1994) Mortality in men with drinking problems: a 20-year follow-up. *Addiction* 89, 1293–8.

Martin, J.E., Calfas, K.J., Patten, C.A. et al. (1997) Prospective evaluation of three smoking interventions in 205 recovering alcoholics: one-year results of project SCRAP-Tobacco. *Journal of Consulting and Clinical Psychology* 65, 190–4.

Merikangas, K.R., Stolar, M., Stevens, D.E. et al. (1998) Familial transmission of substance use disorders. *Archives of General Psychiatry* 55, 973–9.

Posternak, M.A. and Mueller, T.I. (2001) Assessing the risks and benefits of benzodiazepines for anxiety disorders in-patients with a history of substance use or dependence. *American Journal on Addictions* 10, 48–68.

Regier, D.A., Farmer, M.E., Rae, D. et al. (1990) Comorbidity of mental disorders with alcohol and other drug use. *Journal of the American Medical Association* 264, 2511–18.

Rosengren, A., Wilhelmsen, L. and Wedel, H. (1993) Separate and combined effects of smoking and alcohol abuse in middle-aged men. *Acta Medica Scandinavica* 223, 111–18.

Ross, H.E. (1993) Benzodiazepine use and anxiolytic abuse and dependence in treated alcoholics. *Addiction* 88, 209–18.

Ross, J. and Darke, S. (2000) The nature of benzodiazepine dependence among heroin users in Sydney, Australia. *Addiction* 95, 1785–93.

Rounsaville, B.J., Weissman, M.M. and Kleber, H.D. (1982) The significance of alcoholism in treated opiate addicts. *Journal of Nervous and Mental Disease* 170, 479–88.

Sells, S.B. and Simpson, D.D. (1987) Role of alcohol use by narcotic addicts as revealed in the DARP research on evaluation of treatment for drug abuse. *Alcoholism: Clinical and Experimental Research* 11, 437–9.

Sikdar, S. and Ruben, S.M. (1996) Zopiclone abuse among polydrug users (letter). *Addiction* 91, 285–91.

Sokolow, J.K., Welte, J., Hynes, G. and Lyons, J. (1981) Multiple substance abuse by alcoholics. *British Journal of Addiction* 76, 147–58.

Stastny, D. and Potter, M. (1991) Alcohol abuse by patients undergoing methadone treatment programmes. *British Journal of Addiction* 86, 307–10.

Stolerman, I. (2002) Drug stimulus generalisation and Gossop's 'web of dependence'. *Addiction* 97, 152–4.

Sutherland, I. and Shepherd, J.P. (2001) The prevalence of alcohol, cigarette and illicit drug use in a sample of English adolescents. *Addiction* 96, 637–40.

Sutherland, I. and Willner, P. (1998) Patterns of alcohol, cigarette and illicit drug use in English adolescents. *Addiction* 93, 1199–208.

True, W.R., Xian, H., Scherrer, J.F. et al. (1999) Common genetic vulnerability for nicotine and alcohol dependence in men. *Archives of General Psychiatry* 56, 655–61.

Tsuang, M.T., Lyons, M.J., Meyer, J.M. et al. (2000). Co-occurrence of abuse of different drugs in men. The role of drug-specific and shared vulnerabilities. *Archives of General Psychiatry* 55, 967–72.

Tucker, J.A. (2001) Understanding multiple substance misuse: an alternative view from behavioural economics. *Addiction* 96, 776–7.

Vuchinich, R.E. and Tucker, J.A. (1998) Choice, behavioral economics and addictive behavior patterns. In *Treating Addictive Behaviors: Processes of Change*, 2nd edn, ed. Miller, W.R. and Heather, N. New York: Plenum Press, 93–104.

Walsh, D.C., Hingson, R.W., Merrigan, D.M. et al. (1991) A randomized trial of treatment options for alcohol-abusing workers. *New England Journal of Medicine* 325, 775–82.

Warner-Smith, M., Darke, S., Lynskey, M.T. and Hall, W. (2001) Heroin overdose: causes and consequences. *Addiction* 96, 1113–25.

West, R. (2001) Multiple substance dependence: implications for treatment of nicotine dependence. *Addiction* 96, 775–6.

White, J.M. and Irvine, R.J. (1999) Mechanisms of fatal opioid dependence. *Addiction* 94, 961–72.

Woods, J.H., Kate, J.L. and Winger, G. (1988) Use and abuse of benzodiazepines: issues relevant to prescribing. *Journal of the American Medical Association* 260, 3476–80.

10

Physical complications of excessive drinking

Within a total and balanced approach to drinking problems, the physical element must be seen as often very important. Helping services must be so organized as to cope effectively with diagnosis and treatment in the physical domain and, whatever the particular professional affiliation of the person who is working with the problem drinker, there is need for an alertness towards possible physical pathologies. For instance, voluntary workers in a lay counselling centres are, of course, practising their own special types of skill, and no-one would suggest that they should also cultivate a highly specialized knowledge of liver pathology. It is, though, a reasonable expectation that they should know enough about the liver to understand the significance to their client of a diagnosis of cirrhosis, rather than themselves being mystified by this term and consequently deflecting that client from talking about something of vital importance. A polite conspiracy can be set up which pretends that the body does not exist.

Why physical complications matter

Alcohol consumption is a significant cause of physical morbidity and poses a substantial burden on hospital services (Royal College of Physicians, 2001). In Great Britain, approximately 15–30% of male and 8–15% of female admissions to general hospitals in urban areas have alcohol-related problems (Chick, 1994; Canning et al., 1999). The equivalent figure in the USA is 20–40% for both men and women (Lieber, 1995). Alcohol consumption is also responsible for considerable mortality from natural causes and contributes to deaths from accidents, suicide and violence (Edwards et al., 1994; Harris and Barraclough, 1998; Sjögren et al., 2000).

Although physical complications are common in any population of heavy drinkers, early detection and cessation of drinking can lead to recovery. Continued drinking, however, is likely to exacerbate the alcohol-related problem and may seriously threaten life. Physical complications impinge upon all aspects of the problem drinker's life and it is unrealistic to compartmentalize psychological, social and physical disability.

Often physical complications are the main reason for seeking help. If information about the physical symptoms is imparted clearly, so that patients can understand their significance, this information can be used to appraise their position. Thus an understanding of the physical symptoms may have the potential to influence drinking behaviour. As ever, the therapist is the informant, the person who brings up the issue, and who shares and reflects the patient's feelings and concerns, rather than the disembodied pronouncer of facts. The way in which information on physical problems is presented to the patient can be part of therapy. Here are two dialogues which illustrate different ways in which the patient's concern over his physical health can be met at interview. Firstly, and very briefly, a dialogue which is not to be dismissed as caricature.

Patient: What does the doctor mean when he said my liver had been hit by the drinking?
Counsellor: You will have to ask the doctor to explain.
Patient: But he never explains anything.
Counsellor: Well, he's the person to ask.

Secondly, and more constructively.

Patient: What does the doctor mean when he said my liver had been hit by the drinking?
Counsellor: That's something pretty important to talk about. What did you think he meant?
Patient: I suppose I was dead scared. Not sure I believe him, though. He may just be trying to put the frighteners under me. But if what he's really saying is that I'm going to die of cirrhosis, I'll go out in the crest of the all-time greatest booze-up.
Counsellor: I don't think anyone is wanting to scare you in a horror-story sort of way, but it's your own liver and you have a right to know about it.
Patient: So what's the score?
Counsellor: I spoke to your doctor on the phone. You have undoubtedly done your liver some harm, and if you go on drinking you would be risking cirrhosis, and that's a miserable way to die. If you stop drinking, your liver's going to heal. You've a right to know all the facts. It's reasonable to be anxious, but at least there is something positive you can do towards repairing the damage – stop drinking.
Patient: When I was getting that pain, I guessed it must be my liver, but I suppose I have been shutting my eyes, doing the 'it can't happen to me' trick.

The vital question is what any information on physical consequences means to the patient. Too often the results of the physical examination and laboratory tests are left in the case notes, and no-one thinks to ask whether these findings have been shared with the person most intimately affected. Patients and their families are concerned about their physical health, and deserve to be given the facts. Explaining and talking through this information provide an opportunity for the therapist to strengthen the quality of the relationship with the patient.

Some patients stop drinking abruptly when persuaded that alcohol is posing a tangible threat to their physical health. One may suspect, however, that even if the news of physical damage constitutes the turning point, in reality this is only the final event to tip a decision for which the moment for change has been set up by many previous happenings. But using the results of the physical examination or the laboratory tests for crude scare tactics is likely to be counter-productive. The patient may dismiss what he is being told simply because the information is too frightening to be accepted, or he may decide that all is lost and that he may as well drink himself to death.

Causes of physical complications

Heavy alcohol consumption causes physical damage by many direct and indirect effects on the body. Alcohol is a source of calories and therefore displaces normal nutrients, causing malnutrition, in particular deficiencies of folate, thiamine and other vitamins. Pancreatic insufficiency and impaired hepatic metabolism cause malabsorption and secondary malnutrition. Alcohol and its metabolite acetaldehyde are toxic substances which have the potential to cause tissue damage. Cytochrome P450, the key enzyme in the microsomal ethanol-oxidizing system (MEOS), produces a toxic variety of active oxygen which can cause liver damage (Lieber, 1995). In some conditions, both the toxic element and disturbance of nutritional status may be implicated as a cause of damage at the same time. Less is known about the differential risks associated with beverage type, although it has been suggested that the risk of developing certain physical disorders is higher for spirit drinkers (Chou et al., 1998).

What level of alcohol intake constitutes a threshold for physical dangers? The answer must vary according to the particular condition, but in general the evidence points to the probability that risk for many varieties of damage increases in proportion to alcohol intake, even within the ranges of what passes as 'social drinking'. The pattern of drinking is also important. Heavy drinking with frequent intoxication is associated with an increased likelihood of developing alcohol-related medical disorders, such as chronic gastritis, gastrointestinal bleeding, pancreatitis and polyneuropathy (Wetterling et al., 1999). A pattern of heavy weekend or binge drinking, even an amount equivalent to an average of two or three drinks a day, carries risks for physical health. Binge drinkers may be at higher risk of injuries and brain trauma. Paradoxically, light or moderate drinking of one or two drinks per day is likely to reduce the risk of coronary heart disease (CHD) in some populations (see page 159). As we have argued earlier, the issue of level of consumption and risk of physical harm is complex and does not allow for an easy calculation of a 'safe' level.

However, whatever the risks at the relatively lower ranges of intake, by the time someone is drinking in the fashion dictated by the dependence syndrome, the question of whether their level of intake carries dangers hardly needs to be asked. The answer is resoundingly 'yes' for nearly every tissue of the body. Quite apart from any specific tissue damage discussed in this chapter, it should also be remembered that, as a consequence of heavy drinking and dietary neglect, almost every aspect of the body's chemistry may in some circumstances be put out of balance; even such seemingly obscure aspects as serum zinc or magnesium levels may be disturbed.

In the ensuing sections of this chapter, a range of physical complications which can result from excessive drinking is described. This list is comprehensive, but does not claim to be exhaustive. As far as possible, technical language is explained, but, as noted in the Introduction (page xiv), this is a chapter with which the non-medical reader will have to show some forbearance. Box 10.1 lists physical conditions for which particular alertness is appropriate as to the possibility of an underlying drinking problem. However, it must be stressed that basic enquiry into the patient's drinking history should be absolutely routine in medical practice.

BOX 10.1 **Patients presenting to the GP or general hospital with the following should be assessed for an alcohol problem**
- Hepatitis/cirrhosis
- Hypertension
- Stroke
- Cardiac arrhythmias/atrial fibrillation
- Cardiomyopathy
- Pneumonia and tuberculosis
- Myopathy
- Osteoporosis
- Seizures
- Wernicke–Korsakoff syndrome
- Accidents
- Resistant psoriasis and eczema
- Anaemia/raised mean corpuscular volume (MCV)

All patients, whatever their presentation, should, on first contact with medical services, be asked about their drinking.

Acute alcohol intoxication and coma

A life-threatening overdose with alcohol is unlikely to occur with the alcohol dependent person, because of both their experience with handling their drinking and their raised tolerance; that is not to deny the possibility of such a patient at times getting very drunk or drinking to unconsciousness. Drinking to the point of collapse and 'passing out' is more likely to be the result of a casual drinking spree, or a Saturday night celebration, and it is this type of patient who is the familiar late-night visitor to the hospital's casualty department. The tablets which are taken with suicidal intention are sometimes washed down with a quantity of alcohol and a mixed sedative/alcohol overdose then results. Occasionally, a child will overdose accidentally with alcohol, and this is discussed in relation to hypoglycaemia (see page 160).

Intoxication can usually be dealt with on a sensibly conservative basis and patients left to sleep off their binge, with due care being taken to ensure that they do not inhale their vomit; examination must, of course, also ensure that there is no other cause for the unconsciousness. A stomach wash-out may sometimes be indicated. However, with a higher level of intoxication there is a risk of respiratory depression and death. The blood alcohol concentration (BAC) likely to be associated with such a tragedy varies with the individual, but a BAC of 400 mg per 100 ml is usually quoted as the threshold for very serious danger (Peters, 1996). Because of the occasional risk of death from respiratory paralysis, the more common danger from inhaled vomit and the many possibilities of being unwarily caught out by some underlying or complicating condition (head injury, hypoglycaemia, ketoacidosis, systemic infection, overdose of other licit or illicit drugs, for example), the problem set by alcoholic overdose and by the often rather unwelcome visitor to the emergency room should not be too casually dismissed as 'routine'. When coma is thought to be caused by alcohol, it is important that a high alcohol concentration is shown by measurements of breath or blood alcohol. Skull radiography and urine toxicology are other fundamental investigations (Quaghebeur and Richards, 1989). Alcoholic coma has a mortality rate of approximately 5%.

Acute poisoning with methyl alcohol (methanol) is both a rarer and a much more threatening condition than intoxication with ordinary beverage alcohol (ethanol). There are substantial risks of blindness or death and intensive emergency medical care will be required, possibly with dialysis.

Gastroenterological disorders

Alcoholic liver disease

Alcohol misuse is the commonest cause of liver damage in the UK, Europe, the USA and Australia. Rates vary enormously from country to country, but appear to be highest in the wine-growing countries where alcohol consumption is highest. Many studies suggest that women are at greater risk than men for a given level of alcohol consumption (see page 33).

The liver is vulnerable to alcohol-related injury because it is the primary site of alcohol metabolism. Three types of alcoholic liver disease have been described: fatty liver, alcoholic hepatitis and alcoholic cirrhosis. All three may co-exist. Fatty liver is present in up to 90% of persistent heavy drinkers at some time. Alcoholic hepatitis is seen in approximately 40% of individuals with a history of persistent heavy drinking. Between 8% and 30% of heavy drinkers will develop alcoholic cirrhosis, typically after a 10–20-year history of daily heavy drinking. However, not all heavy drinkers develop severe liver disease; some individuals appear to be more susceptible (see page 33). For instance, genetic factors that increase the oxidation of alcohol or reduce the rate of acetaldehyde clearance will increase acetaldehyde levels in the liver and cause greater injury. Women develop cirrhosis at lower levels of alcohol consumption than men. In women, a reduced 'first pass' metabolism of alcohol in the stomach, by gastric alcohol dehydrogenase (ADH), leads to increased blood alcohol levels. This further exacerbates the higher blood alcohol levels in women compared with men, due to their lower body water content and weight.

Environmental factors such as hepatitis B and C may contribute to the development of alcoholic liver disease. Alcohol dependent individuals with hepatitis C infection develop liver injury at a younger age and at a lower cumulative dose of alcohol than those without hepatitis C (Maher, 1997). Continuing heavy alcohol consumption is associated with accelerated progression of liver disease associated with cirrhosis and a higher risk of hepatocellular carcinoma in patients with hepatitis B and C (Sherman and Williams, 1994; James, 1996). Cigarette smoking and coffee consumption also appear to increase the risk of developing cirrhosis in alcohol dependent individuals, although the reasons for this are not known (Maher, 1997). Smoking more than 20 cigarettes per day and drinking four or more cups of coffee per day are associated with a greater risk (Klatsky and Armstrong, 1992). The main features of alcoholic liver disease are summarized in Box 10.2.

BOX 10.2 **Alcohol and the liver**
- Fatty liver rarely causes illness and is reversible with abstinence
- Alcoholic hepatitis may be fatal but can be reversible with abstinence
- Alcoholic cirrhosis is often progressive and fatal but can stabilize with abstinence
- Abstinence is the single most important component of treatment for alcoholic liver disease

---

Fatty liver

The first histological change seen in persistent heavy drinkers is deposition of fat. Although this is usually asymptomatic, patients may present with non-specific symptoms such as malaise, tiredness, nausea, an enlarged, tender liver or abnormal liver function tests. Occasionally, very severe fatty liver can lead to jaundice (obstructive jaundice), liver failure, or death due to a fatty embolism (globules of fat getting into the circulation and obstructing arteries to the brain). Fatty liver is reversible with abstinence.

Alcoholic hepatitis

Minor degrees of alcoholic hepatitis may be asymptomatic and clinically indistinguishable from fatty liver. More severe episodes reflect inflammation and destruction of liver tissue. Scar tissue may begin to replace liver tissue. This process is called fibrosis. Symptoms of alcoholic hepatitis include loss of appetite, abdominal pain, nausea, weight loss, jaundice and fever. Severe alcoholic hepatitis has a mortality of about 60% during the first 6 weeks after hospital admission. Corticosteroids, which suppress the inflammation process, may improve survival in the early stages, but abstinence is the best 'treatment', and is essential for long-term survival. Abstinence leads to reversal of the histological changes, but alcoholic hepatitis almost always progresses to cirrhosis in women, even following abstinence.

Alcoholic cirrhosis

Cirrhosis may arise *de novo* in some cases, without passing through the intermediate state of hepatitis. Here, liver tissue becomes scarred by the development of fibrous septa which link the hepatic veins to portal tracts. This scarring, together with the regeneration of liver tissue, disturbs the normal liver architecture, and the consequences are two-fold. Firstly, the actual loss of functioning liver tissue causes a range of metabolic disturbances and ultimately liver failure may occur. Secondly, and very importantly, the scarring and disorganization lead to the squeezing and blocking off of blood vessels. This physical damming causes a build-up of pressure in the portal venus system (the veins which carry blood from the alimentary tract to the liver), called portal hypertension. This can, in turn, cause bleeding from veins at the lower end of the oesophagus (oesophageal varices), and this bleeding can be severe and fatal.

Cirrhosis can exist in degrees. If the condition is not too advanced, abstinence may lead to stabilization and enhance life expectancy. From the patient's point of view, they may know nothing of this insidious condition until they suddenly become jaundiced, find their abdomen swelling up with fluid (ascites), or have a massive bleed. More often, the diagnosis is picked up at an earlier stage on clinical examination and liver toxicity tests, with confirmation coming from various special investigations. Ultrasound scanning is a relatively easy and non-invasive investigation.

Treatment for cirrhosis is largely directed at relieving symptoms and complications (Krige and Beckingham, 2001). Liver transplantation is increasingly being used as a treatment for end-stage alcoholic cirrhosis, and outcomes are as good as for other liver disease (Martinez-Raga and Marshall, 2002). Psychiatric and specialist alcohol assessments have become an important element of the screening process in many transplant centres, because of the risks of anxiety, depression and relapse to drinking in the post-operative period. If drinking is reinstated, it is usually at lower levels than previously.

Patients with alcoholic liver disease may develop Zieve's syndrome, characterized by a combination of cholestasis, haemolysis (breakdown of red cells) and gross hyperlipidaemia (rise in blood fats).

Acute pancreatitis

Alcohol misuse and biliary disease are the two main causative factors in acute pancreatitis. Individuals with acute alcoholic pancreatitis are likely to be young men, drinking in excess of 80 g of alcohol per day. The most common form of presentation is a sudden onset of severe upper abdominal pain, typically penetrating through to the back, associated with vomiting. The pain lessens in severity over the first 72 hours. Patients with severe acute pancreatitis may be feverish, hypotensive, have rapid breathing and suffer with acute ascites, pleural effusions and paralytic ileus (paralysis of the intestines). The diagnosis is usually made from the clinical presentation and confirmed by gross elevations of amylase and lipase in the blood. The mortality rate is between 10% and 40% (Imrie, 1996).

A businessman aged 52 had a long history of alcohol dependence. On occasion he would stop drinking for a few months, but was never willing to consider long-term abstinence as the goal. One weekend he relapsed once more into drinking with a very heavy binge. On the Sunday night he was admitted as an emergency to his local hospital with appalling abdominal pain radiating through to the back. A raised serum amylase confirmed the diagnosis of acute pancreatitis. Despite the hospital's best efforts he died in shock 36 hours later. Post mortem showed extensive necrosis of the pancreas and some old scarring. There was also evidence of early liver cirrhosis.

Chronic pancreatitis

Heavy drinking is the most frequent cause of chronic pancreatitis in adults, particularly with the calcifying form. It mainly affects men aged 40–50 years who have been drinking heavily. Although the quantity and duration of alcohol consumption are related to the development of this condition, it rarely occurs alongside cirrhosis. The main presenting symptom is severe, dull epigastric (abdominal) pain radiating to the back, which may be partly relieved by leaning forward (Bornman and Beckingham, 2001). The pain is often associated with nausea and vomiting. Steatorrhoea (fat in the faeces making them pale, loose and difficult to flush away), diarrhoea and weight loss also occur. These symptoms occur when over 90% of the functioning exocrine tissue (the tissue which secretes digestive enzymes) is destroyed. Damage to the islets of Langerhans, with consequent failure of insulin secretion and diabetes mellitus, occurs more slowly. Treatment is focused on the management of acute attacks of pain and the other complications such as diabetes mellitus and fat malabsorption. Abstinence from alcohol is the mainstay of treatment, and essential if attacks of pain are to be stopped. Severe and intractable pain may lead to opiate dependence (Toskes, 1996).

Gastritis, peptic ulceration and intestinal symptoms

Alcohol stimulates gastric juice secretion and increases mucosal permeability (Seitz and Homann, 2001). It can cause acute erosive ulcers in the stomach. Chronic, heavy alcohol use favours colonization by *Helicobacter pylori*, which produce ammonia and contribute to chronic gastritis. Heavy alcohol consumption is also thought to contribute to the development of gastric or duodenal ulcers.

Patients presenting to alcohol services commonly suffer from intestinal symptoms such as diarrhoea and malabsorption. The general malnutrition and weight loss seen in these patients are usually due to dietary neglect. Alcohol dependent individuals are therefore at risk of vitamin deficiencies (especially of folic acid, B_1/thiamine and B_{12}). Deficiencies of minerals and trace elements (zinc, selenium) are also possible, again as a result of malabsorption and malnutrition.

Mallory–Weiss syndrome

This syndrome occurs as a result of acute alcohol consumption. Acute, intense vomiting leads to a very high pressure within the oesophagus, which in turn causes a longitudinal tear at its lower end, and consequent vomiting of blood (Seitz and Homann, 2001).

Musculoskeletal disorders

Gout

Gout is a constitutional metabolic disorder characterized by episodic painful swelling of peripheral joints, especially the fingers and toes. Individuals with gout have high uric acid levels, and the joint inflammation is produced by the deposition of uric acid in the joints. Most gout occurs in middle-aged men, who often have a family history of the disorder and drink heavily. Beer is particularly liable to produce hyperuricacidaemia, because of its high purine content (Scott, 1989). Other conditions predisposing to gout include obesity, hyperlipidaemia and hypertension, all of which are independently associated with heavy drinking. Heavy drinking can bring out a latent tendency towards gout or make established gout worse.

Bone disorders

Individuals misusing alcohol have increased rates of osteoporosis (reduction in the amount of bone per unit volume without a change in its composition), osteopenia, an increased frequency of fractures and avascular necrosis (Diamond et al., 1989; Preedy et al., 2001). Do these bone changes occur as a direct result of heavy alcohol use or can they be explained by other disorders associated with heavy drinking such as nutritional impairment (calcium and vitamin D deficiencies), pancreatic or liver disease or endocrine dysfunction? The evidence suggests that alcohol-induced bone disorders occur independently of nutritional status. There may, however, be a link between liver dysfunction and bone disorders, but liver disease is no more common in alcohol dependent individuals with osteoporosis than in their counterparts without osteoporosis (Spencer et al., 1986).

The reduced bone density in alcohol dependence is thought to arise as a result of impaired bone formation (reduced osteoblastic function) and increased bone resorption (increased numbers of osteoclasts). These effects of alcohol on bone metabolism appear to be reversible with abstinence. Heavy drinkers are therefore at risk of fractures, even after minimal trauma. Symptoms of back pain indicative of osteoporosis and possible vertebral collapse should not be overlooked, particularly as these patients are also likely to develop dependence on opiate-based analgesics. Post-menopausal women may be particularly susceptible to the effects of alcohol on bone.

Skeletal muscle myopathy

Acute myopathy, produced by alcohol poisoning, is a condition occurring in less than 5% of alcohol misusers (Preedy et al., 2001). It is characterized by severe pain, tenderness, swelling and weakness of the skeletal muscles. In its severe form, acute rhabdomyolysis is associated with myoglobinuria, renal damage and hyperkalaemia (raised potassium levels). Alcohol consumption reduces the normal metabolic responses of skeletal muscle to the action of insulin by causing an acute insulin resistance (Xu et al., 1996).

Chronic alcoholic myopathy occurs in up to 60% of individuals with long-standing alcohol problems and is easily overlooked or misattributed to poor nutrition (Preedy et al., 2001). As is the case with alcoholic liver disease and brain damage, women are more susceptible than men. Individuals typically present with proximal muscle weakness, pain and abnormal gait, and show evidence of atrophy and loss of muscle fibre in the shoulder and pelvic girdle region. Histology reveals a reduction in the diameters of white (fast-twitch) fibres. The weakness and atrophy tend to improve with abstinence or a substantial reduction in consumption (Urbano-Marquez et al., 1995).

Here is a case abstract which illustrates a fairly typical picture.

A 45-year-old storekeeper who was severely alcohol dependent came along to complain that he had developed 'terrible rheumatics'. There was severe pain and some tenderness and swelling of both upper arms and he could no longer lift his stock down from the shelves. It took about 2 months for him to make a reasonable recovery.

Endocrine disorders

Alcohol-induced pseudo-Cushing's syndrome

Alcohol-induced pseudo-Cushing's syndrome is a term used to describe heavy drinkers who present with a clinical picture similar to that seen in Cushing's syndrome, i.e. truncal obesity with thin extremities, plethoric appearance, 'moon face', bruising, striae, muscle wasting and hypertension (Jeffcoate, 1993). Biochemical abnormalities include elevated urinary and plasma cortisol levels (the latter failing to suppress with dexamethasone) and reduced circadian rhythm of plasma cortisol, and normal or suppressed adrenocorticotrophic hormone (ACTH). The biochemical abnormalities rapidly revert to normal with abstinence from alcohol. The mechanism of this disorder is poorly understood.

Male hypogonadism

Alcohol causes a lowering of plasma testosterone concentrations through a direct toxic effect on the Leydig cells in the testis, where testosterone is synthesized. This effect occurs independently of liver disease and may be related to the total lifetime dose of alcohol consumed.

Cancers

Heavy alcohol consumption is associated with an increased risk for cancers of the oropharynx, larynx, oesophagus (gullet) and liver in men, and possibly with breast cancer in women (Smith-Warner et al., 1998). Most studies show a dose–response relationship. Because heavy drinkers are also heavy smokers, it has been difficult to separate the relative contribution of either alcohol or tobacco in the genesis of certain cancers. Alcohol is not thought to increase the risk of cancers of the stomach, pancreas or lung. However, its role in colorectal cancer is equivocal.

The risk for cancer of the oropharynx is related to the number of drinks consumed per day, even after adjustment for smoking. For cancers of the larynx, the effect of alcohol consumption is exacerbated by smoking (Tuyns, 1991). Alcohol misuse is an important co-factor in the development of primary liver cancer, and liver cancer may arise consequent to alcoholic cirrhosis.

Cardiovascular disease

Alcohol-related arrhythmias

Arrhythmias (disturbances of the normal heart rhythm) may occur as a result of acute alcohol intoxication, or during withdrawal. Binge drinking may be particularly implicated, increasing the risk of arrhythmias whether or not CHD is present. This is commonly called 'holiday heart' because of its association with binge drinking at weekends and holidays (Ettinger et al., 1978). The mildest presentation is that of palpitations, caused by a few extra and irregular beats (extrasystoles). Atrial fibrillation (irregular twitching of the atrial muscle) is the most common arrhythmia associated with alcohol use (Koskinen and Kupari, 1992). It occurs as a result of both binge drinking and heavy consistent alcohol use and resolves with abstinence. Ventricular arrhythmias have also been reported.

Several studies have now documented an association between alcohol use and sudden coronary death in both heavy drinkers and occasional drinkers. It is possible that some of the occasional drinkers were binge drinkers with an increased risk of cardiac arrhythmias leading to sudden death (Puddey et al., 1999).

Hypertension

Over the past 20 years, epidemiological data from cross-sectional, prospective cohort and intervention studies have suggested an association between alcohol consumption and blood pressure (Saunders, 1987; Kaplan, 1995). Chronic excessive alcohol consumption is associated with hypertension (increased blood pressure) in both men and women, independent of age, body weight and cigarette smoking, and is thought to be the second most important non-genetic risk factor for hypertension. Binge drinking may be particularly implicated. Approximately 7–11% of hypertension in men can be attributed to alcohol consumption of over 40 g per day. The figure is nearer 1% in women, because of their lower consumption. Intervention studies indicate that persistent heavy drinkers who cut down on their alcohol consumption, or who abstain, lower their blood pressures. Individuals presenting with hypertension to a general practitioner or physician should always have an alcohol history taken, together with appropriate laboratory investigations, and should be advised to reduce their alcohol consumption.

Cerebral vascular disease or stroke

There are two broad categories of stroke – ischaemic and haemorrhagic. In ischaemic stroke, blockage of brain blood vessels by clot formation or emboli causes cerebral infarction. Haemorrhagic stroke is due to either intracranial haemorrhage or subarachnoid haemorrhage. Alcohol may interact with a variety of risk factors for stroke, including hypertension, cigarette smoking, diabetes and obesity. However, there appears to be an independent, dose-dependent relationship between heavy drinking and the risk of haemorrhagic stroke (Corrao et al., 1999; Mazzaglia et al., 2001). Binge drinkers also have an increased risk of haemorrhagic stroke. The evidence linking heavy drinking and ischaemic stroke is more inconsistent, and it may be that hypertension acts as a mediating risk factor. Light to moderate drinking appears not to confer any protective effect.

Coronary heart disease

There is now strong evidence to suggest that light to moderate alcohol consumption is associated with a lower risk of CHD (Rimm et al., 1991, 1997; Thun et al., 1997; Wannamethee and Shaper, 1997). This 'protective' effect is present in men over 40 and in post-menopausal women. The reduced risk for CHD occurs at alcohol consumption levels of as little as 10 g per day and remains similar up to about 30–40 g per day (beyond about 20–30 g for men and 15–20 g for women, advantages for the heart will be outweighed by other risks). Individuals drinking over this level have an increased incidence of CHD which is dose related (Edwards et al., 1994; McElduff and Dobson, 1997) and a binge-drinking pattern seems to be particularly implicated.

The 'cardioprotective' effect appears to derive from ethanol itself, rather than from any specific beverage type, and the underlying mechanisms are not fully understood. Alcohol may have a partial inhibitory effect on atherosclerosis by increasing levels of high-density lipoproteins (HDLs), which carry cholesterol to different parts of the body. HDLs are associated with a reduced risk of CHD and are thought to protect the arteries from a build-up of cholesterol. Alcohol also reduces platelet stickiness and aggregation, lowers plasma fibrinogen and increases fibrinolysis. A recent meta-analysis concluded that an alcohol intake of 30 g per day would cause an estimated reduction of 24.7% in risk of CHD and that this lower risk was mediated via changes in concentrations of HDLs, fibrinogen and triclycerides (Rimm et al., 1997).

Alcoholic cardiomyopathy (alcohol-induced heart muscle disease)

Chronic, excessive alcohol consumption is associated with dilated cardiomyopathy (Rubin and Urbano-Marquez, 1994). This appears to occur as a result of the toxic action of alcohol on heart muscle. A genetic predisposition may also be an important factor. Previously, alcoholic cardiomyopathy was attributed to thiamine deficiency, but this is probably not the case because it occurs in heavy drinkers who are well nourished. The disorder usually manifests itself between the ages of 30 and 60 years. Although commoner in men, due to their heavier consumption, women seem to be particularly vulnerable (Urbano-Marquez et al., 1995).

Alcoholic cardiomyopathy is characterized by an enlarged, hypertrophied heart. The left ventricle is dilated and there is dysfunction in cardiac contractility, leading to a depressed output (ejection fraction). In the early stages of hypertrophy and dilatation, there may be few symptoms. However, as the disorder progresses, patients develop arrhythmias, including atrial and ventricular tachyarrhythmias and atrioventricular conduction defects. Congestive cardiac failure is another typical form of presentation (breathlessness on exertion, breathlessness at night and peripheral oedema).

Subclinical forms of alcoholic cardiomyopathy are evident in problem drinkers, using non-invasive procedures such as echocardiography. Early detection and abstinence may arrest or reverse the progress of this disorder.

Respiratory disease

Heavy alcohol consumption is associated with defects in the body's immune responses and clinically this is reflected in an excess of lower respiratory tract infections with *Streptococcus pneumoniae*, *Mycobacterium tuberculosis* and *Klebsiella pneumoniae*. Self-neglect and the associated way of life, particularly in the Skid Row drinkers, are also important factors predisposing to infections. Because heavy drinkers may both vomit and become stuporose, they are prone to inhale material into their lungs and hence develop lung abscesses or bronchietasis (dilatation and infection of the smaller bronchi).

Many problem drinkers also smoke heavily. A carcinoma of the lung is not, therefore, an uncommon coincidental finding, sometimes confusing the diagnostic picture. What is thought to be an alcoholic 'dementia' turns out, for instance, to be a secondary cancer of the brain or a severe 'alcoholic' peripheral neuropathy is found out to be a cancer-related (carcinomatous) neuropathy. The simple message is that if a problem drinker presents for an assessment and has not had a recent chest x-ray, such an examination should be arranged.

Metabolic disorders

Hypoglycaemia

Alcohol-induced hypoglycaemia (lowering of the blood sugar) can occur as a result of alcohol intoxication or after a modest intake of alcohol in individuals who are malnourished or fasting (Turner, 1996). Clinically the patient may present as flushed and sweaty with a rapid pulse and the appearance of being 'drunk' and inco-ordinated. An alternative presentation is in coma and hypothermic, without obvious features of hypoglycaemia. Children and adolescents are particularly susceptible to alcohol-induced hypoglycaemia and the condition for them is much more dangerous than in the adult (Lamminpaa, 1995).

Alcoholic ketoacidosis

This is a rare condition and usually arises after an episode of heavy drinking which has been followed by cessation of eating or vomiting. Thus the patient can present drowsy and collapsed, and have a blood alcohol level of zero. Typically, the patient presents with a metabolic acidosis which responds to rehydration and glucose. A metabolic alkalosis may also be evident if there has been vomiting.

Hyperlipidaemia

Heavy drinking is associated with a rise in circulatory blood fats (serum triglycerides). This will only be picked up by laboratory tests, but probably carries implications for enhanced risk of arteriosclerosis.

Haematological effects

Problem drinking gives rise to anaemia, macrocytosis, simple iron deficiency, neutropenia and thrombocytopenia (Weatherall, 1996).

Anaemia

Anaemia is common in problem drinkers and can be caused by a variety of factors, including malnutrition, chronic blood loss, liver disease, malabsorption, chronic infections and the direct toxic effect of alcohol on the bone marrow.

Macrocytosis

Macrocytosis (enlarged red blood cells) is also common in problem drinkers, and an unexplained macrocytosis should always alert clinicians to the possibility of an alcohol problem. If nutrition is adequate, it is probably caused by the direct toxic action of alcohol on the bone marrow. Folate deficiency in malnourished problem drinkers can give rise to a megaloblastic anaemia. However, alcohol may interfere directly with folate metabolism.

Iron deficiency

Iron deficiency among heavy drinkers will probably reflect a poor diet or chronic blood loss due to gastritis or bleeding varices. It may be associated with folate deficiency.

Neutropaenia and thrombocytopaenia

Heavy drinking may cause a neutropaenia (lowering of white cells), either by a toxic effect on the bone marrow or as a result of folate deficiency, and thereby render patients susceptible to infections. Alcohol may also interfere with neutrophil locomotion. Thrombocytopaenia (decrease in platelets) is frequent in heavy drinkers and can account for a susceptibility to bruising. The platelet count usually returns to normal with abstinence.

Neurological disorders

The mechanisms underlying alcohol-related brain damage are complex. Poor nutrition and diminished vitamin reserves predispose to thiamine and nicotinic acid depletion. Alcohol is neurotoxic and acetaldehyde, its main metabolite, may have a similar action. Metabolic factors resulting from acute and chronic intoxication and withdrawal, such as hypoxia, electrolyte imbalance and hypoglycaemia, are also important, as are alcohol withdrawal seizures, hepatic encephalopathy, subarachnoid haemorrhage, haemorrhagic stroke and head injury.

Alcohol withdrawal seizures

Alcohol withdrawal seizures occur in about 5–15% of alcohol dependent individuals, approximately 7–48 hours after cessation of drinking (Brennan and Lyttle, 1987). The seizures are generalized, tonic–clonic (grand mal) and are thus associated with a loss of consciousness, followed by convulsive movements in all four limbs. During a particular withdrawal episode the patient may have only one seizure, but more commonly there will be three or four seizures over a couple of days. Very rarely, status epilepticus will supervene. This is a continuous run of seizures, one merging into another, which is associated with risk to life. Alcohol withdrawal seizures have sometimes been termed 'rum fits', but they are not associated with any one type of beverage.

Predisposing factors to alcohol withdrawal seizures include hypokalaemia, hypomagnesaemia, a previous history of withdrawal seizures and concurrent epilepsy. The EEG is generally unhelpful but a brain scan will help to rule out intracranial lesions (Earnest et al., 1988).

Alcohol dependent individuals who have experienced seizures due to alcohol withdrawal may be more prone to developing further seizures in future withdrawal episodes. Any proposed detoxification for this group should therefore be carried out in an in-patient setting. Patients at risk of alcohol withdrawal seizures should be advised not to stop drinking suddenly, but to continue at the same level of consumption until admission, or to institute an extremely slow reduction.

Tragedies have sometimes occurred when a severely dependent patient has stopped drinking on his or her own initiative and sustained a withdrawal seizure which has led to an accident. For example, the driver of a heavy goods vehicle had, after a long period of sobriety, relapsed into dependent drinking, but after 2–3 months he determined abruptly to put a stop to his drinking. He had a seizure, his truck went out of control and mounted a pavement and killed a woman who was standing by a bus stop. There are thus a number of reasons for taking withdrawal seizures and the risks of such seizures very seriously.

Seizures of other origin

A number of other possible reasons for seizures in patients with drinking problems must be borne in mind, as well as the fact that seizures may be entirely coincidental. Heavy drinking may, for example, lower the threshold in a person with an underlying epileptic tendency of any origin. An epileptic patient who is being treated with anti-convulsants may simply forget to take his tablets when he goes on a drinking binge. Heavy drinking can, as a result of liver enzyme induction, lead to increased metabolic clearance of such medication.

Heavy drinkers are often heavy cigarette smokers and a seizure may on occasion be the first and tragic signal of the secondary spread to the brain (metastases) from a carcinoma of the lung (see page 160). Problem drinkers are prone to accidents and a seizure may be symptomatic of an old or more recent head injury. Alcoholic 'dementia' may sometimes be accompanied by seizures. A rather common cause of seizures is coincidental withdrawal of sedative or hypnotic drugs, particularly chlormethiazole. Rarer causes include alcohol-related hypoglycaemia (lowered blood sugar, see page 160) and fatty emboli lodging in the brain (see page 153).

Peripheral neuropathy

Alcoholic peripheral neuropathy is a sensorimotor neuropathy detectable to some degree among approximately 10% of chronic heavy drinkers. The main aetiological factors are thought to be vitamin B deficiency and the toxic effect of alcohol. The lower limbs are more frequently affected than the upper limbs and the typical presentation is with an insidious onset of weakness, pain, paraesthesiae and numbness in the feet, which progresses proximally and symmetrically in a 'glove and stocking' distribution. Bilateral foot drop and weakness of the small hand muscles and finger extensors may occur. Distal reflexes are usually absent. Treatment includes B group vitamins and abstinence. Recovery is usually slow and incomplete, with residual sensory loss.

Alcoholic cerebellar degeneration

The cerebellum is a part of the brain concerned with balance and motor integration, and it is sometimes the focus for alcohol-related brain damage (Charness, 1993). Alcoholic cerebellar degeneration usually develops insidiously and is characterized by ataxia of gait and inco-ordination of the legs. It is thought to be due to thiamine deficiency, but alcohol neurotoxicity may also be an important factor. Abstinence and treatment with thiamine (vitamin B_1) may halt the progress of the disorder, but the patient may still be left with a disabling condition.

Central pontine myelinolysis

This is a rare disorder of cerebral white matter in the brain stem, which is usually seen in alcohol dependent individuals, but can also occur in malignancy, non-alcoholic liver disease, chronic renal disease, rapid correction of hyponatraemia, hypokalaemia and other debilitating diseases (Charness, 1993). Clinical features include a pseudobulbar palsy and spastic or flaccid quadraplegia which evolves over a few days or weeks, often resulting in coma or death. Lesions can be visualized on magnetic resonance imaging (MRI) but not on computerized tomography (CT) scans. Post-mortem examination reveals demyelination of the pons.

Marchiafava–Bignami disease

This rare disorder of the corpus callosum and adjacent white matter is not confined to problem drinkers (Charness, 1993). A nutritional deficiency or a contaminant of alcohol has been postulated as the cause. Presentation can either be acute with agitation, apathy, hallucinations, epilepsy and coma, or insidious with dementia, spasticity, dysarthria and inability to walk. Lesions can be visualized on scanning, but the diagnosis is usually made only at post mortem.

Alcohol amblyopia

This uncommon condition presents as a gradual bilateral blurring of vision in association with alcohol misuse. It can be accompanied by difficulty in distinguishing red from green. Most patients are also smokers. Testing reveals a central blind spot (scotoma), with the peripheral field of vision intact. The most likely cause is a deficiency of both thiamine and vitamin B_{12}. It responds to treatment with thiamine and B-complex vitamins. The same picture sometimes occurs as 'tobacco amblyopia'.

Hepatic encephalopathy

In heavy drinkers with alcoholic liver disease, the predominant clinical picture can be that of hepatic encephalopathy. This is a chronic, organic reaction with psychiatric and neurological abnormalities which come and go and are extremely variable. The typical features include impaired consciousness (ranging from hypersomnia to coma), delirium, impaired recent memory, mood swings, a flapping tremor, muscular inco-ordination, foetor hepaticus (a characteristic smell on the breath), upgoing plantar responses, and hypoactive or hyperactive reflexes (Krige and Beckingham, 2001). Liver function tests are usually abnormal and the electroencephalogram (EEG) shows a typical picture which can be extremely helpful in diagnosis. Hepatic encephalopathy is a sign of deteriorating liver function. It can be precipitated by alcohol withdrawal and benzodiazepine use.

Foetal alcohol syndrome

That the mother's drinking can cause foetal damage was widely believed in the nineteenth century, but was later to be forgotten or dismissed as temperance scare-mongering. It is only over the last three decades or so that firm evidence has accumulated for the reality of the danger, and even so there are questions remaining as to the level of maternal drinking which carries risk (see page 176). The distinctive syndrome is much more widely prevalent in the USA than in the UK, and it is unclear whether this reflects differing levels of awareness or a real difference in occurrence rate. Estimates even within the USA do, however, vary and the prevalence of foetal alcohol syndrome (FAS) has been put as low as 0.33 cases per 1000 live births (Abel and Sokol 1991), or as high as 1.7–5.9 (Phillips et al., 1989). Rates of FAS vary with ethnicity, socio-economic and medical status. Nutrition, licit and illicit drug use and smoking all contribute to variability in studies.

The fully developed picture of FAS includes (i) pre-natal and post-natal growth retardation; (ii) craniofacial abnormalities of the face and head (a small head, shortened eyelids, underdeveloped upper lip and flattened wide nose); and (iii) central nervous system dysfunction. Associated abnormalities include limb deformities and congenital heart disease. As they grow up, these children remain small for their age and often have significant cognitive impairment. Cognitive deficits, together with concentration, attention and behavioural problems, may handicap education or employment.

Alcohol-related birth defects which do not meet criteria for FAS are referred to as a foetal alcohol effect (FAE). Women who drink heavily during pregnancy also have increased rates of complications of pregnancy and delivery, of spontaneous abortion and stillbirth. The greatest risk to the foetus from the mother's drinking is probably within the first 12 weeks of pregnancy.

The crucial public health question relates to what is meant by 'heavy drinking' in this context. It is not known what levels of pre-natal alcohol exposure produce what intensity of developmental problems. However, there is no doubt that a woman who is drinking at a level which implies she has developed alcohol dependence is at risk of damaging her baby. For any alcohol treatment service, the practical message must be that a woman of child-bearing age who has a serious drinking problem requires very special counselling, and should be discouraged from having a baby until the drinking has been dealt with successfully. One has to think not only of the potential damage to an unborn child, but also of the lifetime guilt of the mother should a deformed child be born.

What is the safe upper limit of drinking for a pregnant woman or a woman intending to have a child? Women who are trying to conceive or who are pregnant should be advised to drink no more than one to two standard drinks (8–16 g) once or twice a week. Low levels of alcohol consumption during pregnancy are not associated with harm to the foetus. Binge drinking should be avoided completely.

Skin disease

Heavy drinkers and individuals misusing alcohol are prone to a variety of skin disorders, including psoriasis, discoid eczema and superficial cutaneous fungal infections such as tinea pedis and pityriasis versicolor (Higgins and du Vivier, 1994). Rosacea and acne may be exacerbated by alcohol.

Psoriasis is an alcohol-related skin condition which deserves special note. The daily alcohol consumption of men with psoriasis is higher than that of men with other skin diseases and heavy drinking appears to be related to the severity of the disease (Poikolainen et al., 1990). In heavy drinkers, psoriasis mainly affects the palms of the hands and the soles of the feet (Higgins and du Vivier, 1994). Alcohol-induced psoriasis responds poorly to treatment unless the patient stops drinking.

The immune system

Chronic excessive alcohol use is associated with suppression of the immune system, leading to high rates of infectious disease in this group (Cook, 1998). Autoimmunity is also triggered by heavy alcohol consumption, contributing to organ damage such as alcoholic liver disease and skin disorders.

Heavy drinkers are at particular risk of respiratory infections and pneumonia, including tuberculosis (TB, see page 160). They are also vulnerable to septicaemia, which can develop from pneumonia, urinary tract infections, bacterial peritonitis and biliary infections. TB has long been the scourge of the chronic heavy drinker. The combination of alcohol dependence and HIV disease puts individuals at particular risk for TB. Unfortunately, there has been a rise in drug-resistant strains of *Mycobacterium tuberculosis* which further compromises immune-deficient populations. Further work needs to be done to elucidate the interaction between alcohol use and HIV disease.

There is some evidence that alcohol dependence predisposes individuals in some way to develop hepatitis C infection, the increased incidence being in the order of 10%. This might reflect an increased susceptibility to hepatitis C in this group or just a lack of knowledge of risk factors.

Although alcohol dependent individuals have increased serum immunoglobulins, they are immunodeficient, because this increase is due to an abnormal regulation of the synthesis of antibodies (Estruch, 2001). They have reduced cell-mediated immunity. Lymphocyte (white cell) numbers are reduced in those with liver disease; although numbers are normal in those without liver disease, alterations in the percentage of various types are seen. B cells are normal or slightly reduced and natural killer cells show reduced functional activity.

Accidents/trauma

Alcohol is an underlying and frequently overlooked risk factor for accidents in the general population, not just in individuals with alcohol problems or alcohol dependence. Ingestion of alcohol causes diminished co-ordination and balance, increased reaction time and impaired attention, perception and judgement, all of which increase accidental injury (Cherpitel, 1993). Road traffic accidents in which alcohol is implicated are more serious than accidents in which it is not, and the risk of being involved in an accident rises as a function of the increased blood alcohol concentration (BAC). Approximately one-third of pedestrians killed in road traffic accidents by day have measurable BACs. Although the literature on alcohol-related accidents has historically focused largely on road traffic accidents and drink driving, accidents in the home, workplace and civil aviation and also leisure accidents such as drownings now receive more prominence. The consumption of more than 60 g of alcohol within a 6-hour period is associated with a significant risk of injury. Alcohol consumption may put women at particular risk for injury because of the greater physiological impact of a given dose of alcohol (McLeod et al., 1999).

Studies from various countries suggest that drinking is involved in 26–54% of home and leisure injuries (Edwards et al., 1994). It is particularly associated with violent family incidents (see page 79) and is implicated in child abuse. Positive blood alcohol levels have been obtained in 40% of fatal industrial accidents and in 35% of non-fatal work-related accidents.

Surgery

Heavy drinking is associated with an increased risk of post-operative complications. This risk is evident in consumption levels of about five drinks ($\geq$ 60 g) per day (Tønnesen, 1999). Complications include prolonged hospital stay, the need for further surgery, infections, cardiopulmonary insufficiency and bleeding. A Danish study has shown that 1 month of pre-operative abstinence (treatment with disulfiram 800 mg twice weekly) reduced post-operative complications in heavy drinkers with colorectal disease (Tønnesen et al., 1999).

It is worth entering a brief general reminder as to the potential importance of the patient's heavy drinking to the work of the anaesthetist both operatively and post-operatively (Payne, 1986). Emergency surgery may, in particular, run into difficulties if intoxication is overlooked and recovery is complicated by a seizure or by other unexpected withdrawal symptoms. Tolerance to alcohol may result in cross-tolerance to certain anaesthetics, notably thiopentone.

The need for two kinds of alertness

This chapter started with the plea that everyone working with problem drinkers should be more aware of the physical element within the assessment and treatment plan. It should similarly be pleaded that everyone who works in the medical field be vigilant as to the possibility of undeclared problem drinking being behind any one of a host of clinical presentations.

REFERENCES

Abel, E.L. and Sokol, R.J. (1991) A revised conservative estimate of the incidence of FAS and its economic impact. *Alcoholism: Clinical and Experimental Research* 15, 514–24.

Bornman, P.C. and Beckingham, I.J. (2001) Chronic pancreatitis. ABC of diseases of liver, pancreas and biliary system. *British Medical Journal* 322, 660–3.

Brennan, F.N. and Lyttle, J.A. (1987) Alcohol and seizures: a review. *Journal of the Royal Society of Medicine* 80, 571–3.

Canning, U.P., Kennell-Webb, S.A., Marshall, E.J., Wessely, S.C. and Peters, T.J. (1999) Substance misuse in acute general medical admissions. *Quarterly Journal of Medicine* 92, 319–26.

Charness, M.E. (1993) Brain lesions in alcoholics. *Alcoholism: Clinical and Experimental Research* 17, 2–11.

Cherpitel, C. (1993) Alcohol and injuries: a review of international emergency room studies. *Addiction* 88, 923–37.

Chick, J. (1994) Alcohol problems in the general hospital. In *Alcohol and Alcohol Problems*, ed. Edwards, G. and Peters, T.J. *British Medical Bulletin* 50, 200–10. London: Churchill Livingstone.

Chou, S.P., Grant, B.F. and Dawson, D.A. (1998) Alcoholic beverage preference and risks of alcohol-related medical consequences: a preliminary report from the National Longitudinal Alcohol Epidemiologic Study. *Alcoholism: Clinical and Experimental Research* 22, 1450–5.

Cook, R.T. (1998) Alcohol abuse, alcoholism, and damage to the immune system – a review. *Alcoholism: Clinical and Experimental Research* 22, 1927–42.

Corrao, G., Bagnardi, V., Zambon, A. and Arico, S. (1999) Exploring the dose–response relationship between alcohol consumption and the risk of several alcohol-related conditions – a meta analysis. *Addiction* 94, 1551–73.

Diamond, T., Stiel, D., Lunzer, M., Wilkinson, M. and Posen, S. (1989) Ethanol reduces bone formation and may cause osteoporosis. *American Journal of Medicine,* 86, 282–8.

Earnest, M.P., Feldman, H., Marx, J.A. et al. (1988) Intracranial lesions shown by CT scans in 259 cases of first alcohol-related seizures. *Neurology* 38, 1561–5.

Edwards, G., Anderson, P., Babor, T.F. et al. (1994) *Alcohol Policy and the Public Good*. Oxford: Oxford University Press.

Estruch, R. (2001) Nutrition and infectious disease. In *International Handbook of Alcohol Dependence and Problems*, ed. Heather, N., Peters, T.J. and Stockwell, T. Chichester: John Wiley and Sons, 185–204.

Ettinger, P.O., Wu, C.F., De La Cruz, C., Weisse, A.B., Ahmed, S.S. and Regan, T.J. (1978) Arrythmias and the 'holiday heart' alcohol-associated cardiac rhythm disorders. *American Heart Journal* 99, 555–62.

Harris, E.C. and Barraclough, B. (1998) Excess mortality of mental disorder. *British Journal of Psychiatry* 173, 11–53.

Higgins, E.M. and du Vivier, A.W.P. (1994) Cutaneous disease and alcohol misuse. In *Alcohol and Alcohol Problems*, ed. Edward, G. and Peters, T.J. *British Medical Bulletin* 50, 85–98. London: Churchill Livingstone.

Imrie, C.W. (1996) Diseases of the pancreas – acute pancreatitis. In *Oxford Textbook of Medicine*, 3rd edn, Vol. 2, ed. Weatherall, D.J., Ledingham, J.G.G. and Warrell, D.A. Oxford: Oxford University Press, 2027–34.

James, O.F.W. (1996) Alcoholic liver disease. In *Oxford Textbook of Medicine*, 3rd edn, Vol. 2, ed. Weatherall, D.J., Ledingham, J.G.G. and Warrell, D.A. Oxford: Oxford University Press, 2080–5.

Jeffcoate, W. (1993) Alcohol-inducted pseudo-Cushing's syndrome. *Lancet* 341, 676–7.

Kaplan, N.M. (1995) Alcohol and hypertension. *Lancet* 345, 1588–9.

Klatsky, A.L. and Armstrong, M.A. (1992) Alcohol, smoking, coffee and cirrhosis. *American Journal of Epidemiology* 136, 1248–57.

Koskinen, P. and Kupari, M. (1992) Alcohol and cardiac arrythmias. *British Medical Journal*, 304, 1394.

Krige, J.E.J. and Beckingham, I.J. (2001) ABC of diseases of liver, pancreas and biliary system. Portal hypertension – 2. Ascites, encephalopathy, and other conditions *British Medical Journal* 322, 416–18.

Lamminpaa, A. (1995) Alcohol intoxication in childhood and adolescence. *Alcohol and Alcoholism* 30, 5–12.

Lieber, C.S. (1995) Medical disorders of alcoholism. *New England Journal of Medicine* 333, 1058–65.

Maher, J.J. (1997) Exploring alcohol's effects on liver function. *Alcohol Health and Research World* 21, 5–12.

Martinez-Raga, J. and Marshall, E.J. (2002) Role of the psychiatrist in the treatment of alcoholic liver disease. In *Ethanol and the Liver: Mechanisms and Management*, ed. Sherman, D., Preedy, V. and Watson, R. London: Taylor and Francis, 568–91.

Mazzaglia, G., Britton, A.R., Altmann, D.R. and Chenet, L. (2001) Exploring the relationship between alcohol consumption and non-fatal or fatal stroke: a systematic review. *Addiction* 96, 1743–56.

McLeod, R., Stockwell, T., Stevens, M. and Phillips, M. (1999) The relationship between alcohol consumption patterns and injury. *Addiction* 94, 1719–34.

McElduff, P. and Dobson, A. (1997) How much alcohol and how often? Population based case-control study of alcohol consumption and risk of a major coronary event. *British Medical Journal* 314, 1159–64.

Payne, J.P. (1986) Anaesthesia and the problem drinker. *Hospital Update* 12, 287–96.

Peters, T.J. (1996) Physical complications of alcohol misuse. In *Oxford Textbook of Medicine*, 3rd edn, ed. Weatherall, D.J., Ledingham, J.G.G., Warrell, D.A. Vol. 3. Oxford: Oxford University Press, 4276–8.

Phillips, D.K., Henderson, G.I. and Schenker, S. (1989) Pathogensis of foetal alcohol syndrome. *Alcohol, Health and Research World* 13, 219–27.

Poikolainen, K., Reunala, T., Karvonen, J., Lauharanta, J. and Karkkainen, P. (1990) Alcohol intake: a risk factor for psoriasis in young and middle aged men? *British Medical Journal* 300, 780–3.

Preedy, V.R., Mantle, D. and Peters, T.J. (2001) Alcoholic muscle, skin and bone disease. In *International Handbook of Alcohol Dependence and Problems,* ed. Heather, N., Peters, T.J. and Stockwell, T. Chichester: John Wiley and Sons, 169–84.

Puddey, I.B., Rakic, V., Dimmitt, S.B. and Beilin, L.J. (1999) Influence of pattern of drinking on cardiovascular disease risk factors – a review. *Addiction* 94, 649–63.

Quaghebeur, G. and Richards, P. (1989) Comatose patients smelling of alcohol. *British Medical Journal* 299, 410.

Rimm, E.B., Giovannuci, E.L., Willett, M.C. et al. (1991) Prospective study of alcohol consumption and risk of coronary heart disease in men. *Lancet,* 338, 464–8.

Rimm, E.B., Williams, P., Fosher, K., Criqui, M. and Stampfer, M.J. (1997) Moderate alcohol intake and lower risks of coronary heart disease: meta-analysis of effects on lipids and haemostatic factors. *British Medical Journal* 319, 1523–8.

Royal College of Physicians (2001) *Alcohol – Can the NHS Afford it?* A Royal College of Physicians Working Party Report. London: Royal College of Physicians.

Rubin, E. and Urbano-Marquez, A. (1994) Alcoholic cardiomyopathy. *Alcoholism: Clinical and Experimental Research* 18, 111–14.

Saunders, J.B. (1987) Alcohol and hypertension. *British Medical Journal* 294, 1045–6.

Scott, J.T. (1989) Alcohol and gout. *British Medical Journal* 298, 1054.

Seitz, H.K. and Homann, V. (2001) Effect of alcohol on the orogastro-intestinal tract, the pancreas and the liver. In *International Handbook of Alcohol Dependence and Problems,* ed. Heather, N., Peters, T.J. and Stockwell, T. Chichester: John Wiley and Sons, 149–68.

Sherman, D.I.N. and Williams, R. (1994) Liver damage: mechanisms and management. In *Alcohol and Alcohol Problems,* ed. Edwards, G. and Peters, T.J. *British Medical Bulletin* 50, 124–38. London: Churchill Livingstone.

Sjögren, H., Eriksson, A. and Ahlm, K. (2000) Role of alcohol in unnatural deaths: a study of all deaths in Sweden. *Alcohol: Clinical and Experimental Research* 24, 1050–6.

Smith-Warner, S.A., Spiegelman, D., Yaun, S-S. et al. (1998) Alcohol and breast cancer in women: a pooled analysis of cohort studies. *Journal of the American Medical Association* 279, 535–40.

Spencer, H., Rubio, N., Rubio, E., Indreika, M. and Seitam, A. (1986) Chronic alcoholism. Frequently overlooked cause of osteoporosis in men. *American Journal of Medicine* 80, 393–7.

Thun, M.J., Peto, R., Lopez, A.D. et al. (1997) Alcohol consumption and mortality among middle-aged and elderly US adults. *New England Journal of Medicine* 337, 1705–14.

Tønnesen, H. (1999) The alcohol patient and surgery. *Alcohol and Alcoholism* 34, 148–52.

Tønnesen, H., Rosenberg, J., Nielsen, H.J. et al. (1999) Effect of preoperative abstinence on poor postoperative outcome in alcohol misusers: randomised controlled trial. *British Medical Journal* 318, 1311–16.

Toskes, P.P. (1996) Diseases of the pancreas: chronic pancreatitis. In *Oxford Textbook of Medicine*, 3rd edn, Vol. 2, ed. Weatherall, D.J., Ledingham, J.G.G. and Warrell, D.A. Oxford: Oxford University Press, 2034–9.

Turner, R.C. (1996) Hypoglycaemia. In *Oxford Textbook of Medicine*, Vol. 2, 3rd edn, ed. Weatherall, D.J., Ledingham, J.G.G. and Warrell, D.A. Oxford: Oxford University Press, 1505–12.

Tuyns, A.J. (1991) Alcohol and cancer. An instructive association. *British Journal of Cancer* 64, 415–16.

Urbano-Marquez, A., Estruch, R., Fernandez-Sola, J., Nicolas, J.M., Pare, J.C. and Rubin, E. (1995) The greater risk of alcoholic cardiomyopathy and myopathy in women compared with men. *Journal of the American Medical Association* 274, 149–54.

Wannamethee, S.G. and Shaper, A.G. (1997) Lifelong teetotallers, ex-drinkers and drinkers: mortality and incidence of coronary heart disease events in middle-aged British men. *International Journal of Epidemiology* 26, 440–2.

Weatherall, D.J. (1996) The blood in systemic disease. In *Oxford Textbook of Medicine*, 3rd edn, ed. Weatherall, D.J., Ledingham, J.G.G. and Warrell, D.A. Vol. 3. Oxford: Oxford University Press, 3676–87.

Wetterling, T., Veltrup, C., Driessen, M. and John, U. (1999) Drinking pattern and alcohol-related medical disorders. *Alcohol and Alcoholism* 34, 330–6.

Xu, D., Dhillon, A.S. and Palmer, T.N. (1996) Metabolic effects of alcohol on skeletal muscle. *Addiction Biology* 1, 143–55.

11

Women with drinking problems

Drinking patterns of women

Women are less likely to drink and to drink heavily than men in most cultures. Those who drink consume alcohol less frequently than men and drink smaller amounts per drinking occasion. Social and cultural factors still exert a powerful influence on the pattern and degree of drinking in women, altering their vulnerability to the development of alcohol problems. Despite social and cultural changes, there is still less social pressure on women to begin drinking and more pressure for them to stop.

However, society is harsh in its judgement of women with drinking problems. They are held in low esteem, are perceived as having deserted the roles of wife and mother and as being vulnerable to sexual promiscuity. Such misperceptions are often mirrored in the attitude of health professionals, who view women with drinking problems in a negative light, as deviant personalities who are particularly untreatable. These attitudes have no place in the treatment setting.

We believe that the role of this chapter is to sensitize as well as inform, and thus to challenge the still too prevalent stereotyping of the woman who has a drinking problem. As for structure, we firstly provide a note on basic epidemiological findings. In the following section a range of factors that can be correlated with drinking problems among women is identified and risk factors across the life course are discussed. Attention is then given, in turn, to physical complications, psychosocial co-morbidity and social complications. The treatment inferences emerging from this factual background are considered. Mention has been made in Chapters 3 and 10 of physiological factors that may predispose women to alcohol-related tissue vulnerability (see pages 33 and 152).

Epidemiology of alcohol problems in women

The five-site Epidemiologic Catchment Area (ECA) study in the USA reported a 4.6% lifetime prevalence of DSM-III alcohol abuse or dependence in women (Helzer et al., 1991). The corresponding figure for men was 23.8%, and rates were highest in the 18–29-year and 30–44-year age groups for both sexes. In Great Britain, the Office for National Statistics (2000) estimates that 15% of adult women drink more than the recommended 'sensible' level of 14 units per week, of whom 2% are drinking very heavily, i.e. more than 36 units per week. There is evidence of a modest decline in drinking amongst women in the USA throughout the 1980s: although the overall drinking rate has changed little, the proportion of heavy drinkers has decreased, and there has been a reduction in heavy episodic drinking.

Correlates of women with alcohol problems – a heterogeneous group

Women with alcohol problems are a heterogeneous population. Drinking behaviour in women is influenced by a number of demographic factors such as age, marital status, employment status and ethnicity (Plant, 1997). These factors interact with other risk factors such as genetic predisposition (Kendler et al., 1995; Prescott et al., 1997), psychological and socio-cultural factors to determine the onset and course of drinking problems (Wilsnack et al., 1994). Risk factors are summarized in Box 11.1.

BOX 11.1 Some risk factors for problem drinking in women

- Positive family history
- Childhood problem behaviours related to impulse control
- Early use of nicotine, alcohol and other drugs
- Poor coping responses in the face of stressful life events
- Depression
- Divorced/separated/cohabiting
- Heavy drinking partner
- Working in a male-dominated environment
- Sexual dysfunction

Age

Younger women have higher rates of heavy drinking and drinking problems than older women.

Marital status

Being single, divorced, separated or co-habiting is associated with heavy drinking (Wilsnack et al., 1994). Divorce appears to put women without a drinking problem at greater risk for increased drinking, but it may also provide a 'remedy' for women with established drinking problems, who appear to reduce their alcohol consumption following divorce (Wilsnack et al., 1994). Co-habitation is strongly associated with problem drinking.

Employment

Contrary to expectation, there appears to be little relationship between full-time employment and alcohol problems in women (Wilsnack et al., 1994). Multiple roles (family, marriage, employment) appear to have a beneficial effect on women, reducing their risk for problem drinking. However, women working in male-dominated environments are more likely to drink heavily and to have drinking problems. Peer influence, increased drinking opportunities and the stress of working in a male-dominated culture have been invoked as reasons for this (Wilsnack and Wilsnack, 1993).

Race and ethnicity

In the USA white women are most likely to drink, African-American women the least likely and Hispanic women are intermediate. Little is known about the cultural and ethnic differences in drinking amongst women in the UK.

Drinking partner

Women appear to be more influenced by the drinking habits of their male partners than *vice versa* (Wilsnack and Wilsnack, 1995).

Childhood sexual abuse and relationship violence

Women with drinking problems have higher rates of childhood sexual abuse and are more likely than other women to have experienced physical violence, as either children or adults (Winfield et al., 1990). Sexual abuse in childhood is strongly associated with the development of alcohol problems/dependence in adulthood (Breslau et al., 1997: Spak et al., 1997; Wilsnack et al., 1997). However, further scrutiny of the backgrounds of such women usually indicates that other factors are also involved, including having a cold and uncaring mother, having an alcoholic partner and a belief that alcohol is a sexual disinhibitor (Fleming et al., 1998). Women are often in violent relationships with men when they enter treatment. Distressing and vivid memories of childhood sexual abuse and rape may resurface during abstinence.

Sexual experience

Sexual dysfunction may contribute to the chronicity of excessive drinking in women. Problem drinking amongst women may be associated with risky sexual behaviour, putting them at high risk for HIV/AIDS. This is particularly true of women with multiple substance use, who may share injecting equipment with their partners and engage in unprotected sex.

Depression

Depression is more likely to be associated with chronicity of problem drinking amongst women than to be a risk factor for the onset of problem drinking (Wilsnack et al., 1991). Depression appears to pre-date alcohol problems in women, but seldom does in men (Helzer and Pryzbeck, 1988).

Stressful life events

Negative life events during childhood and adolescence (death of a parent, economic deprivation, illness in the family, unstable family of origin) may predispose to drinking as a coping style to relieve stress. Women often date the onset of their heavy drinking to a stressful life event, explaining that they used alcohol in order to forget their problems and to increase their social confidence (Copeland and Hall, 1992).

Multiple substance use

Many women with alcohol problems also have significant drug problems and dependence. In the 1970s and 1980s, prescription drugs such as minor tranquillizers and sedatives were typically used, but illicit drugs such as cannabis, cocaine, other stimulants and hallucinogens are becoming increasingly common, particularly in women under the age of 30 years (see also Chapter 9).

Risk factors across the life span

Although most risk factors are relevant to all age groups, some are more specific to certain stages in the life cycle. Peer influence plays a greater role amongst female adolescents than amongst their male counterparts (Wilsnack et al., 1994). Young, single, working women, particularly those under 25 years, drink heavily, possibly for a variety of reasons, including a relaxation in the attitudes to women drinking, greater opportunities to drink, and financial independence. Many women alter their drinking patterns during their twenties and thirties. Infertility, post-natal depression, marital or other relationship breakdown, bereavement and physical illness are all factors which may influence drinking behaviour at this stage. Different stresses influence drinking behaviour in the forties and fifties. Marital or relationship break-up, lack of employment, the departure of children from the family home, bereavement and loss of attractiveness are all important factors. Elderly women with alcohol problems are more likely to be widowed, living alone and depressed.

Physical complications

Although women start to drink heavily at a later age than men, the way in which they metabolize alcohol seems to put them at higher risk of developing physical complications than men, and of developing these complications earlier in their drinking careers: the 'telescoping' effect (Blume, 1997; Randall et al., 1999). Physical complications include alcoholic liver disease, cardiomyopathy, myopathy and brain damage (see Chapters 3 and 10). There is also evidence for a relationship between alcohol consumption and breast cancer (Smith-Warner et al., 1998)

Chronic heavy drinking is also associated with inhibition of ovulation, infertility and a wide variety of gynaecological and obstetric problems (Blume, 1997). Heavy alcohol consumption during pregnancy is associated with spontaneous abortion, intrauterine growth retardation, foetal alcohol syndrome (FAS) and foetal alcohol effects (FAE) (see below). Excessive drinking also leads to diminished libido and has been linked to an early menopause. Treatment programmes must therefore pay special attention to the physical health and pregnancy status of women.

Women with alcohol problems have a considerable excess mortality when compared with the general population and to their male counterparts (Lindberg and Agren, 1988). The causes of premature death include alcohol intoxication and delirium tremens, cirrhosis of the liver, violent death, stroke and breast cancer (Lindberg and Agren, 1988; Lewis et al., 1995).

Pregnancy and childbirth

Women who drink heavily during pregnancy put the developing foetus at significant risk of FAS. Other factors may also be involved, including tobacco, caffeine and illicit drug use, prescribed medication, maternal age, past obstetric history and social class. The estimated incidence of FAS is between one and three cases per 1000 live births. FAS is described in Chapter 10.

Other FAE such as spontaneous abortion, reduced birth weight and behaviour changes are associated with lesser degrees of drinking. The greatest risk to the foetus from the mother's drinking is probably within the first few weeks of pregnancy, even before she knows that she is pregnant. Although low levels of alcohol consumption have not been associated with adverse effects, no safe level of alcohol use in pregnancy has been established. In the UK, the advice is to drink no more than one to two standard drinks once or twice per week during pregnancy. In the USA, abstinence from alcohol during pregnancy is recommended (see Chapter 10).

Pregnant women who are drinking heavily need sensitive and sympathetic treatment. Ideally, they should be followed up by the same midwife and alcohol counsellor throughout the pregnancy, liaison between the two services should be close and pregnant women should be happy with the arrangements. Admission to hospital may be required. At the very least, a comprehensive assessment of alcohol and drug use, past physical, obstetric and psychiatric history and drug use status of the partner is needed. Testing for hepatitis B and C and HIV should be considered in agreement with the woman herself. Child health services also need to be forewarned.

Psychological co-morbidity

Both men and women with drinking problems have high rates of associated psychiatric disturbance (see Chapter 8). A consistent finding of clinical studies is that depression is more commonly diagnosed in women with alcohol problems. Women also have higher rates of anxiety disorder, psychosexual dysfunction and bulimia (Ross et al., 1988), lower self-esteem (Walitzer and Sher, 1996) and borderline personality disorder (Walitzer and Sher, 1996). They are also at higher risk of suicide than women without drinking problems. There is a modest relationship between substance misuse and eating disorder (Schuckit et al., 1996). Psychiatric co-morbidity appears to be associated with a greater severity of problem drinking (Ross and Shirley, 1997). Even socially intact women with drinking problems, early in their treatment careers, have high levels of mood and anxiety disorders (Haver and Dahlgren, 1995). Alcohol problems and post-traumatic stress disorder (PTSD) commonly occur together and the course of the combined disorder appears to be more severe than the course of either disorder alone (Brown et al., 1995).

Psychiatric co-morbidity is often underestimated in women presenting for treatment. Use of the Symptom Check List-90 (SCL-90) may be helpful in identifying those women who need further assessment (Haver, 1997).

Social complications

Women with alcohol problems often drink alone at home, thus reducing the likelihood that their problem will be uncovered, and increasing the risk of social isolation. Women drinkers report more marital problems than their male counterparts. Children are more likely to be taken into care, particularly if the mother is a single parent or her partner is also a heavy drinker.

More women now live independently and own their own cars and drive, and recent studies report an increased crash risk for women who drink and drive. This may be due in part to the fact that women metabolize alcohol differently from men and have higher blood alcohol concentrations (BACs) for a given volume of alcohol consumed (see Chapter 3). It is also possible that women are more sensitive than men to the effects of alcohol on driving performance.

Three clinical vignettes

The illustrations given below point to just three among a host of different ways in which a woman may present with a drinking problem.

Early onset and progression to physical disaster

Ms A was a shy woman from a privileged background. Her father and paternal grandmother were both problem drinkers. When she was aged 15, she began to drink and smoke at her parents' cocktail parties and found that she could tolerate alcohol well and that it gave her confidence. After school she did an Arts degree, and lived student life to the full, drinking most evenings and bingeing at weekends. She married in her mid-twenties, but by this time early signs of alcohol dependence were evident. She had a successful career as a media consultant, but following a series of miscarriages and the breakdown of her marriage, she became depressed and her drinking escalated. She lost her job when she was 35 because of absenteeism and going to work intoxicated. She did not present to the treatment services until she was 40, but by this time she had alcoholic cirrhosis and alcohol-related brain damage and was living in a squat with a partner who also had an alcohol problem. She died of liver failure shortly afterwards.

An alcohol problem following sexual abuse

Ms B, a 32-year-old woman, was referred for treatment by her GP. She was one of nine children and her early life was one of poverty and deprivation. Her mother was an invalid and her father, a labourer, sexually abused her and her two sisters between the ages of 5 and 16 years. She began to drink whisky at the age of 13 and soon found that it anaesthetized her 'raw emotional pain' and made life bearable. She left school at 15 and worked as a waitress in a restaurant. She enjoyed her work and was well liked by patrons. Her drinking, however, increased and by the time she was 25 years old she was drinking every day, both at lunch time and in the evening. She lost her job and began to drink in local parks. Two attempts at in-patient treatment failed because horrific and unbearable memories of her childhood sexual abuse emerged with abstinence.

A problem of later onset

Mrs C, a 56-year-old woman, was referred for treatment by her GP, who reported in the referral letter that her husband, 'a good man', could no longer cope with her drinking and was threatening to leave her. Mrs C was a quiet person who worked as a cleaner. She had been a devoted mother to her three sons and was proud that they were doing well in life. However, their leaving home had left an emptiness and loneliness and she realized that she had little in common with her husband, who was himself a heavy drinker. She had always been close to her mother, who, until her death 5 years previously, had lived nearby. Following her mother's death, she became depressed and began to drink sherry. Her consumption had increased slowly over the years and she was now consuming about one bottle per day.

Treatment issues

Barriers to help-seeking and detection

Although the numbers of women presenting to alcohol treatment services have increased over recent years, they still under-use such resources (Swift and Copeland, 1996). The failure to seek help may reflect barriers, either real or perceived, which are specific to women. Moralistic societal attitudes and the social stigma associated with drinking problems are important. Often women do not see drinking as their primary problem and present with associated health and psychosocial problems, such as depression (Thom, 1986; Plant, 1997). The fear of stigma and social disapproval may prevent them from approaching a general practitioner or local community alcohol team (Copeland and Hall, 1992). Drinking partners may discourage or actively prevent help-seeking. Low self-esteem may lead women with drinking problems to believe that they are not worthwhile. Sometimes their needs are so basic (housing, money, clothing and food) that more specific help is deferred. Lack of resources to arrange childcare and fear of removal of their children are very potent barriers (Swift et al., 1996). All too often, children have been removed already and life is so bleak that treatment seems worthless. Opposition from friends and family and negative professional attitudes can also play a part.

Barriers to engaging in and remaining in treatment

Women with alcohol problems are often regarded as more deviant and personality disordered, more difficult to help and less motivated than their male counterparts. Confrontational techniques may be harmful and compound feelings of anxiety, low self-esteem and depression (Beckman, 1994). Women are likely to receive less support from their partners and families and lack adequate childcare facilities. Often the treatment is not tailored sufficiently to their needs. For instance, a woman with a history of childhood sexual abuse will find it difficult to cope on an in-patient unit where she is the only woman. There is considerable debate as to whether women are better served in a women-only treatment programme or a 'mixed' facility (Dahlgren and Willander, 1989; Hodgins et al., 1997). It is possible that women-only services have a role in attracting women of particular backgrounds into treatment, possibly women with dependent children, lesbians, women with a maternal history of a drug or alcohol problem and those who have suffered childhood sexual abuse (Copeland and Hall, 1992; Copeland et al., 1993).

Treatment outcomes

There is a prevailing assumption that women with alcohol problems have poorer outcomes than men. However, closer scrutiny of the literature reveals that women are under-represented in treatment outcome research (Vannicelli and Nash, 1984) and that outcomes are often similar. There is a suggestion that women do better in the first year after treatment, whereas men have better results at follow-up after 12 months (Jarvis, 1992). Women may be better than men at using self-help material to reduce heavy or problem drinking (Sanchez-Craig et al., 1989). The presence of co-morbid psychopathology is an important factor.

Very few studies have examined the factors that predict outcome in women with drinking problems. Factors from women-only samples associated with poor outcome include marital problems prior to treatment, a dysfunctional relationship with an important person, few primary relationships prior to treatment and multiple life problems (MacDonald, 1987), a history of delirium tremens, early onset of the drink problem, unemployment, antisocial personality disorder and not living with a husband (Smith and Cloninger, 1984). These factors are summarized in Box 11.2. Paradoxically, women with major depressive disorders and alcohol dependence have better outcomes than women with no other psychiatric diagnosis (Rounsaville et al., 1987).

BOX 11.2 **Factors predicting poor outcomes in women with drinking problems**
- Early onset
- Few primary relationships prior to treatment
- Multiple life problems
- Dysfunctional relationship with an important person
- Unemployment
- A history of delirium tremens

Pregnant women may be particularly responsive to advice about drinking. A randomized clinical trial of a brief intervention for pregnant women assigned 247 women attending a Boston maternity unit to either a brief intervention or assessment only (Chang et al., 1999). Both groups reduced their alcohol consumption during pregnancy. A recent primary care study in Wisconsin showed that brief alcohol-focused intervention was associated with reduction in alcohol consumption in women of childbearing age (18–40 years) who were defined as problem drinkers (Manwell et al., 2000). This sample was well educated, and almost 50% reported a history of lifetime depression.

Practical and service issues

Women are not readily attracted into specialist alcohol services – they are more likely to approach generalist services, at least in the first instance. It is therefore vital that primary care workers, general psychiatrists, physicians, parasuicide teams and accident and emergency workers are aware of the special needs of women and help to bridge the gap between generalist and specialist services. Such links are fundamental to early intervention. Women should have more choice in their treatment; specialist services should guarantee that certain women are seen by women counsellors and have access to women-only groups. Where possible, agencies should make it possible for all women, at least in the first instance, to be seen by a woman counsellor. Recommendations for service planning have been described previously (Davison and Marshall, 1996).

Special attention should be given to a history of physical or sexual abuse and its consequences. Comprehensive past medical and psychiatric histories should be taken, and complemented with a mental state assessment and a physical examination. There may be important family issues to uncover. What is the woman's relationship with her partner like? Is the partner drinking? Are there any children and who is minding them? Women with alcohol problems are often burdened by a crippling guilt and low self-esteem, which need to be addressed at the first interview. An empathic and non-judgemental approach is likely to bear more fruit in terms of treatment than a dismissive 'I told you so' style.

Fundamental commonalities

Whatever the differences that men and women bring to the origins and presentations of their drinking problems, whatever the special sensitivities needed to analyse and appreciate the position of the woman with a drinking problem, and whatever the special issues which the treatment of the woman with the drinking problem may raise, there is fundamentally much in common between the man and woman drinker. Men and women equally need individual understanding and individual help unhampered by stereotypes.

REFERENCES

Beckman, J.L. (1994) Treatment needs of women with alcohol problems. *Alcohol Health and Research World* 18, 206–11.

Blume, S.B. (1997) Alcohol and other drug problems in women. In *Substance Abuse, a Comprehensive Textbook*, 3rd edn, ed. Lowinson, J.H., Ruiz, P. and Millman, R.B. Baltimore: Wilkins and Wilkins, 794–867.

Breslau, N., Davis, G.C., Peterson, E.L. and Schultz, L. (1997). Psychiatric sequelae of post traumatic stress disorder in women. *Archives of General Psychiatry* 54, 81–7.

Brown, P.J., Recupero, P.R. and Stout, R. (1995) PTSD, substance use comorbidity and treatment utilisation. *Addictive Behaviours* 20, 251–4.

Chang, G., Wilkins-Haug, L., Berman, G. and Goetz, M.A. (1999) Brief intervention for alcohol use in pregnancy: a randomized trial. *Addiction* 94, 1499–508.

Copeland, J. and Hall, W. (1992) A comparison of women seeking drug and alcohol treatment in a specialist women's and two traditional mixed-sex treatment services. *British Journal of Addiction* 87, 1293–302.

Copeland, J., Hall, W. and Didcott, P. (1993) A comparison of a specialist women's service and other drug treatment service with two traditional mixed-sex services: client characteristics and treatment outcome. *Drug and Alcohol Dependence* 32, 81–92.

Dahlgren, L. and Willander, A. (1989) Are special treatment facilities for female alcoholics needed? A controlled 2-year follow-up study from a specialized female unit (EWA) versus a mixed male/female treatment facility. *Alcoholism: Clinical and Experimental Research* 13, 499–505.

Davison, S. and Marshall, E.J. (1996) Women who abuse alcohol and drugs. In *Planning Community Mental Services for Women*, ed. Abel, K., Buszewicz, M., Davison, S., Johnson, S. and Staples, E. London: Routledge, 128–44.

Fleming, J., Mullen, P.E., Sibthorpe, B., Attewell, R. and Bammer, G. (1998) The relationship between childhood sexual abuse and alcohol abuse in women – a case-control study. *Addiction* 93, 1787–98.

Haver, B. (1997) Screening for psychiatric comorbidity among female alcoholics: the use of a questionnaire (SCL-90) among women early in their treatment programme. *Alcohol and Alcoholism* 32, 725–30.

Haver, B. and Dahlgren, L. (1995) Early treatment of women with alcohol addiction (EWA): a comprehensive evaluation and outcome study. I. Patterns of psychiatric comorbidity at intake. *Addiction* 90, 101–9.

Helzer, J.E., Burnam, A. and McEvoy, L. (1991) Alcohol abuse and dependence. In *Psychiatric Disorders in America: the Epidemiological Catchment Area Study*, ed. Robins, L.N. and Regier, D.A. New York: Free Press, 81–115.

Helzer, J.E. and Pryzbeck, T.R. (1988) The co-occurrence of alcoholism with other psychiatric disorders in the general population and its impact on treatment. *Journal of Studies on Alcohol* 49, 219–24.

Hodgins, D.C., El-Guebaly, N. and Addington, J. (1997) Treatment of substance abusers: single or mixed gender programmes. *Addiction* 92, 805–12.

Jarvis, T.J. (1992) Implications of gender for alcohol treatment research: a quantitative and qualitative review. *British Journal of Addiction* 87, 1249–61.

Kendler, K.S., Walters, E.E., Neale, M.C., Kessler, R.C., Heath, A.C. and Eaves, L.J. (1995) The structure of the genetic and environmental risk factors for six major psychiatric disorders in women. *Archives of General Psychiatry* 52, 374–83.

Lewis, C.E., Smith, E., Kercher, C. and Spitznagel, E. (1995) Assessing gender interactions in the prediction of mortality in alcoholic men and women: a 20-year follow-up study. *Alcoholism: Clinical and Experimental Research* 19, 1162–72.

Lindberg, S. and Agren, G. (1988) Mortality among male and female hospitalised alcoholics in Stockholm 1962–1983. *British Journal of Addiction* 83, 1193–200.

MacDonald, J.G. (1987) Predictors of treatment outcome for alcoholic women. *International Journal of the Addictions* 22, 235–48.

Manwell, L.B., Fleming, M.F., Mundt, M.P., Stauffacher, E.A. and Barry, K.L. (2000) Treatment of problem alcohol use in women of childbearing age: results of a brief intervention trial. *Alcoholism: Clinical and Experimental Research* 24, 1517–24.

Office for National Statistics (2000) *Living in Britain, Results from the 1998 General Household Survey*. London: The Stationery Office.

Plant, M. (1997) *Women and Alcohol: Contemporary and Historical Perspectives*. London: Free Association Books.

Prescott, C., Neale, M.C., Corey, L.A. and Kendler, K.S. (1997). Predictors of problem drinking and alcohol dependence in a population-based sample of female twins. *Journal of Studies on Alcohol* 58, 167–81.

Randall, C.L., Roberts, J.S., Del Boca, F.K., Carroll, K.M., Connors, G.J. and Mattson, M.E. (1999) Telescoping of landmark events associated with drinking: a gender comparison. *Journal of Studies on Alcohol* 60, 252–60.

Ross, H.E., Glaser, F.B. and Stiasny, S. (1988) Sex differences in the prevalence of psychiatric disorders in patients with alcohol and drug problems. *British Journal of Addiction* 83, 1179–92.

Ross, H. and Shirley, M. (1997) Life-time problem drinking and psychiatric co-morbidity among Ontario women. *Addiction* 92, 183–96.

Rounsaville, B.J., Dolinsky, Z.S., Babor, T.F. and Meyer, R.E. (1987) Psychopathology as a predictor of treatment outcome in alcoholics. *Archives of General Psychiatry* 44, 505–13.

Sanchez-Craig, M., Leigh, G., Spivak, K. and Lei, H. (1989) Superior outcome of females over males after brief treatment for the reduction of heavy drinking. *British Journal of Addiction* 84, 395–404.

Schuckit, M.A., Jayson, E.T., Athenelli, R.M., Bucholz, K.K., Hesselbrock, V.M. and Nurnberger, J.I. (1996) Anorexia nervosa and bulimia nervosa in alcohol-dependent men and women and their relatives. *American Journal of Psychiatry* 153, 74–82.

Smith, E.M. and Cloninger, C.R. (1984) A prospective twelve-year follow-up of alcoholic women: a prognostic scale for long-term outcome. *National Institute of Drug Abuse Research Monograph Issues* 55, 245–51.

Smith-Warner, S.A., Spiegelman, D., Yaun, S.-S. et al. (1998) Alcohol and breast cancer in women: a pooled analysis of cohort studies. *Journal of the American Medical Association* 279, 535–40.

Spak, L., Spak, F. and Allebeck, P. (1997) Factors in childhood and youth predicting alcohol dependence and abuse in Swedish women: findings from a general population study. *Alcohol and Alcoholism* 32, 267–74.

Swift, W. and Copeland, J. (1996) Treatment needs and experiences of Australian women with alcohol and other drug problems. *Drug and Alcohol Dependence* 40, 211–19.

Swift, W., Copeland, J. and Hall, W. (1996) Characteristics of women with alcohol and other drug problems: findings of an Australian national survey. *Addiction* 91, 1141–50.

Thom, B. (1986) Sex differences in help-seeking for alcohol problems. I. The barriers to help seeking. *British Journal of Addiction* 81, 777–88.

Vannicelli, M. and Nash, L. (1984) Effect of sex bias on women's studies on alcoholism. *Alcoholism: Clinical and Experimental Research* 8, 334–6.

Walitzer, K.S. and Sher, K.J. (1996) A perspective of self-esteem and alcohol use disorders in early adulthood: evidence for gender differences. *Alcoholism: Clinical and Experimental Research* 20, 1118–24.

Wilsnack, S.C., Klassen, A.D., Schur, B.E. et al. (1991) Predicting onset and chronicity of women's problem drinking: a five year longitudinal analysis. *American Journal of Public Health* 81, 305–18.

Wilsnack, S.C., Vogeltanz, N.D., Klassen, A.D. and Harris, T.R. (1997) Childhood sexual abuse and women's substance abuse: national survey finding. *Journal of Studies on Alcohol* 58, 264–71.

Wilsnack, S.C. and Wilsnack, R.W. (1993) Epidemiological research on women's drinking: recent progress and directions for the 1990s. In *Women and Substance Abuse*, ed. Gomberg, E.S.L. and Nirenberg, T.D. NJ: Ablex Publishing, 62–99.

Wilsnack, S.C. and Wilsnack, R. (1995) Drinking and problem drinking in US women. In *Recent Developments in Alcoholism*, Vol. 12, ed. Galanter, M. New York: Plenum Press, 30–60.

Wilsnack, S.C., Wilsnack, R.W. and Hiller-Sturmhofel, S. (1994) How women drink. Epidemiology of women's drinking and problem drinking. *Alcohol Health and Research World* 18, 173–84.

Winfield, I., George, L.K., Swartz, M. and Blazer, D. G. (1990) Sexual assault and psychiatric disorders among a community sample of women. *American Journal of Psychiatry* 147, 335–41.

12

Some special presentations

This chapter describes a varied set of clinical presentations, identified in Box 12.1. These pictures are selected arbitrarily from a much wider gallery, and anyone who practises in this field will soon themselves begin to identify additional headings. To keep a mental card index which allows one to see patterns of presentation and use the last such case to illuminate understanding of the next will add to the reward and interest of therapeutic work. The only proviso to be borne in mind is the latent danger of forcing people into pigeonholes. Management of the next elderly patient will be helped by thinking through one's previous case experience with individuals in this age group, but each new patient is different.

BOX 12.1 Presentations contained within this chapter

The patient with impaired brain function

The person who is drunk and violent

When a child is at risk

The younger person with a drinking problem

A combined problem with drink and drugs

A drinking problem in later life

Cultural differences

The family member making contact

A patient on a general hospital ward

Dual diagnosis

The very important patient

The patient with impaired brain function

A description of the brain pathologies that can result from excessive use of alcohol is given in Chapter 7. Here, discussion focuses on the everyday clinical implications

of the fact that brain damage will, in some patients, compromise their ability to respond to and engage in the usually available treatment programmes. The following
passage gives a nurse's report on a 50-year-old man with a long history of alcohol
dependence.

> He gets everyone else irritated in the group. He doesn't seem to listen to what other people say
> and then bats in with his own views, saying exactly the same as he said yesterday and the day
> before. Things like 'If you keep yourself tidy and clean you've got no problem'. I don't think that
> after 3 weeks he even knows anyone else's name.

That observation might be evidence of a particular patient's habitual conversa-
tional style, but it must also raise a warning flag as to the possibility of brain damage
(Knight and Longmore, 1994). Subsequent psychological testing with this patient
revealed short-term memory impairment and evidence of frontal lobe impairment.

Gross brain damage is not likely to set difficulties in recognition. What has to
be cultivated is an alertness to lesser but still clinically important degrees of brain
impairment. The problem can present with various severities, but the picture given
by the patient who was having difficulties in functioning in the ward group is fairly
typical. There is often a sense of the patient's social awareness being blunted, of them
not being good at taking in new ideas or information, of their memory for newly
learnt material being impaired (hence that patient's difficulty with remembering
names), and there may also be difficulty in sustaining concentration.

Ward observation and watching the patient's behaviour in groups can be helpful
diagnostically, as can a report from an occupational therapist. In many instances
some recovery in functioning takes place over weeks or months, and serial assessments are therefore needed. Testing carried out immediately after detoxification
can give misleadingly pessimistic results. Beyond the ward observation and routine mental state examination (simple tests of memory and concentration), a full
assessment will involve skilled psychological testing and perhaps also brain imaging.

If testing and a brain scan confirm the presence of significant impairment and
damage and if repeated assessment demonstrates that recovery is likely to be incomplete, the implications for clinical management must be considered. A patient
who is experiencing cognitive difficulties will become frustrated by a demanding
therapeutic regime: the best therapeutic programmes involve a great deal of new
learning, emotional awareness, and social interaction, and it is in exactly the skills
needed to engage successfully in those types of experience in which the brain-
damaged patient may be deficient. If sympathetic note is not taken of their special
needs and handicaps, the patient will either go through the programme without
benefit or, more probably, they will break therapeutic contact.

A programme which acknowledges the needs of this type of patient cannot be
formulated on a one-off basis, but must be designed by interaction with the patient

concerned. Would it be helpful for them to have individual discussions which identify the core simplicities of their personal recovery programme? Would they be helped by written material or by making out checklists?

On return to their own home from the ward, thought must be given to the special aftercare needs of such a patient and their family, as discussed in Chapter 5. The programme should put therapeutic emphasis on the management of external and situational factors such as arranging how money is to be controlled, how time is to be spent, how work or sheltered employment is to be found, and how the local liquor stores are to be persuaded to be proscriptively helpful.

The patient who is drunk and violent

The general issue of the relation between drinking and violence is discussed elsewhere in this book (see Chapter 6 and Graham et al., 1998). Every now and then, a therapist will be faced by the worrying problem set by the patient who repeatedly turns up drunk and violent and demanding to be seen. The safety of staff and other patients may be at risk, and an enormous amount of anxiety can be engendered. If an alcohol treatment service is co-existing closely with other facilities, it will acquire a bad name if disruption is allowed to get out of hand.

A 40-year-old man, after a long drinking history, had been thrown out of his home, and was now drifting around temporary accommodation or sleeping rough. Over a period of 6 months he was twice admitted to hospital, but on each occasion came back drunk onto the ward, assaulted the nurses and smashed the furniture. A few days after his last discharge he came to the hospital late at night and got into a fight with a porter. He then arrived at out-patients drunk and demanding admission, with threats of further violence if admission was not granted.

In such circumstances there are two courses of action which are anti-therapeutic and should not be followed. The first of these is to tolerate further violence or threat of violence. The patient will not be helped, the morale of the treatment service will be torn apart, and staff may indeed be hurt. The second non-answer is to ban the patient from the hospital. Even if the banning is successful, it will only transfer the problem of violence onto someone else's doorstep, and things will not look too good if a week later the man is on an assault charge with the court told that a hospital has abrogated its responsibilities. The principle which guides the therapeutic response to this kind of patient is the realization that violence is often triggered by contextual cues which provoke that reaction (Graham et al., 1998).

Such a problem is dealt with more easily by a treatment service than by anyone working in isolation. A hospital, for instance, ought to be able to meet this type of problem and the general practitioner and other local services will not be grateful if the hospital seeks to pass the buck. What is needed is a firm treatment policy drawn up for the individual, and one which sets explicit limits but which is nonetheless a treatment rather than a mere containment policy. It must reward constructive behaviour and in no way reinforce unacceptable behaviour, and it must be communicated fairly and openly to the patient herself, put at the front of the case notes, and a copy given to all staff who may be involved. It is useful to hold a staff meeting for formulation of the plan so that things go forward by agreement, and with everyone fully in the picture. It may be wise to ensure that the organization's administrative staff are consulted, with a legal opinion obtained if necessary.

On the basis of consultation, a memo such as the following might be put into the case notes of the man whose story has just been sketched.

Mr Smith: agreed treatment plan

So that we can go on helping this patient within a treatment programme, the following guidelines have been agreed by the treatment team, and we would be grateful if everyone will give this plan support.

1. Mr Smith will only be seen by appointment, and if he comes up without an appointment he should be asked to leave.
2. He will then only be seen at appointment if he is not intoxicated. If there is any suspicion of intoxication, he will be asked to leave without being seen further.
3. If Mr Smith refuses to leave when asked, or if he threatens or offers violence, help should be summoned through the hospital's usual emergency system and the police should be telephoned. The number is . . . and the police station has been alerted. On no account should an individual staff member attempt to argue with this patient.
4. Mr Smith has been told that if he commits any chargeable offence on the hospital premises, the hospital will not hesitate to press charges.
5. These ground rules have been explained to Mr Smith personally, and they have been set up not only to protect the staff but also so as to make it possible for us to go on working with this patient within a constructive treatment plan.

Contained within those seemingly harsh guidelines is a plan designed to enable the team to go on offering help to a man who would probably be rejected by many centres as unhelpable. In practice, this drawing of limits is reassuring to the patient himself. A disorganized and inconsistent response, which may even involve a sort of complicity with his violence, is likely to exacerbate anxiety and violence, whereas a firm policy often results in patients showing a capacity to go along with constructive expectations. They are able to come to appointments sober, and make a new and positive therapeutic engagement. Things do not, however, always run smoothly, and if the patient does turn up drunk and tries to hit someone, a charge may have to be brought, for otherwise no learning can take place. To be able to use the police in support of the treatment plan requires careful liaison.

With the immediate threat of violence contained, it should be possible to get down to an individually planned and positive treatment programme. Violence is then no longer the central issue, and the patient's reputation should not be allowed to overshadow therapeutic dealings. There will be a need to talk about the violence, and the patient has to come to terms with the full implications of the fact that alcohol for them releases violent feelings.

The problem has also to be met as to how, flexibly, the stated rules are to be interpreted in certain difficult circumstances. For instance, if there is anxiety about the possibility of head injury, a deterioration in the patient's physical condition, or concern as to whether underlying mental illness is now hidden within the picture, appropriate help should be obtained. There has therefore to be an understanding that individual clinical judgement allows a flexible response to emergency, but the team should, whenever possible, be brought into the decision or promptly informed as to what has been done. There are some patients who pose extreme dangers of violence, and staff safety and public safety should then be the paramount consideration without prevarication or apology.

A child at risk

There has over recent years been a sharp increase in public anxiety about the risks to which children may be subjected as a result of parental violence or sexual abuse. Such anxieties provide the context within which social service departments will deal with the sensitive problems which arise when a parent's drinking appears to put a young child's safety at risk (see also Chapter 5).

Mr and Mrs B had met when they were both patients in an alcoholism treatment unit. He was aged 35, she 30, and they had both experienced deprived childhoods and chaotic adult life histories. In their recovery they gave each other a great deal of mutual understanding, and they started to live together. Seen 3 years later, they reported much improvement but they would still periodically relapse into short bouts of drinking. At these times they were sometimes violent to each other, the furniture was apt to be broken and the police had been called on several occasions. They now had an 18-month-old daughter and the neighbours had reported their concern about the safety of this child to the social services.

The issues which are being dealt with in this section overlap with the previous discussion of the patient who was drunk and violent, but a new and worrying element is introduced when a child is at risk (Sherr, 1991). Every such case must be approached differently, but guidelines can be helpful.

The child's safety and welfare must come first

In any decision-making around this case, that simple rule of priority must never be lost from sight.

Do not panic, but err on the side of caution

No one would wish reflexly to put every child into care where there is a history of parental drinking. But at the same time it would be culpable to engage in an extended process of leisurely assessment rather than taking firm emergency action in those instances in which the safety of the child requires immediate placement in care.

Try to work with, rather than against, the parents

This advice will seem obvious to the experienced case worker. The parents may feel guilty about, and frightened by, their own behaviour and their failure adequately to care for a child who is precious to them. Any threat of having that child taken away is likely to cause a reaction, not only in terms of self-blame, but also of angry projected blame of other people. The parents need therefore so far as possible to be helped into a position in which they can accept that everyone is working constructively together for a resolution of the problem.

Assess the total background family situation and interactions rather than focusing only on the drinking

In the case which has been outlined above, there was evidence that when both parents were sober they cared for their child lovingly and competently. When sober, the relationship between the parents was also a happy one, and whenever they could obtain a baby-sitter they went to Alcoholics Anonymous (AA) meetings together. There was no suggestion of violence other than in the setting of drunkenness.

Assess the parental drinking history and the likely consequences of the drinking for the child

Drinking bouts in this family tended to last about 3–5 days, with one parent's drinking sparking off drinking in the other partner, although sometimes one would drink and the other stay sober. There was evidence that several months (sometimes as long as 6 months) could elapse without a bout occurring. There had never been any indication of intentional violence to the child, but she had on one occasion been accidentally knocked to the floor. She had also been left neglected and crying in a bedroom when both parents were drinking and rowing. Drunken driving may also cause concern when the child is at risk as a passenger.

Examination of the child

Assessment is not complete without a physical and developmental assessment of the child. This is usually best conducted by a child psychiatrist or a paediatrician. A social worker will also usually be involved in assessing the child and the family situation. In the case we are describing, the little girl showed no abnormalities.

Setting up an appropriate level of safeguard and monitoring

The appropriate level of safeguard must depend on the individual situation and can range from the emergency decision to take a child into care to putting that child on the 'at-risk' register, or even some lesser level of intervention. In the present circumstances it was felt that there was a small but real danger of the child coming to accidental harm if the parents continued to drink and fight in this explosive fashion. The parents agreed to strict supervision, and each decided to take disulfiram and attend a hospital outpatient group. It was agreed that their ability to look after their child would have to be viewed as dependent on their continued sobriety. Twelve months later, they had remained abstinent and made good therapeutic progress.

Not every such story has a happy outcome. Circumstances may arise when a child has to be taken into care, but the hope may then still be that a constructive and monitored programme can be set up which allows the parents access and the opportunity to work towards getting their child back.

This discussion has been in terms of a situation in which both parents have a drinking problem. Situations also arise when only one parent is drinking or where there is drinking and a single-parent family.

The young drinker

In many countries a common experience over recent years has been the increasingly frequent presentation of young people (including young women) with drinking problems. 'Young' may, in extreme instances, mean the early teens, but the particular focus of this discussion is on patients in their late teens or early twenties. More significant than the exact boundaries of chronological age is the fact that these are people who, in an important sense, see themselves as *not adult,* and who have not made the social transition from adolescent to adult self-image. The therapist is encountering a person who is still finding a way through adolescent conflicts, and who has not resolved fundamental questions about the balance between dependence on others and independence. For the anxiety, anger and despair which may be generated by these frustrations, alcohol can be a panacea. It temporarily relieves a painful confusion of feelings, provides at the same time a 'high' of optimism and excitement, while in a state of intoxication the aggressive feelings can be liberated and acted out, and with the natural energy and physicality of this age adding intensity to the chaos. Moreover, drinking can give companionship and the approbation of peers.

As for the pattern of alcohol use itself, in most instances the young person will not have had a drinking history of sufficient duration for established alcohol dependence. The picture is of repeated drinking to the point of intoxication, often with experience of amnesias.

Possibilities for growth

There is a common belief that severe personality disorder is likely to be associated with a drinking problem of early onset, and a diagnosis of underlying sociopathy is readily pinned on the patient. But there is the paradox with this type of disturbance that the unformedness of personality can itself bear witness to potential for growth. A uniformly pessimistic attitude towards the prognosis of the young drinker is therefore unjustified, even when their behaviour is flagrantly disturbed. Here is a brief case history of one such young person whose story typifies this kind of presentation.

A 22-year-old man was referred to a counselling centre by the court. He had been charged with assault after a pub fight, and he had also broken a few windows. There had been several suicide gestures. He had been working in a garage but had been sacked. His drinking involved his becoming explosively and obstreperously drunk whenever he had money in his pocket. He had been forced to leave his parental home because of his rowdy drunkenness at the age of 19, and his respectable parents did not want him back. Five years after being seen at the counselling centre he had a steady job in the Post Office and was happily married. He now drank occasionally and moderately. He looked back on his past as distant, and saw it in terms of 'I was all messed up at that time'.

What needs to be emphasized is that, while pessimism is often self-fulfilling, a treatment approach which responds to the needs for growth may catch a moment of possibility. There is no one recipe for treatment in this type of case, and the basic approach will have much in common with what is done to help the patient of any age. This young man discovered a capacity to talk about his problems and was helped by a counsellor, who was able to arrange her schedule so that she had time to see him whenever he dropped in for an hour's talk – he needed to do a lot of talking. During the first 2 years he was a keen AA attender. He also benefited from a 6-month residence in a 'dry' hostel and from a set of friendships which developed from that stay. Later, he was lucky to meet the right partner. In essence, what these various relationships offered, each in their own way, was a series of experiments in facets of growing up. If there are common ingredients in such stories of therapeutic success, they lie in the qualities of the therapist – someone who is specially and evidently warm, who will be able to tolerate projection of unworked-out feelings towards parents, but who will not be manoeuvred into treating the patient as a child. There is also often a need to find a way of helping the young person pull out of a pattern of living (or pattern of drifting) which is a series of makeshifts rather than anything which offers either real demands or real rewards.

Special difficulties

Having taken as illustration a case with a happy outcome, it is necessary also to look at reasons why the story may on other occasions be turbulent or marked by nothing but defeat. One reason may be that the personal handicaps are already more fixed, a matter of psychological damage rather than of frustrated growth. The young man or woman who is profoundly anxious, restless and irritable, who cannot easily use or tolerate a relationship of any kind, who will not stay in a job and who is likely to disappear to another town or go off to sea, is going to be difficult to help. Even so, it is worthwhile holding out the availability of friendship, with the modest expectation of working for small immediate gains and taking a very long-term view.

Another reason for special difficulty, grossly evident or only revealed by assessment, is when excessive drinking in someone of this age is symptomatic of brain damage. A further common diagnostic perplexity is the interpretation to be made when a client in this age group reports 'being depressed'. Usually, this complaint is to be understood in terms of the general lability of mood which so often accompanies problems in development. It is a mistake to over-diagnose depressive illness or inappropriately to prescribe antidepressant drugs. However, there are cases in which recurrent depressive illness may first declare itself at this age, and in which this distress leads to use of alcohol as self-medication.

Yet another type of story is that of the young man or woman who is referred to an alcohol clinic because drinking has been seen as the exclusive problem. It then becomes apparent that one is dealing with a major psychiatric illness, the exact nature of which is perplexingly difficult to diagnose. The picture shifts perhaps from that of depression to a presentation that looks worryingly like schizophrenia. The excessive use of alcohol is no more than a confounding factor in a very complex disturbance.

Taking the problems of the young drinker very seriously

With these young patients, there are a number of reasons for arguing with special force the general position that earlier rather than later intervention is to be preferred. They should be helped before dependence supervenes. The young drinker who is left to run deeper into trouble is in danger of becoming increasingly unemployable. It must also be remembered that it is particularly among young drinkers that mortality rates are elevated, often as a consequence of accident or violence. There are therefore good reasons for taking the young drinker very seriously.

A combined problem with drink and drugs

A woman aged 26 had been given an assessment appointment at the request of her lawyer. She was a single parent, her 6-year-old son had been taken into care, and she wished to contest the decision and regain custody.

The patient arrived with a half-consumed can of lager in her hand and, despite requests not to smoke, she repeatedly lit up a cigarette. She was so excited, irritable and importuning as to make it impossible to proceed with the interview. A few days later she came back in a more co-operative mood and apologized for her previous behaviour – 'Sorry, I'd been snorting cocaine'. Her story was of previous use of injected heroin (she was now on methadone maintenance), intermittent use of cocaine, heavy current use of cannabis, and diazepam swallowed like sweets. Mixed with all this, intermittent heavy drinking was occurring to the point of gross intoxication. She was beginning to experience alcohol withdrawal symptoms. Clearly, it was impossible to support this woman's wish immediately to have her child returned to her care. After some further out-patient visits, she was, at her request, admitted to hospital – 'I can't do it by myself, give me a break'. Six weeks later she came out of hospital off all drugs other than prescribed oral methadone and 30 cigarettes a day, and the social services were, as a preliminary, happy for her to make supervised visits to her son.

Here are some principles which may guide the therapeutic approach to someone exhibiting this sort of chaotic combined use of drugs and alcohol.

- Alcohol and other drugs all need to be responded to with equal and concomitant seriousness. There is a danger that drug treatment services will ignore the alcohol (and perhaps also the diazepam), with risks of fatal overdose from methadone taken in combination with these cerebral depressants (Advisory Council on the Misuse of Drugs, 2000). The drinking cannot safely be regarded as an optional therapeutic target to be left over for a later day.
- Admission to hospital may be needed not once but on a repeated, low-threshold basis for detoxification, renewed goal setting and another start.
- Treatment goals need to be unambiguously defined. Abstinence from alcohol and all other psychoactive drugs other than the prescribed methadone is likely to be the only feasible long-term goal. Tolerance of setbacks and failure, a willingness to accept achievable intermediate goals and policies for harm minimization need to be combined with the maintenance of the long-term effort to help the patient towards being 'clean and sober', with accompanying positive life changes. Therapeutic drift is sadly likely to see death by overdose, hepatitis C, liver damage exacerbated by the drinking, or death by alcoholic cirrhosis 20 years on. The

need to deal with the nicotine dependence should not be ignored (Breslau et al., 1996).

The needs of a patient like the young woman described here may pose a considerable challenge to service organization based on separation of alcohol and drug services, with each type of facility working within its own predelictions and organizational culture. In Chapter 9 we deal with this kind of problem at length.

Alcohol problems in later life

A long-standing history of excessive drinking continuing into old age may often be marked by brain damage and other physical complications, and nutritional neglect is common. The drinking pattern may have become fragmented compared with previous years, and loss of tolerance to alcohol is a frequent manifestation (see Chapter 4).

In contrast is the elderly patient who has taken to excessive drinking as a response to a problem or cluster of difficulties which he or she has encountered only recently. Widowhood, retirement and a general loss of purpose in life are often important factors in the onset of a drinking problem at this age. The possible significance of underlying brain disease or of depressive illness should also be considered as a cause of a late onset problem.

The division of the drinking problems which occur in this epoch of life into those of early and late onset is clinically useful, and carries implications for management of the problem. A not unusual story is of the seemingly late onset condition being found to have a much longer background history on closer enquiry. Many of the basic features can, however, be the same whether the onset of the problem was remote or recent, and one should be aware of elements which can very generally colour the presentation at this age. For instance, there is often the likelihood of social isolation. Delirious states are common in the elderly, and at this time of life depression and a degree of brain impairment often go together. There are often multiple physical pathologies.

Help for the older patient

Basic principles have to be borne in mind, but for patients in this age group special skills will be needed to design a treatment plan which effectively responds to their situation in life (Janik and Dunham, 1983; Hinrichsen, 1984; Koford et al., 1987; Fitzgerald and Mulford, 1992). This implies a knowledge of the local resources which are available to help the elderly, including clubs, day centres, home helps, community nurses, and so on. Mobilizing whatever family support is available can also be important. The patient may be ambivalent about surrendering independence, but sheltered accommodation can provide companionship and enable better adjustment than continued isolation. Initial hospital admission may be needed for diagnosis, but it should not be too prolonged. The sensitivity of the ageing nervous system to drugs should be borne in mind, with tranquillizers or sedatives used only in the short term and with caution. Disulfiram is too dangerous at this age. Some older people will join AA, but that kind of group experience is usually difficult to utilize at this age.

Whatever the specifics of therapy, the non-specifics are again important, including the warmth, the hopefulness and the goal-setting. An old person may need things explained slowly, positions explored, and solutions negotiated at an acceptable pace. Abrupt and clumsy interference will be met deservedly with tetchiness, and there will be no therapeutic gain.

The approach to old-age drinking problems still tends sometimes to be negatively influenced by a gulf in understanding: 'Well, drink is all she's got, and if she drinks herself to death...'. Such attitudes are unjustified. Elderly people with drinking problems can be helped, with large benefit in terms of health, enjoyment of life and dignity.

The patient from a cultural background other than the therapist's

'I don't understand him at all', said the Community Psychiatric Nurse (CPN) who was reporting on a visit to her patient's home. 'He's a Pakistani who owns a fruit shop, aged about 60, very much the head of the family, two grown-up sons who help in the business and take orders from their father. He and his wife still have only a rather poor understanding of English. He has a bottle of whisky at the back of the shop, and swigs at it steadily throughout the day. When I went round I was treated with kindness, loaded with presents of fruit, and met with massive denial. He says that he uses a little whisky now and then for medicine.'

The CPN had the openness to admit that she did not understand this patient's cultural position, and no doubt the shopkeeper was puzzled as to the role, credentials and purpose of this person whom his doctor had asked to call.

The cultural meaning of the drinking itself can be puzzling. What does 'normal' drinking mean within a particular culture, and how are religious prohibitions interpreted in practice? What are the legitimate functions of alcohol and its symbolism? What are the culturally determined ideas which define 'drinking too much' and, if there is a concept equivalent to 'alcohol dependence', with what adverse connotations is that idea loaded? The questions which relate to difficulties in understanding the drinking itself constitute only a small part of the total cross-cultural puzzle. The essential background problems relate to such issues as understanding of personality, family and family roles, religion, social class and status, and who has a right to say what to whom (Heath, 1993; Blane, 1993). Different cultures will carry different assumptions as to what constitutes 'treatment', the primacy given to the prescription of medicines, or the degree of directiveness which is expected (Edwards and Arif, 1980).

The case of that shopkeeper is one example of the many and varied cross-cultural problems in understanding which can be met whatever the country in which the therapist is practising (Brisbane and Womble, 1985; Collins, 1993). The presentation may be the recently immigrated family, the postgraduate student from abroad, the immigrant labourer who is today part of the workforce in many parts of the world, or the patient of the therapist's own culture but with regional or social class identity different from the therapist's. The problems set by the extreme cases of cultural difference can, in fact, serve as a useful reminder of the need for a more general awareness of the culture clash which is often present in many 'ordinary' therapeutic encounters.

There can be no one formula for dealing with such situations. It is important to be alert to the need for understanding, and hence to avoid those clumsy errors which come from assuming that everyone else is like us, or that there is something odd about others if they do not comply with our own, parochial expectations. Treatment services are still often too ethnically insensitive.

Every such case has to be seen as an exercise in building bridges. With the fruit-shop owner it may, for instance, be possible to find a second-generation member of the family who can be a broker in understanding. The patient's son may identify the key figures within the extended family network who have a right to advise and intervene. It may also be possible to find a professional within the local agencies or hospitals who speaks the language and understands the culture, and who can help with an assessment or perhaps take over the case.

The family member as intermediary

Anyone working in this field will from time to time receive the following type of letter or a phone call of similar nature.

I wonder whether you can possibly help. It is not about myself but it's my daughter who needs assistance. She will not take any notice of me, but I know she is an alcoholic.

The letter may be from a mother about her son or daughter, a husband about his wife, a divorced wife about her ex-husband, or reflect any one of a wide range of other possible combinations. The common theme is that a concerned family member is seeking help on behalf of someone who is not themselves at that moment of a mind to do so.

Helping agencies ought to have the capacity to meet such requests, at least by offering a preliminary evaluation session. The principle which guides response to this type of proxy consultation is that there may be fruitful possibilities of working with the person who is actually in the room (the intermediary), rather than the therapist being lured into the impossible position of trying to find instant solutions for the person who is absent (the problem drinker).

For instance, the mother who has come to talk about her daughter's drinking may in fact be wanting to talk about her own sense of guilt, anger or frustration, or about her need to control, or her difficulty in 'letting go'. More than one session may be required. Information about AA can be timely.

Secondly, there are possibilities of the encounter with the intermediary leading to help for the individual who is drinking. Information can be passed on about treatment services and AA, or an open and unthreatening invitation can be offered for the drinker to come along to discuss whether there is anything to talk about. Beyond that level of information giving, there may also be indirect ways of working with the drinker through changing the behaviour, attitudes and level of confidence of a key family member. In terms of family systems theory (Bennett and La Bonte, 1993), one is introducing movement into a system which is otherwise going to maintain the drinking. One should also be aware that this kind of approach can at times be manipulative and an attempt to establish blame, and one does well not to be lured into secret contracts.

A presentation on a general hospital ward

This is an account of a late-night happening on a surgical ward.

A woman had been admitted 3 days earlier with an abdominal emergency. A diagnosis of acute pancreatitis had been made and the patient had spent the first 2 days in intensive care. With her physical condition stabilized, she was back in a surgical bed. That evening, at about midnight, she pulled out her intravenous line, made for the door of the ward and said she was going home in a taxi. She drifted into the belief that she was in a hotel, but then suggested that her husband was hiding in a gas cylinder.

Delirium tremens (see Chapter 7) is not infrequently precipitated by a medical or surgical event, with consequent admission to hospital and abrupt withdrawal of alcohol. The condition is often satisfactorily treated in that kind of general ward setting, but sometimes there are difficulties. The case history outlined above reflects the situation in which a surgical team is suddenly faced by a dangerous alcohol-related emergency. It is the danger which needs to be emphasized. If she is allowed to run off the ward, she may get lost in the hospital grounds and die of exposure, or walk into traffic and be killed. If the patient is brought back onto the ward without a safe nursing environment established and appropriate medication given, there is a danger of a fall from a window or other accident.

When a surgical or medical team is confronted by this kind of presentation, there are three golden rules. First, the patient must by all means possible be kept on the ward and their physical safety ensured. Second, psychiatric advice should immediately be obtained. Third, adequate and appropriate medication should be given to bring the disturbance under control as quickly as possible, but with care taken not to induce overdose. A later response may need to be a review of staff training and procedures.

Dual diagnosis

Every type of psychiatric illness known to the textbooks may at some time or other be the diagnosis accompanying a drinking problem, and there are again here important questions for treatment services organization (Drake et al., 1998). In Chapter 21, a case is described of a patient with a drinking problem and schizophrenia, illustrating the need for alertness to these kinds of joint presentations. Here, let us briefly sketch three variations on the dual diagnosis theme.

A 40-year-old lawyer was persuaded by his colleagues to seek help because they thought his excessive drinking was making him unpredictable and bad tempered. At interview it became clear that he was in the hypomanic swing of a bipolar illness. His generally heavy background drinking was apt to go out of control during this kind of episode. With lithium instituted and his own decision that drinking was 'best cut out', he returned to practice.

A 35-year-old woman with her own home-based design consultancy was narrowly saved by her partner from death by hanging. Her family history showed a heavy loading, with both depressive illness and alcohol dependence, and she undoubtedly was suffering from both problems. She responded well to a maintenance antidepressant and accepted that she had to stop drinking.

A dental surgeon aged 50 came to disciplinary attention because he had been found to be injecting himself with diazepam obtained from his practice. Assessment revealed a long-standing drinking problem. He then began to talk about 'hearing voices'. Over the next few months, it became evident that he was developing a severe schizoaffective illness. The clinical course was stormy, with continued drinking. He had to cease practising.

Dual diagnosis is a common rather than an exceptional problem and services must be geared to cope with this fact (Moggi et al., 1999; Moos et al., 2000). Only if the psychiatric problem is treated will there be hope of therapeutic progress with the drinking problem. Chapter 8 discusses such matters in detail.

The 'very important patient'

Frequently, and despite every supposed personal advantage, the man or woman with a large public reputation is the person whose alcohol problem is likely to be mishandled. Because of the aura of prestige, no-one quite dares make the diagnosis or take a firm line. Phone calls are made in the middle of the night, a quick visit is demanded to a hotel room, and instead of a full history there is a superficial and interrupted conversation, and everything is a whispering game. Therapists may need considerable confidence to stand their ground when dealing with the demands and expectations of the tycoon, the politician, the famous actress, the judge or the distinguished surgeon, but, unless they are willing to hold to a therapeutic position, their patient will not be well served. Paradoxically, the rich and famous may be as much at hazard of receiving inadequate treatment as the drinker on Skid Row.

The key to dealing with such problems is to act with an awareness that this person, as much as the vagrant or any other patient who comes one's way, is indeed to an extent a 'special case'. However, at the same time one has to hold to the commonalities and the basic working rules of the therapeutic approach. These two ideas need to be discussed briefly and separately.

As regards the 'specialness' of this type of patient, the situation may be clouded by fear of public revelation. For instance, the politician will be concerned about the damage to their reputation and electoral chances from any rumour that they are an 'alcoholic'. Advice that they should attend AA, where their face will be recognized, may in these circumstances be impractical, and anxiety about the dangers of 'the newspaper getting hold of things' may consequently so dominate their thinking as to block every effort to help them. The truth of the matter can be that their drinking habits are already public knowledge and a known embarrassment to their colleagues – and news that they are getting help can only do good, not harm. The extent to which it is possible for someone in this position to admit publicly that they have had to deal with a drinking problem must vary from country to country and across professions. In the USA, for example, such openness is increasingly and beneficially possible (Hughes, 1997).

There are certain other rather typical features. The pressure under which such people are living and working can be extreme and engender a great deal of tension, with alcohol used as self-medication. Fear of failure may be potently linked to this stress, with an uncertain personal sense of worth and security despite every public success. The lifestyle may involve frequent entertaining and thus pressures to drink. Marriages are often under strain.

With this kind of patient, there may sometimes be difficulty in initiating effective therapy because the patient claims that they are too important to waste their time on treatment: there is a film to make, a business meeting to be attended on the other side of the world, an invitation to Downing Street which must take priority.

So much for a brief consideration of what may be 'special'. It must, however, be obvious that what has been instanced as special could be turned around and argued the other way. There is nothing unique about fear of public exposure, and it may affect the driver of the company car as well as the company president, while stress and fear of failure are common themes whatever the stratum from which patients are drawn. Although it is necessary to be alert to the intensity and clustering of certain factors that affect the 'special' patient, one is soon brought back to the need to hold on to the basics of the therapeutic approach. A full assessment must, for instance, be carried out, rather than the argument accepted that the patient is too busy for proper time to be given to this task. The formulation has to be discussed, the diagnosis agreed and goals appropriately set. Also, as always, the quality of the relationship is fundamental. At one level the encounter may be between public figure and psychiatrist or counsellor, but, more fundamentally, it is between a patient or client with a drinking problem and a person seeking as best possible to offer help.

All presentations are special presentations

Every presentation sketched out in this chapter might be met any day in clinical practice. We are not describing the exotic, but the extraordinary texture and variety of the common and ordinary. Good clinical practice in this arena is rooted in the capacity to respond flexibly to a vast spectrum of presentations, with the response fitted to very different needs and circumstances – one formula will never do.

REFERENCES

Advisory Council on the Misuse of Drugs (2000). *Reducing Drug-related Deaths*. London, The Stationery Office.

Bennett, L.A. and La Bonte, M. (1993) Family systems. In *Recent Advances in Alcoholism*, Vol. 11, *Ten Years of Progress*, ed. Galanter, M. New York: Plenum Press, 87–95.

Blane, H.T. (1993) Ethnicity. In *Recent Advances in Alcoholism*, Vol. 11. *Ten years of progress*, ed. Galanter, M. New York: Plenum Press, 109–23.

Breslau, N., Peterson, E., Schultz, L., Andreski, P. and Chilcoat, H. (1996) Are smokers with alcohol disorders less likely to quit? *American Journal of Public Health* 86, 985–90.

Brisbane, F.L. and Womble, M. (1985) *Treatment of Black Alcoholics*. New York: Haworth Press.

Collins, R.C. (1993) Sociocultural aspects of alcohol use and abuse: ethnicity and gender. In *Innovations in Alcoholism Treatment: State of the Art Reviews and their Implications for Clinical Practice*, ed. Connors, G.J. New York: Haworth Press, 89–116.

Drake, R.E., Mercer-McFadden, C., McHugo, G.J. et al. (eds) (1998) *Readings in Dual Diagnosis.* Columbia, MD: International Association of Psychological Rehabilitation Services.

Edwards, G. and Arif, A. (eds) (1980) *Drug Problems in Socio-Cultural Perspective.* Geneva: World Health Organization.

Fitzgerald, J.L. and Mulford, H.A. (1992) Elderly vs younger problem drinkers 'treatment' and recovery experience. *British Journal of Addiction* 87, 1281–91.

Graham, K., Leonard, K.E., Room, R. et al. (1998) Current directions in research on understanding and preventing intoxicated aggression. *Addiction* 93, 659–76.

Heath, D. (1993) Anthropology. In *Recent Advances in Alcoholism*, Vol. 11. *Ten years of progress*, ed. Galanter, M. New York: Plenum Press, 29–45.

Hinrichsen, J.J. (1984) Toward improving treatment services for alcoholics of advanced age. *Alcohol Health and Research World* 8, 31–9.

Hughes, H. (1997) Journal interview. *Addiction* 92, 137–49.

Janik, S.W. and Dunham, R.G. (1983) A nationwide examination of the need for specific alcoholism treatment programs for the elderly. *Journal of Studies on Alcohol* 44, 307–17.

Knight, R.G. and Longmore, B.E. (1994) *Clinical Neuropsychology of Alcoholism.* Hillsdale, NJ: Erbaum.

Koford, L.L., Tolson, R.L., Atkinson, R.M., Toth, R.L. and Turner, J.A. (1987) Treatment compliance of older alcoholics: an elder-specific approach is superior to a mainstreaming. *Journal of Studies on Alcohol* 48, 47–51.

Moggi, F., Ouimette, P.C., Finney, J.W. and Moos, R.H. (1999) Effectiveness of treatment for substance abuse and dependence for dual diagnosis patients: a mode of treatment factors associated with one year outcomes. *Journal of Studies on Alcohol* 60, 856–66.

Moos, R.H., Finney, J.W., Federman, E.B. and Suchinsky, R. (2000) Speciality mental health care improves patients' outcome: findings from a nationwide program to monitor the quality of care for patients with substance use disorders. *Journal of Studies on Alcohol* 61, 704–13.

Sherr, K.H. (1991) Psychological characteristics of children of alcoholics: overview of research methods and findings. In *Recent Advances in Alcoholism*, Vol. 9, *Children of Alcoholics*, ed. Galanter, M. New York: Plenum Press, 301–26.

13

Drinking problems and the life course

Meaning can be given to the phrase 'longitudinal perspective' through a presentation which took place at a postgraduate teaching forum. At this session, the decision was made to review a bundle of case notes from 20 years previously, and to use this material for discussion around issues of prognosis. A psychiatric registrar (resident) had gone through these notes and summarized the patient's case history as follows.

Mr A was aged 42 at the time of his admission to this hospital 20 years previously. His father had been an army officer, his mother had died young, and his childhood had been loveless and arid. After boarding school, he had been commissioned into his father's regiment and had for a time done well and been decorated for bravery. However, by his mid-thirties, his drinking was becoming notorious and he was faced with the choice of forced discharge or resignation. Back into civilian life and with a wife and two children to support, he went into a security business, which was soon insolvent. By the time of the hospital admission he had severe alcohol dependence and most aspects of his life were in ruin – he was separated from his family, heavily in debt and facing prosecution for financial irregularities. It was unclear whether he had a depressive illness, but he confessed to having at times strong suicidal ruminations and said, 'I wonder if I've always been depressed'. The last entry in the notes read, 'Removed from ward today by police on charge of fraud.'

The consultant chairing this clinical conference next invited a short presentation from another registrar on the literature dealing with prognosis in alcohol dependence (Lindquist, 1973; Gibbs and Flanagan, 1977; Edwards et al., 1988; Monahan and Finney, 1996). It was agreed that Mr A's life expectation would probably have been severely curtailed by his drinking (Marshall et al., 1994): it was all too likely that in a drunken state he would have acted out his suicidal fantasies. If, however, he had survived, it was probable that he would have continued to drink (Edwards et al., 1983). One of the nurses present offered the image of 'a shabby and maudlin habitué of a Chelsea pub cadging drinks off other people and still wearing his regimental tie'.

At 11 a.m. precisely, a well-dressed man entered the conference room and was introduced by the consultant chairing the meeting as his former patient. Mr A had recently got in touch by letter and wanted to express his personal thanks for the help and kindness he had received all those years back. He had not drunk since the day he left the ward and he gave a detailed, insightful account of recovery in terms not only of abstinence but also of changes within himself, changed relationships and a new marriage and the ability to love, and business success as creative fulfilment. He remembered acutely certain things which had been said to him on that hospital admission by the psychiatric registrar who was at that time on the firm: 'She said that I had a right to be depressed, don't know why, that was some kind of turning point'.

An abstract discussion of case notes transmuted into empathetic reality by a patient walking into a room is a special kind of event, which in acute and theatrical form makes a general point. Therapists working with drinking problems needs to cultivate a sense of the longitudinal play, to see their patients' lives not just in terms of the immediate clinical encounter and the immediate problems and anxieties, the snapshot, but also in terms of the moving picture show (Vaillant, 1983, 1995; Edwards, 1984, 1989; Ludwig, 1988). Whatever the statistics may say at the aggregate level, it is extraordinarily difficult to foretell at baseline what will have happened 20 years later to the individual person.

Research exists, however, which can support our understanding of the drinker's life course. There are literatures which deal with change and stability in drinking behaviour and problem experience within general populations (Cahalan et al., 1969; Cahalan, 1970; Cahalan and Room, 1974; Fillmore and Midanik, 1984; Fillmore, 1987a, 1987b). Valuable insights have come from follow-up studies on cohorts of subjects recruited not for their drinking but for some other purpose, but with the ensuing drinking behaviour then prospectively explored (McCord and McCord, 1960; Vaillant, 1983, 1995). Another type of study has dealt with the long-term follow-up of patients treated for their drinking problems (Taylor, 1994). Other work has focused specifically on mortality (Sundby, 1967; Marshall et al., 1994). This chapter gives an account of the core conclusions to be drawn from this research background in a statement which is necessarily selective rather than all-inclusive. With the research picture thus sketched, the final section returns to questions of how linkage is to be made between research findings and clinical insights.

Stability and change in drinking behaviour: the significance of general population surveys

Population surveys of drinking behaviour provide a context within which to understand what happens to clinical populations over time. There are likely to be differences between cultures and the sexes, but the general finding is that young people in their twenties are the section of the population who do a lot of drinking, frequently get drunk, and notch up a tally of often drunkenness-related drinking problems (Cahalan and Room, 1974). Their drinking patterns reflect the lifestyle, exuberance and irresponsibility of youth, and much which at the time looks like 'drinking pathology' will 10 years later be found to have ameliorated or faded away (Room, 1977). What is remarkable about this kind of behaviour is its flux rather than its fixity, but the dangers which can attach to youthful heavy drinking should not be ignored: what for the most part may appear to be no more than innocent experimentation and transient excess can carry enhanced risk of accident, trauma and death (Andréasson et al., 1988). Thus a balance should be struck between, on the one hand, an awareness that much drinking in the twenties can be seen as a stage of evolution towards more restricted and sensible drinking and, on the other, the realization that excessive drinking at this age can carry significant and age-related risk of accident (especially motor vehicle accident) and death by violence. What needs to be emphasized is that the drinking itself can carry risks, rather than the problem being defined solely in terms of detecting early signs of alcohol dependence.

What this body of research tends to show is that in middle age the prevalence and incidence of heavy drinking or drinking problems are less than in earlier decades, but the chronicity of problematic drinking at this age is greater (Fillmore, 1987a). Fewer people are now drinking heavily, but those who do so are more likely to go on doing so rather than moving casually in and out of the problem-drinking sector of experience. The explanation is no doubt in part that, at this phase in the life course, the significance of alcohol's dependence potential is becoming manifest.

The question has also been examined as to whether surrounding changes in society will influence evolution in drinking, so that cohorts recruited and followed over different time periods might show different patterns of change. By and large, the age effect appears to be dominant and generalizable whatever the population studied (Fillmore, 1987a).

Alcohol dependence: the long-term outcome

Percentage achieving abstinence and the stability of abstinence

Here, different samples recruited at different times and followed up for different periods show widely varying outcomes. Much must depend on sample character-istics, the outcome definition which is employed and completeness of follow-up (Vaillant, 1995). Less is known about female than male drinkers. Reported rates of abstinence have varied from a high of 64% in a Norwegian sample at 20–35-year follow-up (Sundby, 1967), to 13% in a Norwegian 10-year study (Bratfos, 1974). Most, but not all, reports describe an intermediate category of 'social' or 'asymptomatic' drinking lying between abstinence and continued problemtatic drinking. These subjects are probably a mix of patients who were never severely dependent, those who are sliding towards relapse, and those drinking with lowered tolerance to alcohol (Edwards et al., 1983, 1986). That drinkers interviewed at follow-up do not necessarily tell the truth is a fact which has sometimes been overlooked (Edwards, 1985), with consequently inflated estimates of 'return to normal drinking'.

Research suggests that over the course of any one follow-up year, there will be considerable movement of subjects between abstinence and troubled drinking, with individual patterns gradually becoming more stable over time (Taylor, 1994). Two or 3 years after initial treatment contact, it will be possible to identify a sub-group of patients whose abstinence is likely to remain stable in the long term. There will also be a group of patients whose troubled drinking is relentlessly continuous.

First seen 25 years previously on an alcohol treatment unit, a doctor saw this now 70-year-old patient again for a consultation on a general hospital ward. The original notes had described him as 'blaming everyone but himself'. A quarter of a century later, he complained about 'everyone letting him down'. His alcohol intake was now restricted because of physical illness and lack of resources, but after a stroke he still continued to drink to staggering incapacity as often as his welfare payments would allow.

Alcohol dependent patients do not necessarily 'mature out of dependence', even after many years (Vaillant, 1995).

Recovery from the drinking problem is generally, but not universally, associated with consequent improvement in health, social functioning and quality of life (Duckitt et al., 1985; Vaillant, 1995). 'Good outcome' among severely dependent drinkers more often involves a degree of dysjunction between stopping drinking and in improvement in health and adjustment (Taylor et al., 1986), but there are many subjects who have dealt with severe dependence and have gone on to establish a resoundingly positive life adjustment.

Within all this human variation, any statement on 'average' outcome expectations must be guarded. With that proviso underlined, it is likely that if 100 patients treated for alcohol dependence who were aged 45 at the intake point were followed for 20 years, about 40% would have died by the 20-year anniversary (Box 13.1).

BOX 13.1 **Likely overall long-term outcome**

For patients entering treatment at an average age of 45 years and followed for 20 years, division between outcome categories will be approximately thus:

- 40% dead
- 30% still drinking destructively
- 30% in stable abstinence or drinking moderately without trouble

Depending on the study cohort, alcohol dependent subjects have about a 3.3–5.6 times excess mortality compared with age-matched controls, and excess mortality is probably greater among more dependent drinkers (Rossow and Amundsen, 1997; Finney and Moos, 1991, 1992; Marshall et al., 1994; Öjesjö et al., 1998), and among younger drinkers attending for treatment (Banks et al., 2000). In a Finnish study, excess mortality was correlated with lower socio-economic status (Mäkelä, 1999). Of the remaining subjects, over 30% will still be experiencing continued or intermittent trouble with their drinking and rather less than 30% will be abstinent or engaging in trouble-free drinking. An impaired social support network may be a factor contributing to excess mortality among dependent drinkers (Lewis et al., 1995).

In his most recent report on a study in which he followed up an inner-city cohort of men with drinking problems for 20 years and a parallel group of Harvard graduates with drinking problems for 30 years, Vaillant found some outcome differences between the two samples (Vaillant, 1996b). At follow-up, college subjects were more frequently still engaging in problem drinking than the core city men (59% versus 28%). There were also, however, some important commonalities: after 5 years of maintained sobriety, relapse was unlikely, return to controlled drinking without further trouble was not common, while a further and dominant common feature was the fact that, in many instances and whichever the cohort, disruptive drinking continued remorselessly over the years.

Alcohol dependence: what aids recovery in the long term?

Researchers have found it difficult to identify any strong and consistent baseline pointers to favourable long-term outcome (Lindquist, 1973; Gibbs and Flanagan, 1977; Edwards et al., 1988). Conventional wisdom has it that the patient with better initial social support, less severe dependence and more stable personality will do better than the subject who is not so favoured, but it would be difficult to find conclusive research support for that assertion. There may well be different significant baseline pointers for different subgroups, and in particular for the more and less dependent subjects. In some circumstances, severe baseline dependence and severe problems may actually constitute a favourable prognostic pointer because continued drinking for that person is becoming too punishing (Edwards, et al., 1988).

Besides the none-too-fruitful attempt to identify prognostic indicators, investigators have also examined the change processes which over the long term are associated with achievement and maintenance of sobriety – an attempt, as it were, to understand the dynamics of recovery. The strongest conclusion must be that there is no single pathway to recovery and that people find many different individual paths out of drinking. With the crucial fact of variation stressed (100 different drinkers will have 100 unique life stories), certain recurrent findings can be seen as emerging from research (Vaillant, 1983; Edwards et al., 1987, 1992), and these findings are summarized below (see also Box 13.2).

> BOX 13.2 **Alcohol dependence: what influences recovery in the long term**
> - *Baseline patient characteristics*: It is difficult to identify consistent baseline pointers significant for recovery in the longer term.
> - *Accepting an appropriate treatment goal*: For severe dependence, abstinence is likely to be the appropriate goal, but not always or necessarily so for lesser degrees of dependence.
> - *Treatment and AA involvement* can significantly help recovery in terms of pointing up, nurturing and nudging along the potential for self-determined change.
> - *'Natural processes of recovery'* are of vital importance to initiation and support of sobriety. Treatment must work in sensible alliance with these processes.

Acceptance of the abstinence goal

Recovery from severe alcohol dependence almost inevitably involves personal acceptance of an abstinence goal. Without that crucial cognitive shift, the individual will struggle on and on self-defeatingly against the odds. Insight may come from the buffeting of experience, from what is heard at an Alcoholics Anonymous (AA) meeting, or from professional advice. The importance of goals and goal-setting is obvious but easily forgotten.

Trigger or 'Damascus' events

A frequent story given by recovered drinkers is that they owe their sobriety to a memorable and emotionally laden event which for them constituted a turning point (Tuchfield, 1981). Here is such an instance as reported in a 10-year follow-up study (Edwards et al., 1992).

> . . . a place in Ireland called Knock where the Virgin appeared . . . I visited the place, atmosphere, and I knew I would never drink again or smoke.

Events as trivial as being teased in the street for a dishevelled appearance, or as major as drunken carelessness causing the death of a child, illustrate a spectrum of happenings which drinkers may see as responsible for their abrupt and permanent switch towards sobriety. Both negative and positive life events may be precursors to the achievement of sobriety (Edwards et al., 1992). Many other similar events occurring over time will be without impact or produce only a brief false dawn. Furthermore, attribution should not be confused with cause. Although a 'Damascus' event may stand out in an individual's memory as the unique and immediate cause of a radical change in drinking behaviour, it is more likely that such an event will have triggered or supported cognitive processes which were the preparatory background to a change finally precipitated by the acute event. The personal reality of this kind of event and the potential significance of such phenomena for processes of recovery do, however, suggest that the therapist should be aware of their possible occurrence and be ready therapeutically to capitalize on these events when they occur (see Chapter 17).

The consolidation of sobriety

As emphasized above, although dramatic events may assist or precipitate change, sobriety is usually best conceived as something built and secured over time rather than as a state achieved on a particular day (Moos et al., 1990). Important questions therefore attach to the understanding of what in the individual's life may most effectively support sobriety. In sum, research suggests that sobriety is most likely to be held onto in the longer term when the sober state is felt to be rewarding. The negative reinforcement relating to the possible pains of any further drinking are not as potent as the enhancement in quality of life which can stem from what AA calls 'contented sobriety' (Vaillant, 1983; Edwards et al., 1992). A prime example of this kind of positive influence is the reward which can come from a loving relationship and the discovery of a capacity for altruism, and an ability to give to other people is often associated with the achievement of sobriety. Meaningful employment, energies put into creating a business, hobbies, home-making, house decoration, further educational involvements and enjoyment of holidays provide additional examples of the kinds of activity which can provide substitution for rewards previously found only in drinking (Chapter 17).

One may suspect that the final arrival of a stable and rewarding sobriety after many years of turmoil will also quite often be related to processes of psychological maturation (Vaillant, 1977). People who experience drinking problems are likely as the years go by to undergo the same kinds of maturations and life-cycle changes as other people, albeit perhaps delayed or overlaid by the drinking. Maturation may make sobriety more possible and the continuing destructiveness of drinking less bearable. Within this complex lies the intangible reality of what some people will want to call the growth of spiritual awareness. To shut off that aspect of people's lives when trying to understand processes of recovery is unwise, but that does not imply any likely benefit from moralizing at the drinker.

What the long-term perspective suggests about the significance of treatment or AA involvement

Long-term research gives messages which are by no means nihilistic in terms of the contribution treatment can make to recovery from alcohol dependence. However, within this kind of timeframe, treatment takes its place as one kind of interactive influence within the play of many other self-determined, other-determined and accidental forces. As with the case conference example with which this chapter opened, there is evidence that many years later people will remember 'what a psychiatrist said or did' or the intervention of some other professional as being significantly related to recovery (Edwards et al., 1987). It is the nudging of the person towards a more constructive way of seeing things, the encouragement of self-actualization and the enhancement of self-efficacy, help with choice of appropriate goal, the alliance between therapeutic intervention and natural processes of change which research suggests are in the long term the most potent contributions which treatment can make to recovery. There is no evidence that intensive psychotherapy aids long-term recovery (Vaillant, 1983). Research also again points to the reality of between-person variation: what one person takes from therapy may be different from someone else's gain. Treatment is in retrospect likely to be seen as having been more influential by the more dependent sector of drinkers (Edwards et al., 1987).

As regards the long-term significance of AA involvement in the achievement and stabilization of recovery (Edwards, 1996), the impact of AA on drinking behaviour is notoriously difficult to assess in any controlled sense and even in the short term (see Chapter 18). Long-term research in this arena provides more hints than firm conclusions. Within a British sample at a 10-year follow-up point, about one-third of alcohol dependent patients spoke positively of some aspect of AA involvement: 'hearing other people's stories at AA' and 'friendship through AA' were for these people particularly favoured elements, whereas the religious element in AA rated relatively low (Edwards et al., 1987). Also, degree of dependence enters the equation once more here, with evidence that it is the more dependent subjects who will probably find AA more helpful in the long term.

Recovery without treatment

There is an expanding literature on so-called 'spontaneous' or 'natural' recovery from alcohol and other drug problems (Sobell et al., 2000; Klingemann, 2001). Neither of those terms is altogether satisfactory. At the end of the day, every recovery is made by the individual concerned and is 'natural' to that person's capacities and choice, and at the same time probably every recovery is influenced by cues and context rather than being 'spontaneous' in an out-of-a-clear-blue-sky kind of way (Tuchfield, 1981). That said, it is important to note that many troubled drinkers never contact, or break from contact, with treatment agencies and AA, and yet recover. If the events and processes around those sorts of recovery were to be better understood, they might offer insights into how formal interventions could be better attuned to patient need. The issue goes wider than alcohol (Stall and Biernacki, 1986).

Some idea about the likely outcome for problem drinkers over time can be found in a recently published US study (Timko et al., 2000). These researchers took into their study a large group of previously untreated subjects from the community who were identified as having drinking problems. At 8-year follow-up, 17% had contacted neither AA nor a treatment agency, 15% had been in contact with AA only, 16% had been in contact only with an agency, whereas the largest proportion (52%) had been in contact with both AA and an agency. Those results will reflect the availability of AA and treatment facilities in the geographical area of the study and would not necessarily generalize to other epochs or locations. Indeed, in another American study (Dawson, 1996), lower rates for entry into treatment were found, with only 42% of men and 36% of women with a DSM-IV diagnosis of alcohol dependence entering treatment over a 30-year period.

It seems likely that recovery without treatment can occur in drinking problems of any degree or severity, but is less likely the more severe the problem (Cunningham, 1999; Timko et al., 1999). Causation should not be unquestioningly assumed, but people who go into treatment or affiliate to AA have higher recovery rates than those who try to manage on their own, and getting into treatment earlier is associated with a better prognosis than later-stage enrolment (Timko et al., 1999).

Research evidence and clinical insight

In the paragraphs above, the attempt has been to summarize findings about what happens to drinkers as the years go by, and the parallel findings about what explains the observable changes and transitions. The importance of the clinical sensitivity which can be developed from taking the life-course view of dependence is now brought into focus in this final section of the chapter.

The insights for therapy which can be derived from this long-term view can be ordered under two headings. First there is the benefit which comes from the pervasive impact on the therapeutic position once we comprehend the significance of the truth that our interventions, although often valuable, are part of a longer, broader play (Vaillant, 1988, 1996a, 1996b; Sobell et al., 1991). That view is an antidote to therapeutic arrogance and any tendencies towards a belief in our omnipotence. Therapy does matter and can contribute, but only insofar as the therapist respects, is intrigued by and cultivates awareness of how patients themselves effect change in the context of their ongoing lives. Another aspect of this kind of broad perspective-setting which derives from the longitudinal view is the impact that long-term follow-up data may properly be expected to have on the therapist's personal balance of optimism. On the one hand, the data show that alcohol dependence is a potentially destructive condition, and awareness of the multiple threats which are posed by this condition should never be staled by familiarity. An equally fair conclusion is, however, that dependence is recoverable and that no-one should ever be discarded because of presumed unfavourable baseline prognostic loadings. For patient and therapist alike, there is never any reason not to try, and to deny anyone the possibility of help is wrong.

The second summary heading on clinical relevance relates to the more point-by-point application of this perspective to treatment strategies. What may be profitably emphasized again here is the importance of proposing the appropriate drinking goal, willingness therapeutically to exploit naturally occurring potential change points, the awareness that recovery is process rather than event, the willingness to encourage and support strategies such as substitution of positive and rewarding activities, and the awareness that rather than there being any one unique pathway to recovery there are different paths for different people. The therapist's job is that of assisting each patient to identify their own pathway to recovery and find the means to stay on course.

REFERENCES

Andréasson, S., Romelsjö, A. and Allebeck, P. (1988) Alcohol and mortality among young men: longitudinal study of Swedish conscripts. *British Medical Journal* 296, 1021–5.

Banks, S.M., Pandiani, J.A., Schacht, L.M. and Gauvin, L.M. (2000) Age and mortality among white male problem drinkers. *Addiction* 95, 1249–54.

Bratfos, O. (1974) *The Course of Alcoholism, Drinking, Social Adjustment and Health.* Oslo: Universitets Forlaget.

Cahalan, D. (1970) *Problem Drinking: a National Survey.* San Francisco: Jossey Bass.

Cahalan, D., Cisin, I.H. and Crossley, H.M. (1969) *American Drinking Practices: a National Survey of Behaviour and Attitudes.* Monograph No. 6. New Brunswick, NJ: Rutgers Center for Alcohol Studies.

Cahalan, D. and Room, R. (1974) *Problem Drinking Among American Men.* New Brunswick, NJ: Rutgers Center for Alcohol Studies.

Cunningham, J.A. (1999) Resolving alcohol-related problems with and without treatment: the effects of different problem criteria. *Journal of Studies on Alcohol* 60, 463–6.

Dawson, D.A. (1996) Gender differences in the probability of alcohol treatment. *Journal of Substance Abuse* 8, 211–25.

Duckitt, A., Brown, D., Edwards, G., Oppenheimer, E., Sheehan, M. and Taylor, C. (1985) Alcoholism and the nature of outcome. *British Journal of Addiction* 80, 171–83.

Edwards, G. (1984) Drinking in longitudinal perspective: career and natural history. *British Journal of Addiction* 79, 175–83.

Edwards, G. (1985) A later follow-up of a classic case series: D.L. Davies's 1962 report and its significance for the present. *Journal of Studies on Alcohol* 46, 181–90.

Edwards, G. (1989) As the years go rolling by. Drinking problems in the time dimension. *British Journal of Psychiatry* 154, 18–26.

Edwards, G. (1996) Alcoholics Anonymous as mirror held up to nature. In *Psychotherapy, Psychological Treatments and the Addictions*, ed. Edwards, G. and Dare, C. Cambridge: Cambridge University Press.

Edwards, G., Brown, D., Duckitt, A., Oppenheimer, E., Sheehan, M. and Taylor, C. (1986) Normal drinking in a recovered alcohol addict. *British Journal of Addiction* 81, 127–37.

Edwards, G., Brown, D., Duckitt, A., Oppenheimer, E., Sheehan, M. and Taylor, C. (1987) Outcome of alcoholism: the structure of patient attributions as to what causes change. *British Journal of Addiction* 82, 533–45.

Edwards, G., Brown, D., Oppenheimer, E., Sheehan, M. and Taylor, C. (1988) Long-term outcome for patients with alcohol problems: the search for predictors. *British Journal of Addiction* 83, 917–27.

Edwards, G., Duckitt, A., Oppenheimer, E., Sheehan, M. and Taylor, C. (1983) What happens to alcoholics in the long term? *Lancet* ii, 269–71.

Edwards, G., Oppenheimer, E. and Taylor, T. (1992) Hearing the noise in the system. Exploration of textual analysis as a method for studying change in drinking behaviour. *British Journal of Addiction* 87, 73–81.

Fillmore, K.M. (1987a) Prevalence, incidence and chronicity of drinking patterns and problems among men as a function of age: a longitudinal and cohort analysis. *British Journal of Addiction* 82, 77–83.

Fillmore, K.M. (1987b) Women's drinking as compared to men's: a longitudinal analysis. *British Journal of Addiction* 82, 801–11.

Fillmore, K.M. and Midanik, L. (1984) Chronicity of drinking problems among men: a longitudinal and cohort analysis. *Journal of Studies on Alcohol* 45, 228–36.

Finney, J.W. and Moos, R.H. (1991) The long-term course of treated alcoholism. I. Mortality, relapse and remission rates and comparisons with community controls. *Journal of Studies on Alcohol* 52, 44–54.

Finney, J.W. and Moos, R.H. (1992) The long-term course of treated alcoholism. II. Prediction and correlates of 10-year functioning and mortality. *Journal of Studies on Alcohol* 53, 142–53.

Gibbs, L. and Flanagan, J. (1977) Prognostic indicators of alcoholism treatment outcome. *International Journal of Addiction* 12, 1097–141.

Klingemann, H. (2001) Natural recovery from alcohol problems. In *International Handbook of Alcohol Dependence and Problems*, ed. Heather, N., Peters, T.J. and Stockwell, T. Chichester: John Wiley and Sons, 649–62.

Lewis, C.E., Smith, E., Kercher, C. and Spitznagel, E. (1995) Predictions of mortality in alcoholic men: a 20-year follow-up study. *Alcoholism: Clinical and Experimental Research* 19, 984–91.

Lindquist, G.A.R. (1973) Alcohol dependence. *Acta Psychiatrica Scandinavica* 49, 332–40.

Ludwig, A.M. (1988) *Understanding the Alcoholic's Mind: the Nature of Craving and how to Control it*. New York: Oxford University Press.

Mäkelä, P. (1999) Alcohol-related mortality as a function of socio-economic status. *Addiction* 94, 867–86.

Marshall, E.J., Edwards, G. and Taylor, C. (1994) Mortality in men with drinking problems: a 20-year follow-up. *Addiction* 89, 1293–8.

McCord, W. and McCord, J. (1960) *Origins of Alcohol*. Stanford: Stanford University Press.

Monahan, S.C. and Finney, J.W. (1996) Explaining abstinence rates following treatment for alcohol abuse: a quantitative synthesis of patient, research design and treatment effects. *Addiction* 91, 787-805.

Moos, R.H., Finney, J.W. and Cronkite, E. (1990) *Alcoholism Treatment: Context, Process and Outcome*. New York: Oxford University Press.

Öjesjö, L., Hagnell, O. and Otterbeck, L. (1998) Mortality in alcoholism among men in the Lundby community cohort, Sweden: a forty year follow-up. *Journal of Studies on Alcohol* 59, 140–5.

Room, R. (1977) Measurement and distribution of drinking patterns and problems in general populations. In *Alcohol Related Disabilities*, ed. Edwards, G., Moser, J., Gross, M., Keller, M. and Room, R. WHO Offset Publication No. 32. Geneva: WHO, 61–8.

Rossow, I. and Amundsen, A. (1997) Alcohol abuse and mortality: a 40-year prospective study of Norwegian conscripts. *Social Science and Medicine* 44, 261–7.

Sobell, L.C., Sobell, M.B. and Toneatto, T. (1991) Recovery from alcohol problems without treatment. In *Self Control and the Addictive Behaviors*, ed. Heather, N., Miller, W.R. and Greeley, J. New York: Pergamon, 198–242.

Sobell, L.C., Ellingstad, T.P. and Sobell, M.B. (2000) Natural history from alcohol and drug problems: methodological review of the research with suggestions for future directions. *Addiction* 95, 749–64.

Stall, R. and Biernacki, P. (1986) Spontaneous remission from the problematic use of substances: an inductive model derived from a comparative analysis of the alcohol, opiate, tobacco, and food/obesity literatures. *The International Journal of the Addictions* 21, 1–23.

Sundby, P. (1967) *Alcoholism and Mortality*. Oslo: Universitets Forlaget.

Taylor, C. (1994) What happens over the long term? In *Alcohol and Alcohol Problems*, ed. Edwards, G. and Peters, T.J. British Medical Bulletin Vol. 50. Edinburgh: Churchill Livingstone, 50–60.

Taylor, C., Brown, D., Duckitt, A., Edwards, G., Oppenheimer, E. and Sheehan, M. (1986) Alcoholism and the patterning of outcome: a multivariate analysis. *British Journal of Addiction* 81, 815–23.

Timko, C., Moos, R.H., Finney, J.W. and Lesar, M.D. (2000) Long-term outcome of alcohol use disorders: comparing untreated individuals with those in Alcoholics Anonymous and formal treatment. *Journal of Studies on Alcohol* 61, 529-40.

Timko, C., Moos, R.H., Finney, J.W., Moos, B.S. and Kaplowitz, M.S. (1999) Long-term treatment careers and outcomes of previously untreated alcoholics. *Journal of Studies on Alcohol* 60, 437–47.

Tuchfield, B.S. (1981) Spontaneous remission in alcoholics: empirical observations and theoretical implication. *Quarterly Journal of Studies on Alcohol* 42, 626–41.

Vaillant, G.E. (1977) *Adaptation to Life*. Boston: Little Brown.

Vaillant, G.E. (1983) *The Natural History of Alcoholism*. Cambridge, MA: Harvard University Press.

Vaillant, G.E. (1988) What can long-term follow-up teach us about relapse and prevention of relapse in addiction? *British Journal of Addiction* 83, 1147–57.

Vaillant, G.E. (1995) *The Natural History of Alcoholism Revisited.* Cambridge, MA: Harvard University Press.

Vaillant, G.E. (1996a) Addiction over the life course: therapeutic implications. In *Psychotherapy, Psychological Treatments and the Addictions,* ed. Edwards, G. and Dare, C. Cambridge: Cambridge University Press, 3–18.

Vaillant, G.E. (1996b) A long-term follow-up of male alcohol abuse. *Archives of General Psychiatry* 53, 243–9.

II

Screening, assessment and treatment

14

Case identification and screening

Excessive drinking is frequently and in many settings overlooked. Only about a quarter of 'high-risk' or 'excessive' drinkers are correctly identified by primary care physicians (Wallace and Haines, 1985; Reid et al., 1986). Even in the hospital setting, where one might imagine more time was available for enquiry and investigation, the problem often goes unrecognized (Farrell and David, 1988; Canning et al., 1999). The detection rate in the social work setting has not been adequately investigated, but there can be little doubt that the contribution made by drinking to all manner of social presentations is passed by. Every therapist needs to cultivate a more alert eye, and aim at earlier and more complete diagnosis. If the element of drinking is allowed to remain hidden, it will defeat our plans to help that patient or client. The 'depression' will not respond to the prescribed antidepressant, a stomach ulcer will fail to heal, a family's situation will deteriorate, and we will be left puzzled and frustrated. Treatment which is blind to the drinking problem may indeed do actual harm rather than simply fail in its goal, whereas early diagnosis which can lead to help before dependence is advanced, or irreversible damage established, is very much in the patient's best interests.

This chapter looks at the barriers to the detection and diagnosis of drinking problems and considers ways in which rates of detection may be enhanced. Special consideration is also given to the use of laboratory tests and questionnaires in screening and diagnosis.

Why the diagnosis is frequently missed

There are various reasons why drinking problems so often remain under cover, and several of these reasons may conspire together. They can be listed as follows.

Not knowing what is being looked for

Diagnosticians may only be attuned to looking for alcohol dependence or the extreme case (with their ideas even on these presentations no more than vaguely formed), but with no real knowledge of the many different types of alcohol-related problems which may be daily impinging on their work. They must be familiar with the common diagnostic clues. Neither alcohol dependence nor alcohol-related problems necessarily declare themselves in direct terms, and the shrewd diagnostician has to be familiar with the wide range of signs and symptoms (physical, psychological and social) which can hint at the underlying drinking problem.

Lack of vigilance

The possibility of a drinking problem should always be borne in mind, for otherwise even the person who is armed with all the necessary book learning is at risk of missing the obvious case (Farrell and David, 1988).

Embarrassment at asking questions

The therapist may experience a certain degree of social inhibition in asking about drinking problems, very much related to society's general difficulty in facing up to such matters (Thom and Téllez, 1986). This may be especially so if the doctor knows the patient socially.

Not knowing what to do if the case is uncovered

If therapists lack confidence in their ability to respond to a drinking problem, if and when it is uncovered, they may be reluctant to make enquiries which threaten to put them in an uncomfortable position.

The patient's denial or evasion

A patient who is ashamed of their drinking will have difficulty in bringing the problem forward, perhaps especially so if the patient is a woman. That difficulty will only be overcome if the therapist can convey the message that no-one is sitting in judgement. It must be safe to talk.

These five subheadings together point to a need for investment in relevant professional training, by educators who are themselves close to the realities of practice.

Enhancing recognition rates

The headings above, which outline common reasons for failure in recognition, point to how the barriers to diagnosis need to be overcome. The practical business of diagnosis will be aided by consideration of the following issues.

The use of disarming questions

It is useful to have as one's personal stock-in-trade a few disarming questions about drinking problems which can be fed into any history-taking in almost throwaway fashion. The scene is often best set by a casual introductory remark, such as, 'I always ask everyone about drinking – it can be important to feel that one can talk about one's drinking without being got at'. The implication is that it is routine to question in this area, rather than the patient being singled out as a special case, and this is coupled with an immediate indication that anything the patient reveals will be sympathetically heard. The questions which follow are then usually best phrased in very open terms, for instance, 'Tell me, have you ever been worried about your drinking? Ever? In any way? I mean, has it led to any rows or troubles at home or at work? Health troubles? Ever thought you ought to cut down? Anyone criticized your drinking?'

Questions which thus feel out the possibility of worry or trouble are more likely to provide a way into fruitful dialogue than mechanistic questions along such lines as 'How much do you drink?'. The latter type of interrogation does not immediately reach across barriers towards what the patient is feeling and experiencing. It is too readily deflected by a bland answer, such as 'Just socially'. But if the preliminary questions about worries and troubles suggest that enquiry has to be taken further, it is then essential to construct the outlines of a 'typical drinking day' (see Chapter 15) and go fully into quantity and frequency of drinking.

Remembering who may be specially at risk

To bear in mind a list of who may be especially at risk is useful, provided the therapist does not as a result become blinkered to the wider truth that drinking problems can affect both sexes and, either directly or indirectly, people of any age and every occupation. With that proviso, an awareness of particular occupational hazard is then important (see Chapter 2). The single person, the separated or divorced, those who are considered to be at risk of suicide, and the recently bereaved also go in this 'at-risk' list. Certain ethnic groups are more at risk of drinking problems, with the Irish providing a familiar example. The person who is homeless and drifting might almost be presumed to have a drinking problem until proved otherwise.

Common social presentations

One should always be on the look-out for a hidden drinking problem with the client or patient who is frequently changing house, changing jobs or changing relationships. Family presentations are common – marital disharmony or family violence, the wife presenting with depression or the children with truanting, school failure, antisocial behaviour or neurotic symptoms. Criminal offences also suggest the need to ask about drinking.

Common psychiatric clues

Here, the essential background list derives from Chapters 7 and 8. In particular, one should be alert to the possibility of a drinking problem when the patient or client complains rather non-specifically of 'bad nerves', insomnia or depression. Phobic symptoms, pathological jealousy, paranoid symptoms and dementia or delirium may all at times be alcohol related. A drug problem may also often be associated with a drinking problem. A suicidal attempt or gesture always demands enquiry into drinking.

Common medical clues

An account of the medical complications of heavy drinking is given in Chapter 10. In practical terms, one should be particularly on the alert if a patient repeatedly asks for a 'certificate', is a frequent visitor to the doctor's office on a Monday morning, is suffering from malnutrition or obesity, is complaining of any gastrointestinal disorder or liver problem, has otherwise unexplained heart trouble, or presents with 'epilepsy' of late onset. Bruising may be a clue, or burns which have resulted from a cigarette being dropped on the skin while the drinker is intoxicated. Accidents of any sort may be alcohol related, and 20% of those involved in road traffic accidents may be classified as problem drinkers (Mayou and Bryant, 1995).

Not overlooking the obvious

The patient may declare the diagnosis by the smell of alcohol on their breath, by the bottle sticking out of their pocket, by their flushed face and bloodshot eyes, or by their tremor, but even the fact that they are obviously intoxicated can be overlooked if the possibility of drinking is not held in mind. The patient who makes jokes about their drinking should have those jokes taken seriously. Similarly, obvious presentations may be seen on a visit to the home: bottles and glasses lying around; decoration neglected and furniture reduced to a few sticks; the home may be a sad parody of a stage-set portraying decay. It would, however, be a mistake to think only in terms of such flagrant presentations and therefore overlook lesser clues.

Having a word with the spouse or partner

If there is any cause to suspect excessive drinking, a word privately with the spouse is essential, and particularly so if the patient says that 'the wife's too busy to come along'. It cannot be automatically assumed that the spouse will be ready and willing to talk about a family drinking problem; loyalty, fear of reprisal, embarrassment or a determined unwillingness to face up to the painful truth may all stand in the way.

Much the same sort of tactful and open questioning may therefore be needed as with the partner who is drinking.

Laboratory tests

Several laboratory tests are useful in the screening of clinical populations for possible drinking problems – within, for instance, a routine medical examination when staff are recruited or undergo annual health checks. These tests can also be confirmatory in the individual case when excessive drinking is suspected but has not been admitted. No one test by itself is of as much value as a battery of investigations, and it seems likely that a properly chosen array of tests should today detect over 80% of patients with an at least moderately severe drinking problem (Chan, 1990). A negative result does not rule out the possibility that excessive drinking has begun adversely to affect the individual's life, and false positives also occur. Laboratory tests therefore need to be interpreted shrewdly and no test results stand by themselves; they can only be read in the context of all the considerations that have been listed above.

Sensitivity and specificity

Before listing the individual tests that may be used, it is helpful to identify two characteristics of such tests which provide a guide to their usefulness in making a diagnosis. The *specificity* of a test is a guide to the extent to which a positive result is indicative of the condition of interest. In this case, the condition of interest may be heavy drinking, drinking problems or alcohol dependence, depending upon the circumstances and reasons for screening. A non-specific test for heavy drinking, for example, would show a positive result not just in heavy drinking, but also in a range of other unrelated disorders as well. The ideal test would be 100% specific, indicating that it only became positive as a result of heavy drinking. The *sensitivity* of a test indicates the extent to which it reliably detects every case of the condition of interest. For our present purpose, we would like a 100% sensitive test, which would always be positive, and never negative, in every case of heavy drinking, drinking problems or alcohol dependence (as appropriate).

To date, no one has devised a 100% specific and 100% sensitive test for heavy drinking, drinking problems or alcohol dependence. Different tests are more or less specific and more or less sensitive. The extent to which these tests will serve practical diagnostic needs depends upon the prevalence of heavy drinking, drinking problems or alcohol dependence in the population in which they are being used. In order to understand this better, let us consider a fictitious illustration.

A new test for heavy drinking, 'alcoholin' has 95% specificity and 60% sensitivity. It is used to screen 1000 apparently healthy employees at their annual medical review. Let us assume that 10% of these employees are actually drinking sufficient amounts of alcohol to be a cause for concern. How useful will the new test be?

Out of 1000 employees, 10% ($n = 100$) are drinking too much, and 60% of these ($n = 60$) will be correctly identified by the test as being 'heavy drinkers'. However, out of the whole group of 1000, 5% ($n = 50$) will be identified as positive due to non-specific (i.e. not alcohol related) results of the test. Therefore, a total of 110 people will be identified by the test, and only 60 of these (55%) will actually be drinking too much. The 'alcoholin' test is therefore of limited usefulness, and must be followed by other tests and by more detailed enquiries in order to confirm whether or not each of the individuals testing positive actually is drinking too much. Furthermore, 40 people who are drinking excessively will not be identified by the test.

The problems illustrated by this example become more severe the rarer is the disorder. Thus, if the prevalence of heavy drinking were only 1%, only one in nine of those who tested positive with the same test would actually be heavy drinkers. Conversely, if used in a population in which almost everyone had a drinking problem (say in an alcohol problems clinic), then more than nine out of ten of those who tested positive would be heavy drinkers.

Screening tests for heavy drinking

Let us now give consideration to the actual tests that are used to screen for heavy drinking. The most useful tests are as follows.

Mean corpuscular volume

This is a measure of the size of red blood cells, which may increase in response to heavy drinking. Sensitivity is 20–50% and specificity 55–100% (Conigrave et al., 1995). Mean corpuscular volume (MCV), if it has been elevated as a result of heavy drinking, will remain raised for several months after a reduction or cessation of alcohol consumption. This is because of the relatively long life of red blood cells (about 120 days).

Liver function tests

Serum gamma glutamyl transferase (GGT), serum aspartate aminotransferase (AST) and serum alanine aminotransferase (ALT) are all indicators of alcoholic hepatotoxicity, which may be elevated as a result of heavy drinking. Of these, GGT is generally considered to be the most useful as a screening test for heavy drinking. However, with a sensitivity of 20–90% and specificity of 55–100% (Conigrave et al., 1995), it is of debatable value in this role and its true usefulness has been questioned (Penn and Worthington, 1983). If GGT has been elevated due to drinking, it will fall again after abstinence is established. This is more rapid than the restoration of MCV, but may still take several weeks to return to normal, depending upon the level to which it has been raised. With more serious liver damage, other biochemical parameters, such as alkaline phosphatase and bilirubin, will also be altered and in such cases there may be enduring abnormalities of some enzyme levels, even after prolonged abstinence.

Carbohydrate-deficient (asialylated) transferrin

This is a variant of a serum protein which transports iron. Levels are increased in response to heavy drinking. Its sensitivity as a test of heavy drinking is probably about 60–70%, but may be less, and its specificity is about 95% (Conigrave et al., 1995; Godsell et al., 1995). Carbohydrate-deficient transferrin (CDT) is arguably better than most other tests, and it is now considered by some to be the best available screening test for heavy drinking. However, it is probably not much better than GGT.

Blood alcohol concentration

Blood alcohol concentration (BAC) returns to zero quickly with abstinence: in humans, the average rate of clearance of alcohol from the blood is 15 mg/100 ml per hour. This results in a fairly low sensitivity when used as a screening test for habitual heavy drinking. Depending upon the time and context of testing, as well as the threshold alcohol concentration used to define a positive result, moderate social drinkers will also be detected, thus making BAC fairly non-specific as well. Blood alcohol (or breath alcohol as an indirect measure) is therefore not often used as a screening test in the way that GGT or CDT may be used. However, BAC is known to be related to impairment of psychomotor performance and therefore provides a particularly valuable measure in the workplace, or in other safety-sensitive contexts such as driving. BAC may also have an underestimated utility as a screening test in the clinical setting (Wiseman et al., 1982).

Even if not used as a screening test, BAC may be a useful confirmatory investigation. A patient may say, for instance, that he 'only had a few drinks' the previous evening, but at 9 a.m. next morning he still has a blood alcohol level of, say, 60 mg/100 ml, suggesting much heavier consumption. The finding of a high BAC in the absence of evident intoxication suggests a high level of tolerance and is therefore important presumptive evidence for habitual heavy drinking.

Other tests

Although rarely used specifically as screening tests for heavy drinking, uric acid, cholesterol and a variety of other markers all show alterations in response to heavy drinking and may therefore be helpful indicators, particularly in combination with the results of other tests (Chan, 1990).

It will be apparent that none of the tests mentioned above offers improvement over the fictitious 'alcoholin' test. In fact, 'alcoholin' could easily be GGT or CDT. All these tests are limited in their usefulness as screening instruments and in some

Table 14.1 Advantages and disadvantages of different screening procedures

Procedure	Advantages	Disadvantages
Clinical interview	Flexibility Potentially high specificity Potential to detect cases that laboratory tests or questionnaires will miss	Subjectivity Dependent upon clinical skill and time/trouble taken Poor sensitivity if the subject is embarrassed or covering up Can be time consuming
Laboratory tests	Objective Quick and convenient for screening large numbers of subjects If positive, useful to monitor subsequent progress Detect heavy use/some tissue toxicity (e.g. liver/blood)	Limited sensitivity and specificity (CDT arguably best, but GGT not much worse) CDT is expensive (GGT much cheaper) Do not detect social/ psychological problems
Breath alcohol estimation	Objective Cheap and convenient Good for detecting drinking in safety-sensitive context (e.g. drinking and driving) Useful to confirm history and monitor progress	Rapid clearance of alcohol from the blood/breath limits sensitivity Detects alcohol use, not problems *per se* (i.e. poor specificity)
Questionnaires	Standardized and more objective than clinical interview Cheap and convenient	Subject to honesty of the respondent Limited sensitivity and specificity (but better than laboratory tests)

circumstances medical history and clinical signs will do better (Skinner et al., 1986). In one recent study, the calculated sensitivities of laboratory tests (including MCV, GGT and CDT) were so low (7–41%) as to lead the authors to the conclusion that they are of no value at all for screening for alcohol abuse or dependence in a primary care setting (Aertgeerts et al., 2001). However, the sensitivity and specificity of laboratory tests as screening instruments may be improved when they are used in combination. A profile of, for example, MCV, GGT, CDT and other biochemical tests is of considerably more value than any of these tests in isolation, (Table 14.1).

Diagnosis and monitoring

Laboratory tests may also prove useful in other situations. Comment has already been made regarding the usefulness of a confirmatory BAC in the clinical context. Similarly, laboratory tests can be helpful in confirming a diagnosis and, where there is clinical suspicion but initial denial from the patient, the feeding of test results into discussion may help the development of insight. Once an abnormal result on one of these tests has been identified, and assuming that this is attributable to heavy drinking, repeat measures over time can also be useful in monitoring clinical progress.

Reference ranges

When laboratory tests are employed in screening, diagnosis or clinical monitoring, the question arises as to what results might be considered 'normal'. The provision of an answer to this question is less simple than might be imagined. Firstly, for at least some tests, different laboratory conditions and methods will result in different results being obtained from identical specimens. Secondly, the 'normal' populations against which abnormal results are compared are in practice often not screened to exclude cases of heavy drinking, drinking problems or alcohol dependence. It is therefore more appropriate to talk about the 'reference range', rather than the 'normal range', for each test. For similar reasons, reference ranges often vary somewhat from one laboratory to another.

Table 14.2 provides a ready guide to the reference ranges for tests most commonly used in the screening, diagnosis, assessment and monitoring of patients with drinking problems.

Screening for drug misuse

A proportion of people with drinking problems will also be using other prescribed psychotropic drugs, 'over the counter' medicines or illicit drugs on a regular or intermittent basis (see Chapter 9). The pattern, dosage and manner of using these drugs may in themselves constitute a problem of drug misuse or dependence. Although it will not always be necessary to conduct screening for such problems, it may be appropriate to screen those at greatest risk and/or those who reveal signs or symptoms of other forms of drug misuse. A urine drug screen is the most appropriate investigation, and is readily available at most clinical pathology laboratories. It is usually appropriate to screen for a range of commonly misused drugs, including benzodiazepines, opioids, cannabinoids, cocaine and amphetamine. However, specialist advise may be required in respect of positive results, as prescribed medication, and even food ingredients, can cause a 'false-positive' result with some tests.

Table 14.2 Reference ranges for laboratory tests used in screening, assessment, diagnosis and monitoring of drinking problems

Test	Abbreviation	Reference range	Comments
Mean corpuscular volume	MCV	<92 fl	Most laboratories quote <96 fl, but reference ranges do not relate to abstinent subjects
Gamma glutamyl transferase	GGT	<50 IU/l	Many laboratories quote <60 IU/l or even higher upper limits
Alanine aminotransferase	ALT	<50 IU/l	
Aspartate aminotransferase	AST	<50 IU/l	
Bilirubin		3–20 mmol/l	
Carbohydrate-deficient transferrin	CDT	<5%	Some laboratories quote <6% The percentage form of the test is to be preferred to the absolute CDT level
Cholesterol		<5 mmol/l	<6 mmol/l often quoted Low-density lipoprotein (LDL) cholesterol may be a better indicator than total cholesterol
Uric acid		0.1–0.4 mmol/l	
Blood alcohol concentration	BAC	<5 mg/dl	In theory, BAC should clearly be 'zero' Many laboratories quote <5 mg/dl as 'negative' It is claimed that some individuals produce small amounts of endogenous alcohol by autofermentation in the bowel

Laboratory tests: an overall judgement

The overall judgement on the value of laboratory tests might therefore be that they are of assistance to therapist and patient if used with discrimination; in this field of practice there are skills to be learned in using this technology to best advantage.

Screening questionnaires

Numerous screening questionnaires have been devised which are intended to aid in the detection of heavy drinking or alcohol-related problems. The test which has been most widely researched for its reliability and validity is the 25-item Michigan Alcoholism Screening Test, or MAST (Selzer, 1971), which has also been published in a shorter 10-item form (Pokorny et al., 1972). The CAGE questionnaire is even briefer, containing only four items (King, 1986). These tests generally tend to pick up the more extreme rather than the early case. The MAST, for instance, has among its items delirium tremens and hospital admission for drinking. However, the screening questionnaires show remarkably good sensitivity and specificity, for 'excessive drinking' as well as 'alcoholism', and may be superior to laboratory tests when used as screening instruments (Bernadt et al., 1982).

Such instruments are therefore of value for routine screening, for example in a hospital setting (Bernadt et al., 1982), where there is a more or less captive population which is reasonably attuned to the idea of filling in questionnaires. Questionnaires may also be of value in primary care, although usefulness in this setting is more debatable (King, 1986). However, these tests in general have found more application as research tools than in the front-line medical and social settings, where a paper-and-pencil test provides no substitute for vigilance, sympathetic questioning and the very real skills needed for identifying drinking problems of all manner of degree, type and hiddenness.

In this context, the development of a more recent instrument, the Alcohol Use Disorders Identification Test (AUDIT), is of interest. The AUDIT was developed by an international group of investigators, at the request of the World Health Organization (Babor et al., 1989). It was designed for use by health care workers in developed and developing countries. It is useful in screening for both currently harmful and potentially hazardous drinking, shows good sensitivity and specificity and can identify mild dependence. Potentially, this is the screening questionnaire which should be of most future value to clinicians and researchers in primary care.

The AUDIT is administered as a brief (ten-item) structured interview or self-report questionnaire which includes questions about recent alcohol consumption (three items), alcohol-related problems (four items), and alcohol dependence (three items) (Babor et al., 1992). It is also available as an even briefer five-item questionnaire which has almost 80% sensitivity and 95% specificity in screening for hazardous alcohol intake and alcohol disorders (Piccinelli et al., 1997).

Screening in high-risk populations

In some circumstances, the identification of heavy drinkers and of those with drinking problems or alcohol dependence may be of such importance as to warrant a formal and systematic screening programme. Given the benefits of brief interventions for those who are drinking in a 'risky' fashion, this might occur in primary care (Babor and Higgins-Biddle, 2000). However, it will more frequently be seriously considered in settings in which there are particular safety considerations relating to the health-impairing and performance-impairing effects of alcohol, such as commercial transportation (Cook, 1997) and other areas of industry (Smith and Cook, 2000). In such circumstances, it will often be combined with a screening programme to test for use of other psychoactive drugs.

Screening might be considered as a routine prior to employment for new recruits, on a random basis for all employees, or following specific circumstances which might give cause for concern (e.g. accidents or other adverse incidents which might be alcohol related). In each case, it is important that there is a clear policy in place to govern how positive screening tests will be responded to. It is likely that the response will include a medical and an administrative component, and it should be made clear in the policy documents as to how these will inter-relate. For example, will opportunity be given for treatment and rehabilitation followed by a return to work? If so, what measures will be taken to ensure early detection of any relapse that might subsequently occur? Such screening programmes are surrounded by a minefield of ethical and legislative considerations, and occupational physicians, or others involved with them, are strongly advised to familiarize themselves with their statutory and professional responsibilities.

Choice of the most appropriate screening tools will need to take into account the considerations outlined above, in respect of the available questionnaires and laboratory and other tests. It will usually be the case that a combination of tools will be employed, so as to maximize the overall sensitivity and specificity of the screening programme. However, assuming that the prevalence of heavy drinking or drinking problems will actually be relatively low in most such populations, particular consideration must be given to the probability that positive test results will frequently be 'false positives'. This will least frequently be a problem when breath alcohol testing is employed to detect intoxication within a safety-sensitive context. It will most frequently be a problem when blood tests are used to screen for heavy drinking or drinking problems.

Screening for psychiatric co-morbidity

Assessment of patients with a suspected or confirmed drinking problem should also include consideration of the possibility of co-morbid psychiatric diagnosis (see Chapter 7). There are few blood tests which will assist in this process, and in practice even standardized questionnaires are of limited value. However, some questionnaires may be of assistance in routine use, including, for example, the

General Health Questionnaire (Goldberg, 1972). Patients should routinely be asked about their past or present contact with psychiatric services and about any treatment for psychiatric problems which they might have received from their primary care physician. In cases of high suspicion or concern, a referral to psychiatric services will always be the safest and best option.

Practical conclusions

The relative utility of the various procedures described above, for the detection and diagnosis of heavy drinking and drinking problems, is summarized in Table 14.1. To a large extent, their utility for detection and screening is determined by their sensitivity, and their utility for diagnosis depends upon their specificity. However, both parameters are important in both contexts. Cost, convenience and flexibility are also important.

There is no substitute for careful clinical enquiry as a means for detecting heavy drinking, drinking problems or alcohol dependence, either in specialist practice or in primary care or other generalist settings. Information gained in this way may valuably be supported by the discerning use of appropriate laboratory investigations, breath alcohol testing and questionnaires.

Where a large, healthy population must be screened, as, for example, in the occupational setting, even a brief clinical interview may not be possible and questionnaires are therefore advantageous. However, when the follow-through of detection includes disciplinary procedures or other adverse consequences, responses to questionnaires may not be reliable. In such circumstances, laboratory tests such as GGT, MCV or CDT can give useful information. Where ensurance of a safety-sensitive environment is of concern, such as drinking and driving or certain work settings, blood or breath alcohol testing may also constitute cost-effective technology.

REFERENCES

Aertgeerts, B., Buntinx, F., Ansoms, S. and Fevery, J. (2001) Screening properties of questionnaires and laboratory tests for the detection of alcohol abuse or dependence in a general practice population. *British Journal of General Practice* 51, 206–17.

Babor, T.F., de la Fuente, J.R., Saunders, J. and Grant, M. (1989) *AUDIT The Alcohol Use Disorders Identification Test: Guidelines for Use in Primary Health Care.* Geneva: World Health Organization.

Babor, T.F., de la Fuente, J.R., Saunders, J. and Grant, M. (1992) *AUDIT The Alcohol Use Disorders Identification Test: Guidelines for Use in Primary Health Care.* Geneva: World Health Organization.

Babor, T.F. and Higgins-Biddle, J.C. (2000) Alcohol screening and brief intervention: dissemination strategies for medical practice and public health. *Addiction* 95, 677–86.

Bernadt, M.W., Mumford, J., Taylor, C., Smith, B. and Murray, R.M. (1982) Comparison of questionnaire and laboratory tests in the detection of excessive drinking and alcoholism. *Lancet* 1, 325–8.

Canning, U.P., Kennell-Webb, S.A., Marshall, E.J., Wessely, S.C. and Peters, T.J. (1999) Substance misuse in acute general medical admissions. *Quarterly Journal of Medicine* 92, 319–26.

Chan, A.W.K. (1990) Biochemical markers for alcoholism. In *Children of Alcoholics*, ed. Windle, M. and Searles, J.S. New York: Guilford Press, 39–72.

Conigrave, K.M., Saunders, J.B. and Whitfield, J.B. (1995) Diagnostic tests for alcohol consumption. *Alcohol and Alcoholism* 30, 13–26.

Cook, C.C.H. (1997) Alcohol policy and aviation safety. *Addiction* 92, 793–804.

Farrell, M.P. and David, A.S. (1988) Do psychiatric registrars take a proper drinking history? *British Medical Journal* 296, 395–6.

Godsell, P.A., Whitfield, J.B., Conigrave, K.M., Hanratty, S.J. and Saunders, J.B. (1995) Carbohydrate deficient transferrin levels in hazardous alcohol consumption. *Alcohol and Alcoholism* 30, 61–6.

Goldberg, D. (1972) *The Detection of Psychiatric Illness by Questionnaire.* Maudsley Monograph No. 21. Oxford: Oxford University Press.

King, M. (1986) At risk drinking among general practice attenders: validation of the CAGE questionnaire. *Psychological Medicine* 16, 213–17.

Mayou, R. and Bryant, B. (1995) Alcohol and road traffic accidents. *Alcohol and Alcoholism* 30, 709–11.

Penn, R. and Worthington, D.J. (1983) Is serum gamma-glutamyltransferase a misleading test? *British Medical Journal* 286, 531–5.

Piccinelli, M., Tessari, E., Bortolomasi, M. et al. (1997) Efficacy of the alcohol use disorders identification test as a screening tool for hazardous alcohol intake and related disorders in primary care: a validity study. *British Medical Journal* 314, 420–4.

Pokorny, A.D., Miller, B.A. and Kaplan, H.B. (1972) The brief MAST: a shortened version of the Michigan alcoholism screening test. *American Journal of Psychiatry* 129, 342–5.

Reid, A.L.A., Webb, G.R., Hennrikus, D., Fahey, P.P. and Sanson-Fisher, R.W. (1986) Detection of patients with high alcohol intake by general practitioners. *British Medical Journal* 293, 735–8.

Selzer, M.L. (1971) The Michigan alcoholism screening test. *American Journal of Psychiatry* 127, 1653–8.

Skinner, H.A., Holt, S., Sheu, W.J. and Israel, Y. (1986) Clinical versus laboratory detection of alcohol abuse: the alcohol clinical index. *British Medical Journal* 292, 1703–8.

Smith, G. and Cook, C.C.H. (2000) Alcohol and drug misuse. In *Fitness for Work: the Medical Aspects.* 3rd edn, ed. Cox, R.A.F., Edwards, F.C. and Palmer, K. Oxford: Oxford University Press, 480–93.

Thom, B. and Téllez, C. (1986) A difficult business: detecting and managing alcohol problems in general practice. *British Journal of Addiction* 81, 405–18.

Wallace, P. and Haines, A. (1985) Use of a questionnaire in general practice to increase the recognition of patients with excessive alcohol consumption. *British Medical Journal* 290, 1949–53.

Wiseman, S.M., Tomson, P.V., Barnett, J.M., Jenns, M. and Wilton, J. (1982): Use of an alcometer to detect problem drinkers. *British Medical Journal* 285, 1087–90.

15

Assessment as the beginning of therapy

Case history as initiation of therapy

Taking a history from a patient should not be a matter only of obtaining facts to be written down in the case notes. It is an interaction between two people, and ought to be as meaningful for the person who answers the questions as for the questioner. The patient should be invited to use the occasion as a personal opportunity to review his or her past and present, and to make sense of what may previously have been a chaotic array of happenings. There is research evidence which demonstrates the potential power of the initial clinical encounter to change the drinker's attitudes, enhance commitment and clarify goals (Thom et al., 1992).

Assessment is therefore the beginning of therapy (Novey, 1968). The relationship between patient and therapist begins to be determined at this moment and, if the occasion is mishandled, the patient may not attend for a second appointment. A positive relationship has been shown between the perceived quality of the initial assessment and subsequent willingness to engage in treatment (Hyams et al., 1996).

This chapter seeks to cover practical issues related to the art and technique of history-taking. The earlier chapters have sought to lay out the general ground-work of understanding, and we now have to explore how that understanding is to be addressed to practical ends. The present chapter is cast in the form of a series of working guidelines. The framework builds on the general format for the psychiatric history-taking which has for many years been employed at the Maudsley Hospital, London (Departments of Psychiatry and Child Psychiatry, The Institute of Psychiatry and the Maudsley Hospital London, 1987). This assessment should be conducted in a carefully created setting which should make open self-appraisal possible.

History-taking is a rewarding aspect of therapeutic work, and the reader should not be daunted by the details of this presentation. Anyone coming to this type of work for the first time should not attempt to absorb everything that is being said here at one sitting.

With the format for the patient interview outlined, the chapter describes a parallel approach to history-taking from the spouse or 'significant other'. Tables provide a summary of the key points in history-taking, both for the person presenting with the problem and the spouse. Finally, a scheme for the construction of a case formulation is given.

Our concern here is with clinical interviewing. Structured approaches to the alcohol research interview are provided by relevant sections of the Diagnostic Interview Schedule (DIS: Griffin et al., 1987; McCrady et al., 1992), and the Structured Clinical Interview for DSM-III-R (SCID: Kranzler et al., 1996; Segal et al., 1994). Another widely used approach is the Comprehensive International Diagnostic Interview (CIDI: Cottler et al., 1989; Cottler and Compton, 1993; Comptom et al., 1996). A comparison of five types of diagnostic interview has been given by Hasin (1991).

Setting the tone

Handling the initial contact with someone who has a drinking problem does not stand entirely apart from work with any other type of patient, but it may have been especially difficult for this person to get so far as to recognize that they have a need for help, and then to keep the first appointment. To admit that they are not fully in control of their drinking can be felt by the patient to be admitting failure, and they may be highly ambivalent about walking into the consulting room.

It is therefore worthwhile for the therapist to ensure that they are not taking their own goodwill as self-evident. Special care must be put into showing ordinary courtesies: to walk up the corridor with the patient rather than five paces in front, to take a coat and hang it up, to show the person towards a comfortable chair are small but telling gestures. It may be useful to say, 'I'm glad you've decided to come, and I hope that this afternoon will be helpful for you'.

Case notes have to be recorded and a semi-structured approach is useful. There is a way of handling this procedure which makes it informal and unthreatening. The first question should always be something like, 'Tell me what it is that we should talk about'. There should then be a willingness to listen to the answer, while looking at the person who is talking. The answer may be discursive or brief, may bear on the drinking or deal with other issues, but the patient is setting the scene in the way that he or she finds helpful. It can be useful to explore the circumstances that have led to this appointment being made.

The therapist then has to introduce the fact that they are going to take a history. A statement such as the following can be made.

I've listened to what you are saying carefully. If you don't mind, it would help if I asked you some questions and made notes. I'm going to assume that all your answers are as honest and open as you can possibly make them. If there's anything too difficult to talk about, let me know, and I'll respect your feelings.

This might seem to be emphasizing the ordinary assumption of the therapeutic position in a way which is overdrawn. But if history-taking is clumsily handled and the initial relationship not sympathetically established, the interview will be interpreted as attack, and defences will rapidly be brought into play. The stereotype of the drinker as someone who 'never tells the truth' will have been confirmed. The disadvantages which stem from a neglect of the dynamic interactions of the initial interview are not only that the information obtained will probably be incomplete and inaccurate, but also that damage will be done to what should have been the initiation of therapy.

How much time for history-taking?

The scheme described in this chapter for the patient's history-taking envisages two parts to the reconstruction – the background history and the drinking history. To cover all the matters which lie in either area, and to conduct the interview at a pace which allows useful pauses and human interactions, clearly means that the process cannot be accomplished in a few minutes. The general practitioner may know that 15–20 minutes is the most that can be allowed for a consultation. It could therefore seem impractical to lay out a scheme for history-taking which may on occasion require 2 hours for completion.

The causes for believing that it is reasonable primarily to set things out in this way are several. There need be no apologies for the worth of investing time in thorough initial history-taking (especially if this is also seen as the start of therapy, and therapeutic time well spent). The only problem is how that time is to be found. In some settings it may not be out of step with usual practices to expect that considerable time can be found for the initial history – a hospital in-patient unit, for instance. In other settings it may be feasible to take part of the history and then ask the patient to come back so that the work can be completed. It is often possible to find a point at which the history-taking can temporarily be interrupted, and the patient may return for the second session with some reflective working-through accomplished meanwhile, and an enhanced ability to join in the work of historical review.

Another consideration is the usefulness of extended history-taking for training. The process of taking, say, five to ten histories at full length and with supervision and feedback can mean the acquisition of very worthwhile skills. With trained practice, an interview may then be conducted more quickly than had previously seemed feasible (and without an undue sense of hurry). To acquire skill in handling such an enquiry, and then to design for oneself a shorter approach based on what has been learnt and the needs of a particular setting or agency, is better than starting out with a greatly abbreviated approach. Once familiar, the essential framework of this scheme is, moreover, not overwhelmingly complex.

With the reasons for setting out a full-length approach to history-taking thus stated, we also give as a heading 'What might go into a 15-minute assessment'. In the paragraphs which follow, the discussion first focuses on the meeting with the patient or client and then turns to the interview with the spouse.

Background history

It is assumed that anyone coming to this work will already have developed their own general style of case history taking, or that the agency in which they operate will have its preferred format. Emphasis will instead be placed on elucidating those features of background history which are likely to be especially relevant to the understanding of drinking problems.

In taking this history, a habit that may be useful is to check what is coming in from the questioning by mentally pausing now and then, to ask oneself whether one can imagine what the patient was experiencing at the point in their life now reached by the history. What did their parents' house look like, and how would it have felt for a small child to be walking in at the front door? In what sort of street did that house stand and what kind of a street was it to play in? At school, would that child have been standing in a corner of the playground or joining in a game? A striving to understand the culture and the social environment cannot be separated from the attempt to empathize with the individual.

Background history and drinking history are intimately related. In the *background* section, many matters are touched on which will inevitably elicit information on drinking and drinking problems, and such information should be jotted down, rather than discarded or ignored because it does not come tidily at the right moment. The *drinking* section, as well as eliciting further new information, then gives an opportunity to bring together and *explore the relevance of* material which the patient has given earlier.

Family history

1. *For both parents.* Age, health (and mental health) and occupation; date and cause of death if deceased. Quality of relationships offered to patient in childhood;

parents' drinking and drinking attitudes and drinking problems and their use of drugs; psychiatric illness. Present relationship with parents. Enquiry may also be needed into drinking problems and psychiatric illness in the wider family.

2. *Siblings.* Basic information, social and personal adjustment or maladjustment (including drinking and use of drugs), present contact with patient and quality of relationship.

3. *Childhood environment.* Reconstruction of the home atmosphere during childhood, and the social and cultural milieus to which this home related. Parental discord, separations.

The purpose of this section is to obtain a preliminary understanding of the crucial early relationships and experiences which have contributed to the shaping of the individual's strengths or vulnerabilities, the possible dynamic meaning of alcohol (the meaning attached to alcohol because of parental drinking), and the cultural symbolism of alcohol.

Personal history

1. *Birth.* Date of birth; any evidence of birth trauma which might result in brain injury.

2. *Adjustment in childhood.* Evidence of neurotic symptoms in childhood; difficulty in relating to other children; conduct disorder; and childhood illness. Questioning around this area may help understanding as to whether the patient has exhibited lifelong traits of anxiety or difficulty in adjustment, and it is useful to go back to a period before the personality picture was overlaid by the drink.

3. *Schooling.* Information on schooling, with particular reference to social adjustment at school – how the patient got on with other children and with teachers, school refusal or truancy, certificates obtained. To ask 'What were you best at?' will help confer a sense of self.

4. *Technical or university qualifications.*

5. *Occupational history and present occupation.* Chronological information on jobs held; the alcohol-exposed nature of any occupation; problems which drinking has caused.

6. *Sexual orientation and adjustment,* and the impact of drinking.

7. *Relationships and marriage.* Marriage and the general implications of drinking for the family have already been discussed in Chapter 5. Information should be gathered on previous relationships and marriages and reasons for breakdown.

8. *Children.* Age and sex; closeness of the patient to children and parenting abilities; perceived impact of drinking on the children and their reaction to the drinking.

9. *Finances and housing and the impact of drinking.*

10. *Leisure.* The way in which the person usually spends his or her leisure; involvement of drinking in leisure pursuits; the degree to which leisure activities have been curtailed by drinking; and the rewards of leisure.

11. *Forensic history.* Enquiry should be made regarding public drunkenness offences, drink driving and all other convictions or pending court appearances. The relationship between the drinking and offending may need to be explored.

Social support, friendship networks and the quality of life

The aim here is to let patients sense and speak about the overall security, extent and rewardingness of their engagement with the social world around them. What other than alcohol makes life rewarding for them? Do they have friends who are not drinking friends?

Previous illnesses

1. *Physical illness, operations and accidents.*
2. *Psychiatric illnesses.*

Information is needed under both sub-headings, with emphasis on the identification of alcohol-related health problems. Under the heading of psychiatric illness, specific enquiry should always be made for any history suggesting the experience of depressive illness or pronounced mood swings, generalized or situational anxiety, obsessional disorder, pathological jealousy, suicide attempts and drug taking.

Personality

Here, what is required is a description of personality prior to drinking or in periods of sobriety – 'the real you'. Information is usefully elicited by open-ended questions such as:

What is the *real* you like?
What are your good points?
What are your bad points?
What do you want out of life?
What do you expect of friends?
What sort of things worry you or upset you?
What really makes you happy?

Prompts such as 'Go on. Tell me a bit more' will often give revealing information at a point where the patient at first believes that there is nothing to add. An indication should be obtained on at least the following aspects of personality: self-esteem; ability to experience warm feelings and to relate to others; self-control, explosiveness, irritability; social conformity, rule-breaking, deviance; outgoingness, introversion; drive, ambition, passivity; habitual ways of coping with stress or adversity.

Drinking history

Evolution

It is unnecessary to obtain a detailed account of everything that has happened over a lifetime's drinking, but we are seeking here to understand the individual's drinking in longitudinal perspective (Vaillant, 1983; Edwards, 1989; see Chapter 13). It is necessary to identify important milestones, and to understand the phases of the drinking career and the broadly related influences on it. This picture needs to be built up through exploring four different but closely related dimensions to the person's life, as follows.

1. *The evolution of drinking.* The task is to chart the major phases in drinking quantities and patterns, from first experiences of alcohol to the present. Useful questions may relate to such issues as:

   first drinking other than the occasional sip in childhood;
   first buying own drink;
   first drinking most weekends;
   first drinking spirits;
   any periods completely off drinking;
   first drinking every day;
   first drinking 8 pints of beer at a sitting, or half a bottle of spirits;
   first drinking in present pattern.

2. *Evolution of drink-related problems.* Apart from noting objective impacts on health and social functioning, there are two special questions which are often useful:

   When did you yourself first *realize drinking was a problem?*
   Looking back now with greater understanding, when in fact do you think drinking *really became a problem?*

   With hindsight, patients will nearly always distinguish between the first self-admission of there being a problem (precipitated, perhaps, by some catastrophic event) and an earlier date now recognizable as the period when drinking was undramatically beginning to, say, erode the happiness of a marriage or interfere with work.

3. *Evolution of dependence.* Here, the task is to date the onset of a gradual or sometimes rather abrupt shift in the individual's overall relationship with alcohol, their realization that they could no longer control their drinking, that they were 'hooked'. Enquiry can then also be made as to the approximate date of onset for specific dependence symptoms such as morning shakes or morning relief drinking.

4. *Evolution of pressures and circumstances.* The dimension which has to be charted under this heading is concerned with an understanding of the pressures and

circumstances which have caused, contributed to or shaped the evolving drinking patterns, dependence and problem experience. Questioning has to sense out influences which were already operating when the patient began to drink (parental example, peer group pressures, cultural influence, and so on), and then go forward to understand the subsequent impact of environment, life events, personal relations, mental state and other relevant factors. A few examples of questioning are:

> How did your drinking alter:
> > when you first left home?
> > at college?
> > when you were married?
> > after the children were born?
> > when the children left home?
> > when you were promoted to manager?
> > when you worked abroad?
> > after your spouse left you?
> > after you developed depression?

The typical recent heavy drinking day

Review of the evolution in drinking history seeks to build understanding which is *longitudinal* – the present is understood in its historical perspective. Reconstruction of the typical drinking day focuses exclusively on the present and on the cross-sectional rather than the longitudinal view (Dunn et al., 1992). The styles of enquiry are correspondingly different. When reconstructing the evolution of the problem, it is the broad sweep which is important, and the reconstruction of how drinking has interacted with a life path. Analysis of the typical day requires, in contrast, a minute and focused enquiry directed at present behaviour. This understanding should be so exact that in the mind's eye it is possible to play out a videotape of the patient's day.

1. *Establishing the notion of 'typical'.* Firstly, the concept which is involved has to be conveyed to the patient. He or she is asked to identify a *recent period* when drinking was, in terms of their own definition, *heavy*, with the drinking then of a kind which they would generally consider to be *typical* of their recent drinking. The patient has to identify the exact period they have in mind – 'the way I was drinking until 2 weeks ago when I lost my job and had to cut down'. What has to be emphasized is the actuality, rather than any generalized abstractions which have no real time base. Most patients find it possible to identify such a period, but for others there is so much variability in their drinking pattern that what is typical is difficult to define, and this in itself is a reality which has to be described.

2. *Waking and events around waking.* Having explained the ground rules, it is necessary to establish at what time the patient usually wakes. Enquiry is then made as to the events immediately around the time of waking, for it is here that evidence will be obtained of withdrawal symptoms, withdrawal relief drinking, and other signs and symptoms which help to elucidate the patient's degree of dependence.

3. *Subsequent hour-by-hour timetabling.* The patient is then taken through a reconstruction of the day, as follows.

    (i) *The background structure of daily activities.* For instance, what time they leave the house in the morning, what train they catch, what time they get to work, when they take their lunch break, and so on.

    (ii) *The timetabling of drinking.* With the framework now provided by the structure of the day, the next task is to fit in a full description of the day's drinking. What time does the patient take their first drink, how much do they drink and over what duration? This enquiry is then taken forward step by step, through the day. To a description of actual alcohol intake is in each instance added a note of where the drinking takes place, and with whom (if anyone) the patient is drinking. Note also has to be made of the patient's ideas as to the determinants of each drinking occasion – whether to relieve or avoid withdrawal symptoms, to relieve anxiety or other unpleasant inner feelings, whether in the setting of business or for the companionship of the pub, or for any other reason. A final aspect of drinking which has to be timetabled is the experience of intoxication, and whether at any point of the day the patient would consider that drink is interfering with ordinary functioning.

Influence of drinking on personality

Some patients are not aware that drinking alters their personality, while others will state that 'I'm an entirely different person when I've been drinking – Jekyll and Hyde'. The issue has to be examined, both in terms of positive and negative effects. Positively, some patients may, for instance, see themselves as more outgoing, confident and assertive when drinking. On the negative side, the effect may be irritability and loss of control over temper (including violence), suspicion, moroseness, self-pity or lack of feeling for others.

Probing and checking

The following dialogue shows how an important aspect of the drinking history can be elucidated by careful probing.

Therapist: All right, you say you have three pints of lager at lunchtime. How long do you spend in the bar at lunchtime?

Patient: Twelve noon till 2 p.m., sometimes 3 p.m.
Therapist: More often 2 p.m. or 3 p.m?
Patient: Say 2.30 p.m.
Therapist: Three pints in two-and-a-half hours seems quite slow drinking.
Patient: If I'm there 12 to 2.30, I suppose it would be 4 or 5 pints. I was thinking of when I have a short lunch break. It's more often a long liquid lunch these days.
Therapist: You say 4 or 5 pints – could it be more?
Patient: No, I'd get too bloated. I don't think I'd ever go above 5 pints.
Therapist: Anything else besides lager at lunch-time?
Patient: Probably have a couple of whiskies.
Therapist: Why 'a couple' – could it be more?
Patient: No, I'll have just a couple of whiskies to round things off when I've finished with the lager. Not more than a couple.
Therapist: Double or single measures?
Patient: Doubles.
Therapist: Ever leave out the whisky?
Patient: No, it's pretty regular.

Putting quantity consumed against time spent drinking, sometimes checking stated consumption against money usually spent, testing the stated upper limit by offering a higher or lower one, going through alcoholic beverages other than the one first named, relating the stated drinking to the company and other circumstances – all these provide useful methods for checking which can help to build up a valid picture.

Totalling the daily intake

Information on quantity drunk throughout the day can be summed to total daily intake. Because of uncertainties in size of drink poured, broad variations in alcohol content for drinks within any beverage type (beer, wine or spirits), and international differences as to the size of a standard drink, the summated figure is an approximation rather than an exact index (Turner, 1990; Miller et al., 1991). For research purposes, the most satisfactory approach is to express the total in terms of grams of absolute alcohol, but in the clinical setting the idea of *units* provides a useful basis. A unit of intake can be defined approximately thus:

One glass (half pint) of medium strength beer	1 unit
Large can of strong lager	3–4 units
One glass of wine	1 unit
One measure of fortified wine (port or sherry)	1 unit
One measure of spirits	1 unit

A standard bottle of wine is likely to contain about 6–8 units and a bottle of spirits 30–32 units. A British unit thus defined corresponds to about 8–10 g of absolute alcohol. American units or 'standard drinks' contain more alcohol (11–12 g) than a British unit, and in the USA the unit concept has not gained as much popularity as in the UK. A Canadian unit is probably about 13–14 g and an Australian unit 10 g. Various questionnaires exist specifically for recording alcohol consumption (Witte and Haile, 1996).

Bringing together the evidence for dependence

Much information relevant to establishing the degree to which the patient is alcohol dependent will have been obtained from questioning in the areas of *evolution* and *drinking day*. It is, however, necessary to have in the history a place where evidence on dependence is reviewed and brought together.

The picture of the dependence syndrome and its degrees of variation have been fully discussed in Chapter 4 and the headings used in that chapter to describe the core elements of the syndrome provide the framework for this section of the history-taking. Brief notes are added below on the practical approach to questioning in each instance.

1. *Narrowing of the drinking repertoire.* Useful questions relate to the sameness or otherwise of drinking during weekdays as opposed to weekends, or during the working year as opposed to holidays.

2. *Salience of drinking.* Reconstructing the evolution of the patient's drinking will have implicitly provided an account of the progressive importance of alcohol in their life, and their progressive ability to discount other considerations. An attempt should also be made to explore with the patient how salient drinking has become in the here and now. Useful questions are, for instance:

   Just how important has drinking become for you?
   Is drinking more or less important for you than eating?
   Is drinking more important than people?

   A particular phrase in the patient's answers may suddenly and empathetically convey the reality of their drink-centredness: 'When my wife said she would leave me if I went on drinking, I had the sly thought, well, if she leaves me, there will be more time and money for drinking.'

   Here it is often useful to ask a question like, 'What are the good things that drinking does for you?' In this way one gains a sense of the functional significance of alcohol for that patient – whether, for example, they see themselves as drinking for company and the pleasures of the bar-room environment, or for the 'high' state and directly pleasurable effects of intoxication, or for relief of unpleasant feelings, or for a combination of these reasons. The dependent drinker may insist that they have ceased to get any pleasure out of drinking, or even say that they hate every drink – they are caught on a tread-mill.

3. *Increased tolerance (or evidence of decreased tolerance)*. Most patients will say that they can 'drink a lot without getting drunk', and the quantity which is habitually taken is itself evidence of tolerance. If at a later stage in the drinking career a severe *decline in tolerance* is being experienced, this is often reported as a worrying happening (see Chapter 4).

4. *Withdrawal symptoms*. Questioning has to deal with the frequency and intensity of the commoner withdrawal symptoms – tremor, nausea, sweating, mood disturbance. These symptoms may be experienced not only on waking, but also with partial alcohol withdrawal during the waking day. Any history of subacute hallucinatory experiences, delirium tremens or withdrawal fits should also be noted.

5. *Relief or avoidance of withdrawal symptoms by further drinking*. Questioning must cover the frequency with which the patient drinks to relieve or avoid withdrawal, and the perceived urgency for such a drink.

6. *Subjective awareness of compulsion to drink*. Matters that may bear on the assessment of subjective experience are discussed in Chapter 4. Craving may be most intense during withdrawal, but there may be rumination on drink and the need to protect the drink supply pretty well throughout the day.

7. *Reinstatement after abstinence*. Questioning should focus on the actualities of what happened on recent occasions when the patient was off drink and went back to drinking again – when they came out of prison, perhaps, or when they came out of hospital, or when after a period of involvement with Alcoholics Anonymous they 'had a slip'. How quickly were they again experiencing withdrawal symptoms or needing to take a morning drink?

Standard diagnostic systems for alcohol dependence

DSM-IV (American Psychiatric Association, 1994) and ICD-10 (Word Health Organization, 1992) criteria for diagnosis of alcohol dependence are reproduced in Boxes 15.1 and 15.2 respectively. These approaches are of great value in standardizing diagnostic practice, nationally and internationally, and they carry authority. Their drawback from the clinician's point of view is that they both picture dependence as an all-or-none rather than dimensional state. Categorical formulae are proposed at the cost of clinical subtlety. The DSM-IV and ICD-10 approaches are in many ways similar. In the accompanying text, ICD mentions 'narrowing of repertoire' and 'subjective awareness of compulsion to use', but does not include these elements in its diagnostic rubric. If a history has been taken in the detail outlined above, sufficient information will have been gathered to enable formal diagnostic decisions to be made within either official system.

> BOX 15.1 **DSM-IV criteria for substance dependence**
>
> A maladaptive pattern of substance use, leading to clinically significant impairment or distress, as manifested by three (or more) of the following, occurring at any time in the same 12-month period:
>
> (1) tolerance, as defined by either of the following:
>   (a) a need for markedly increased amounts of the substance to achieve intoxication or desired effect
>   (b) markedly diminished effect with continued use of the same amount of the substance
> (2) withdrawal, as manifested by either of the following:
>   (a) the characteristic withdrawal syndrome for the substance . . .
>   (b) the same (or a closely related) substance is taken to relieve or avoid withdrawal symptoms
> (3) the substance is often taken in larger amounts or over a longer period than was intended
> (4) there is persistent desire or unsuccessful efforts to cut down or control substance use
> (5) a great deal of time is spent in activities necessary to obtain the substance . . .
> (6) important social, occupational, or recreational activities are given up or reduced because of substance use
> (7) the substance use is continued despite knowledge of having a persistent or recurrent physical or psychological problem that is likely to have been caused or exacerbated by the substance (e.g., current cocaine use despite recognition of cocaine-induced depression, or continued drinking despite recognition that an ulcer was made worse by alcohol consumption).
>
> American Psychiatric Association (1994), reproduced by kind permission.

Questionnaires for measuring dependence

A number of standardized instruments have been designed which can be used to rate the individual's degree of alcohol dependence (Skinner, 1981; Skinner and Allen, 1982; Hesselbrock et al., 1983; Davidson and Raistrick, 1986; Davidson et al., 1989). The practitioner will do well to gain a working familiarity with just one such approach so that scores can be readily related to their clinical meaning. The Severity of Alcohol Dependence Questionnaire (SADQ: Stockwell et al., 1979) has been widely employed both for clinical and research purposes. On the SADQ's 60-point scale, scores of around 20–30 suggest that the patient is entering a range of severe dependence. A questionnaire has been developed for rating severity of dependence as represented in patient records (Månsson et al., 1993).

Bringing together the evidence for alcohol-related disabilities

Questioning in this section should be aimed at involving the patients themselves in an audit. Each relevant fact is adduced with the patients' exploration of the

---

BOX 15.2 **ICD-10 criteria for substance dependence**

Diagnostic guidelines

A definite diagnosis of dependence should usually be made only if three or more of the following have been experienced or exhibited at some time during the previous year:

(a) a strong desire or sense of compulsion to take the substance;

(b) difficulties in controlling substance-taking behaviour in terms of its onset, termination or levels of use;

(c) a physiological withdrawal state . . . when substance use has ceased or been reduced, as evidenced by: the characteristic withdrawal syndrome for the substance; or use of the same (or a closely related) substance with the intention of relieving or avoiding withdrawal symptoms;

(d) evidence of tolerance, such as that increased doses of the psychoactive substance are required in order to achieve effects originally produced by lower doses . . .

(e) progressive neglect of alternative pleasures or interests because of psychoactive substance use, increased amount of time necessary to obtain or take the substance or to recover from its effects;

(f) persisting with substance use despite clear evidence of overtly harmful consequences, such as harm to the liver through excessive drinking, depressive mood states consequent to periods of heavy substance use, or drug-related impairment of cognitive functioning; efforts should be made to determine that the user was actually, or could be expected to be, aware of the nature and extent of the harm.

World Health Organization (1992), reproduced by kind permission.

---

significance of the fact and the degree to which alcohol was involved. The list ends up as their audit, rather than being the therapist's private clinical note.

Testing each item: the agreed audit

The introduction to this section of history-taking could be as follows.

Let's try to bring together the ways in which alcohol may have been having any sort of bad effect on your life – on your physical health or your nerves or your job or your marriage, or anything else. You've already told me a lot about separate problems, but now let's try to make out the whole list.

If, for example, the impact of drinking on the patient's marriage were to arise in a particular case, the discussion might be as follows.

Therapist: You told me that your wife walked out on you because of your drinking.
Patient: If it hadn't been for the drinking we might have made a go of it. I'm not saying we *would* have made a go of it. We *might* have made a go of the marriage.

There is a question here which could be explored with this patient later at greater length, but for the purposes of this initial history it is sufficient to establish that the patient accepts as a fair assessment that without the drinking he 'might have made a go of the marriage'. A clumsy interrogation that faced him with no more than a sort of yes/no alternative would not have given him an opportunity to convey and define in a personally meaningful way the impact of drinking on marriage.

The patient should then be played back a summary of what seems to have been established – either fully established or accepted only with reservations. The summing-up has to be made with the opportunity for interruptions and discussion.

A standardized questionnaire for measuring intensity of problem experience

The Alcohol Problems Questionnaire (APQ: Drummond, 1990) is a standardized inventory which exists in a fuller version and which includes sections on marriage, children and employment, and in a shorter form which excludes those areas. The APQ can make a useful contribution to the overall assessment, with the meaning of any scored items discussed with the patient.

Questionnaires to measure craving

The Alcohol Use Questionnaire (AUQ: Bohn et al., 1995) is a useful short questionnaire to measure craving; the 36-item Desires for Alcohol Questionnaire (DAQ: Love et al., 1998) gives scores within three sub-areas. An 'impaired control' scale is also available (Heather et al., 1998).

History of help-seeking for drinking problems and assessment of motivation

Enquiry should be made about both help sought by the patient in the past and help being given at present. It is then essential to understand the patient's reasons for coming to this present consultation – the pressures they see themselves as experiencing (a court order or threats from a spouse, for instance), what crisis may suddenly have precipitated the immediate help-seeking, or what inner sense of need is driving the motivation. Once more, the process of history-taking is an experience for the patient as well as giving information to the therapist. The patient is exploring the question of why he or she is in this room, and trying to understand the ambiguous, confused or contradictory motivations which have brought them here. Such knowledge is an important basis for later work. The history has to be taken with awareness that motivation is always ambivalent: the patient both wants to go on drinking and wants to stop drinking. It is these conflicting forces that have to be identified, rather than the reality of conflict being evaded.

Prochaska and DiClemente's concept of 'stages of change' (Prochaska and DiClimente, 1984) has been appreciated by many clinicians as providing a useful framework when assessing the individual's motivation; Rollnick et al. (1992) have developed a 'readiness to change' questionnaire. Read simply, this approach suggests that it is possible to place patients in one of the four change categories of pre-contemplation, contemplation, action and maintenance. We return to these issues when discussing how psychological interventions may be used to enhance motivation for change.

Physical examination and investigations

Physical examination and laboratory investigations will be part of the assessment routine in a medical setting. In a social work or probation office, this aspect of assessment is not within expected practice, but there will be advantage in such agencies ensuring that the patient receives a physical examination from a doctor, with the results fed back. This insistence on the importance of making a medical connection may go against the usual working methods of some non-medical agencies and be seen as burdensome. However, the likelihood of physical disorder in the patient with a drinking problem puts that person in a different category from many other social work clients.

History-taking with the patient: the essential framework

In Table 15.1 the essential structure for history-taking is laid out. In the first column, major areas of enquiry are tabulated, using the same headings employed previously. The second column seeks to help the practical business of history-taking by providing a few important reminders as to what has specially to be kept in mind during the process of interview – a series of working notes on technique. The third column provides reminders as to the purpose of the whole exercise and of individual sections. If the sense of purpose is lost, there is danger both of the history becoming inordinately long and at the same time of its failing in its essential goals.

What might go into a 15-minute assessment

The way that short time is best used must to an extent be patient and agency specific. The following notes offer some general suggestions.

1. Despite pressures of time, do not lose sight of the fact that assessment should be an initiation of therapy. Give the patient initial free time to talk, try to understand why this person has come to see you, respond to them positively and give encouragement, round off the interview and identify productive next steps.
2. Concentrate on the present. Try to get a sense of present drinking level, present and recent problems with drinking, present life situation and recent help-seeking.
3. Estimate degree of dependence on alcohol. Information on presence and intensity of withdrawal symptoms can provide a useful short cut.
4. Set proximate goals in relation to moderation of drinking or abstinence.

Table 15.1 Summary scheme for history-taking with the patient

Area of enquiry	Matters to be kept in mind	Essential purposes
The whole exercise	History-taking is conducted within a patient–therapist *interaction*. The quality of this interaction must purposively be developed so as to *invite the surrender of defences*.	
	A history must *serve the needs of both therapist and patient*.	**For the patient**: *the initiation of therapy*, in terms of (i) the accomplishment of a self-review which *factually arrays and inter-relates a wide variety of experiences* (with drinking and its impact placed in context), and (ii) an *undefended exploration of the meaning of those facts*, together with (iii) laying the *foundations of a therapeutic relationship*.
		For the therapist: (i) the provision of initial understanding which will be the basis for *developing with this patient the treatment goals and treatment programme*, (ii) building the relationship, and (iii) a basis for *therapeutic training* and the continued *growth of awareness and skills*.
		Overall: to provide (i) essential understanding of *the person in their own right, of their present* as continuous with *their past*, and (ii) the *context for understanding* the drinking history.
Family history Both parents, childhood environment	*To search after* what the home felt like and looked like and who was there: 'the street in which it stood'.	Preliminary understanding of crucial early relationships and experiences which may have contributed to the individual's strengths and vulnerabilities, the

Table 15.1 (*cont.*)

Area of enquiry	Matters to be kept in mind	Essential purposes
		way they will relate to people, and the dynamic and cultural meaning they will give to alcohol; understanding of possible genetic influences.
Personal history Birth, adjustment in childhood, schooling, occupational history sexual adjustment, marriage, children, finances and housing, leisure, forensic history	. . . what it feels like to have lived this life . . .	Serving the overall purpose of this dialogue while in passing some information will be obtained on drinking and its consequences, which has later to be ordered.
Previous illness Physical and psychiatric		Serves the overall purpose as above
Personality	. . . and to be this person	Crucial explorations to serve the overall purpose.
Social support	Friendship networks, faith and belief	How does this person engage with life?
Drinking history	**Throughout** – put drinking against background history.	
Evolution	Four strands of enquiry: 1. drinking pattern 2. dependence 3. drink-related problems 4. pressure and circumstances.	To sense the broad dynamic of an evolving story: *the longitudinal perspective.*
Typical recent heavy drinking day Waking and events around waking: the timetable of drinking, influence on personality, totalling the daily intake	1. Establish the *notion* of the typical day 2. The need to focus down on small actualities 3. The need to check and probe.	To understand the present in fine detail: *the cross-sectional view.*
Bringing together the evidence for dependence Narrowing of repertoire	To look for *coherence.*	An understanding as to whether dependence is *present*, and if so its *degree.*

Table 15.1 (*cont.*)

Area of enquiry	Matters to be kept in mind	Essential purposes
Salience of drinking		
Tolerance		
Withdrawal symptoms		
Relief drinking		
Subjective awareness of		
compulsion		
Reinstatement		
Bringing together the evidence for *alcohol-related disabilities*	Testing each item for the patient's agreement.	Building a broad and comprehensive picture of the way in which alcohol has adversely affected the patient's life – a *shared audit*.
Physical health, mental health, social functioning, and functioning within the family		
History of help-seeking for *drinking problems: motivation*	Motivation is a matter of ambivalence.	To understand why the patient is in this room and the work on motivation that will have to be done.
Past and present		

5. Always seek to identify any possibility of dual diagnosis. Concomitant depression, anxiety and drug taking should always be on the checklist.
6. In a medical setting carry out blood tests (see Chapter 14). A quick physical examination may be needed.
7. Make another appointment, keep in touch, monitor progress, offer to see the spouse, network with other agencies.

Initial assessment with the spouse or partner

We now come to discussion of why it is important to interview the spouse or significant other as part of the initial assessment procedures, how this interview is to be handled, and its content. It is often helpful if the drinker can be interviewed by one member of the team while the spouse is being seen by another, with the information and perspectives then later brought together for joint appraisal and formulation. If that kind of support is not available, the therapist may decide to see both husband and wife at this early stage in assessment. There can be advantages in seeing them separately rather than somewhat uncertainly fusing two accounts. Later, however, added insights may be gained through a joint interview.

An outline of the scheme is given in Table 15.2, and again the detail should not be allowed to intimidate the therapist who is working under extreme constraints

Table 15.2 Summary scheme for history-taking with the spouse or partner

Area of enquiry	Matters to be kept in mind	Essential purposes
The whole exercise	Establishing the objective facts is important	*For the spouse or partner* 1. The review of happenings and feelings in a way that begins to make sense and to have shape
	Feelings and interactions also matter	2. Awareness of self as more than passive participant or victim 3. Laying the foundations for future therapeutic work
		For the therapist 1. Further understanding of the needs of the spouse 2. Further understanding of the marital interactions 3. Collateral information
Personal history of the spouse	A history has to be taken of this person in their own right; to know who this person is; where they are coming from, what is brought to the marriage	Understanding how these heritages interact with current problems and determine present needs
The drinking problem	The objective facts are only to be sensed through the colouring which this witness must bring to a situation in which he or she is personally involved	To sense the outlines and dynamics of the drinking story, the picture of the present drinking, and the extent of hardship
	The account given by the spouse of hardships experienced needs different headings from the patient's account of alcohol-related problems	To enable the spouse to express grief and anger and ambivalences of feeling, and to know that it is safe to share these experiences
Coping	The range and mixture of mechanisms which are being deployed	Understanding the stage of development in the marital interaction and possibilities for more constructive response

of time. With practice, things are simpler than they first seem. Given that many of the issues to be discussed in this part of the chapter parallel those considered earlier with the patient, the emphasis will, as far as possible, be on brevity.

Although this chapter deals with the spouse or partner, the value of at times also obtaining a story from other informants should be remembered – from another family member, from a friend or from an employer. Permission has always to be obtained from the patient.

Making contact

The spouse who is asked to come for interview may be glad to attend or may come along only with reluctance. A wife may herself have formed the view that her husband's drinking is in some sense a 'family problem', whereas another woman may see the problem as being solely in her husband's behaviour and be resistant to seeing herself as other than passive victim. Before the therapist starts to guide the discussion into a loosely formal structure, the spouse or partner should be given time to talk freely and to feel assured that their personal needs are going to be listened to attentively.

It is useful to be alert to some of the commoner ways in which the spouse's account may deviate from anything which could fairly be considered the independent and objective truth. For example, spouses will be found who will exaggerate their partner's drinking, either because of a conscious wish to blackguard a reputation, or because of a profound anxiety about drinking and drunkenness. At the other extreme, a wife or husband may in the face of their partner's appalling and long-continued drinking insist that all is well, either because they are frightened of the drinker's anger if they divulge the truth, or because of subconscious reasons. The more bizarre distortions are not common, but they can give rise to a great deal of puzzlement when they occur. It may be months before the treatment team tumbles to the fact that the client's plaintive insistence on their sobriety is valid, and the partner's account is based on a desire to obtain a divorce. The issue raised here is important, not only in relation to the possibility of extreme distortion. With every case and far short of the extreme, the therapist is being presented with accounts coloured by the active involvement in the story of each person (patient or partner) who is talking. That is both the value and the limitation of this kind of material, but do not expect the abstract truth.

Personal history of the spouse

Family and personal history

The worth of routinely making such enquiry (and the handicaps which result from not asking such questions) is illustrated by the following dialogue.

> *Therapist:* How much did your parents drink?
>
> *Wife:* I went through in childhood everything I'm going through now. How my mother put up with it none of us ever understood. I'd say for years my father never came home sober, and my mother put up with it. He'd come home blinding and swearing and just looking for a fight, and my mother took it year in and year out.

The extent to which this woman is acting out her mother's role is a question vital to any understanding of her (and her husband's) present position, and yet if no one bothers to ask about her parents, she may feel that it is not relevant to tell anyone about her childhood.

Spouse's account of the partner's drinking history
Evolution

The spouse's picture of the evolution of the patient's drinking problem may be the same as the patient's account, or they may be able to offer additional insights.

> He won't tell you this, but I've always felt that he's never liked the attention I've given to the children. I think it was soon after our first son was born that I noticed my husband's drinking. He didn't know how to fit back into the family. Sounds funny, but I've always thought *he* wanted to be the baby in the family.

Present pattern of drinking

To suppose that the spouse can be the independent informant who can give a print-out on the quantity and frequency of the patient's drinking is usually unrealistic. What the spouse can in fact usefully describe is the frequency with which the patient behaves in a way which can be summarized as 'unacceptable' (Orford and Edwards, 1977). A spouse may be able to identify withdrawal symptoms and know that the patient is shaky and retching in the morning or these symptoms may go unobserved.

Problems and hardships

The spouse may or may not be in a position to know what alcohol-related problems the patient has experienced, but it is worthwhile to ask in outline about such matters as illnesses, accidents, lost jobs, debts, forensic involvement, and so on. There is, however, a range of other matters relating to the patient's drinking which the spouse may be uniquely well equipped to speak about, and these concern the direct impact of the drinking on the family and the spouse themselves – the *hardships* which are being experienced (Orford and Edwards, 1977).

Here are some indications as to the areas of questioning which may be useful.

1. *Has drinking made the patient unreliable?* The word 'unreliable' may, for the spouse, exactly catch the frustration of what has been experienced, and a question

phrased in this manner then leads directly into matters they want to talk about.

> Yes. That's it exactly. It's everything from you have the dinner ready and she's not there to eat it, to that dreadful time last year when we were all lined up for the summer holiday and she disappeared. You can never believe what she's telling you, never trust her to do what she says she is going to do.

2. *'Rowing on and on'*. Here, the typical story is of the husband coming home after pub closing time, waking his wife up, and then embroiling her in a smouldering row which goes on for hours. She learns to expect these recurrent scenes in which he recapitulates all her faults and shortcomings, and with the wife knowing of no way to cut into or terminate these dreary replays. Jealous accusations are often part of the content.

3. *'Turning nasty'*. The spouse may come to recognize that at a predictable stage of intoxication *bonhomie* suddenly passes over to a mood of anger or violence. They may know that in such moods the patient will start breaking up the home, or assaulting the spouse or the children.

4. *Money*. Commonly, the financial hardships and uncertainties experienced by the spouse are part of the chronic strain of living with someone with a drinking problem. It may be a matter of taking money from a purse, the housekeeping money not being provided or of the bills not being paid. Possessions may have been sold or pawned.

5. *'Useless in the evening'*. The story here is of the drinker who gets home in the evening and who does not engage in rowing or violence, but who pushes aside the supper and then night after night slumps drunkenly asleep in an armchair. They may be found there in the morning.

6. *Wetting the bed*. Bed-wetting is a not uncommon feature of a drinking problem, and in an advanced stage patients may soil themselves. Also, in a state of drunken confusion they may get up and urinate in a corner of the bedroom.

Coping

The *coping mechanisms* which the spouse may employ are discussed in Chapter 5. Enquiry should be made into the ways in which the spouse is dealing with the patient's drinking and the types of mechanism which they are deploying. It is useful to think in terms of different styles, such as circumvention, attack, manipulation, spoiling, constructive management and constructive help-seeking, although it is likely that in many instances some mixtures of styles will be perceived (Orford and Edwards, 1977; Orford et al., 1998; Orford et al., 2001). This type of understanding can provide a useful basis for later therapeutic work. The spouse begins to see patterns in their own behaviour, and to realize the degree to which they may be persevering in unproductive or counter-productive responses, and the possibilities of more constructive reaction.

Rounding off the interview with spouse or partner

It must be stressed again that any assessment interview is properly a therapeutic encounter, whether that interview is with the person with the drinking problem or with the spouse. For the spouse, the interview should be an opportunity to bring order and understanding to muddled and painful happenings, the chance to discover or express feelings and often a conflict of feelings, a confirmation of worth as an individual, and a sensing of ways in which they may have compounded the problem. When this interview is being rounded off, it is necessary to show an empathetic response to the feelings that have been awakened.

Patient and spouse: assessment as asset

The assessment procedures both with the patient and the spouse constitute a considerable investment of their time and that of the people conducting these procedures. Significant work has been accomplished in terms of building relationships and self-understanding, and the material gathered constitutes an essential base for planning and action. These initial assessments are designed to provide insights and information to be used, and to be employed in guiding the practical next steps forward. A well-conducted assessment is an immensely valuable therapeutic asset on which to build further.

The case formulation

The diagnostic interview or interviews with the patient, interviews where possible with the spouse or additional informants, reports from other agencies, the results of laboratory tests, and any other enquiries will together provide a mass of information. That information has to be synthesized into an initial case formulation. Lots of separate pieces may give many separate and partial insights, but it is crucial that the attempt should then be made to stand back and perceive the whole predicament. Formulation is the attempt to *understand*, and a well-constructed formulation is a creative act of empathy rather than just an ordering of information under headings.

There are several reasons for believing that this additional investment of time is worth the demand. The therapist is directionless until the formulation is made. Furthermore, even if after data gathering has been completed and the therapist has a good grasp of the case, when the patient re-attends, perhaps after a gap of weeks, that sense of close understanding may have faded somewhat: a formulation can serve as a personal *aide-memoire*. The original formulation will also be of great use if a case is reopened after a gap of a year or two, or if the patient's therapy is eventually taken over by someone else. Construction of a detailed formulation is invaluable as a training exercise.

Besides these various ways in which the formulation is of use to the therapist or therapeutic team, it is equally to be conceived as a basis for discussion with the patient and partner.

A formulation should not be of inordinate length or it defeats its purpose. The format proposed here is to be taken only as a starting point, to be amended or scaled down according to individual professional needs and feasibilities.

Headings for a formulation

Diagnosis

It is preferable that this heading should be taken as an invitation to a *full listing* of diagnoses rather than just a statement of 'the' diagnosis. The necessary sub-headings are as follows.

1. Alcohol dependence: its presence or absence and, if present, its degree of development, with an outline of the supporting evidence.
2. All alcohol-related disabilities (medical, psychological and social).
3. Ancillary diagnoses, including underlying or accompanying psychiatric conditions and physical disorders.

Description of personality

It is preferable to attempt a brief description of personality, rather than to use such phrases as 'personality disorder' within the diagnostic listing above. The aim is to summarize provisional insights regarding both personal strengths and vulnerabilities.

Present social situation

1. Marital status or relationship, rewardingness of the relationship, partner's coping, and role of children in the present situation.
2. Employment.
3. Accommodation.
4. Leisure.
5. Religious involvement.
6. Forensic status.

Drinking

1. History of the drinking problem: synopsis.
2. Aetiology of the drinking, in terms of both more distant determinants and more recent influences.
3. The typical drinking day: summary description and estimate of usual daily intake.

4. The balance of present motivations: appraisal of patient's current losses and gains from drinking, and degree of motivation.

5. History of help-seeking.

The family's health and well-being

The problems currently affecting the patient's spouse or children.

Further information needed

A list, for instance, of what further information has to be sought from the patient or other informants, other agencies to be contacted, specialist opinion to be obtained, or specialized diagnostic procedures to be arranged.

Goals

On the basis of what has already been laid out in the preceding sections of the formulation, it should be possible to set up a series of specific treatment goals. As with diagnosis, what is required is a list rather than a single monolithic statement.

Action steps

Under this heading are set out in objective terms the steps which have to be taken to achieve the stated goals. The actualities should be listed, rather than any vague generalizations such as 'treat the alcoholism'. This is an aspect of the formulation which must be designed in co-operation with the patient and his or her family.

Prognosis

Prognosis should be written in terms of an informed, balanced and well-argued weighing of probabilities.

The formulation as shared exercise

Reference has already been made to the necessity of the formulation serving the needs of the patient as well as of the therapist. Before making final notes on the formulation, there should have been an interchange in which the therapist says, 'What we have talked through is valuable ... I see it this way ... What we ought to do is perhaps this ... How do you see it? ... Can we agree then ... ?'. Such discussion ensures that not only is the therapist standing back from the data and gaining a whole view, but also the patient is doing the same, and they are doing so together.

Assessment: the essential business

Assessment is a process which, if skilfully and humanely conducted, should be both rewarding and challenging for the person who has come into the room. It should allow them to see their life as evolutionary and their drinking as it has evolved within their life course. It may strip some defences and denial, but it must at the same time give hope. Assessment is at best a small but important new step in a longer journey, but it should help the patient leave the room with the crucial sense that they are beginning to understand what needs to be done for them to make changes and that change is possible.

REFERENCES

American Psychiatric Association (1994) *Diagnostic and Statistical Manual of Mental Disorders*, 4th edn. Washington, DC: American Psychiatric Association.

Bohn, M.J., Krahn, D.D. and Staehler, B.A. (1995) Development and initial validation of a measure of drinking urges in abstinent alcoholics. *Alcoholism: Clinical and Experimental Research* 19, 600–6.

Compton, W.M., Cottler, L.B., Dorsey, K.B., Spitznagel, E.L. and Mager, D.E. (1996) Comparing assessment of DSM substance dependence disorder using CIDI-SAM and SCAN. *Drug and Alcohol Dependence* 41, 179–88.

Cottler, L.B. and Compton, W.M. (1993) Advantages of the CIDI family of instruments in epidemiological research on substance use disorders. *International Journal of Methods in Psychiatric Research* 3, 109–19.

Cottler, L.B., Robins, L.N. and Helzer, J.E. (1989) The reliability of the CIDI-SAM: a comprehensive substance abuse interview. *British Journal of Addiction* 159, 653–8.

Davidson, R., Bunting, B. and Raistrick, D. (1989) The homogeneity of the alcohol dependence syndrome: a factor analysis of the SADD questionnaire. *British Journal of Addiction* 84, 907–15.

Davidson, R. and Raistrick, D. (1986) The validity of the Short Alcohol Dependence Data (SADD) questionnaire: a short self-report questionnaire for the assessment of alcohol dependence. *British Journal of Addiction* 81, 217–22.

Departments of Psychiatry and Child Psychiatry, The Institute of Psychiatry and the Maudsley Hospital London (1987) *Psychiatric Examination: Notes on Eliciting and Recording Clinical Information in Psychiatric Patients*. Oxford: Oxford University Press.

Drummond, D.C. (1990) The relationship between alcohol dependence and alcohol-related problems in a clinical population. *British Journal of Addiction* 85, 357–66.

Dunn, J.N., Seilhamer, R.A., Jacob, T. and Whalen, M. (1992) Comparisons of retrospective and current reports of alcoholics and their spouses on drinking behaviour. *Addictive Behaviours* 17, 543–55.

Edwards, G. (1989) As the years go rolling by. Drinking problems in the time dimension. *British Journal of Addiction* 154, 18–26.

Griffin, M.L., Weiss, R.D., Mirin, S.M., Wilson, H. and Bouchard-Voelk, B. (1987) The use of the Diagnostic Interview Schedule in drug dependent patients. *American Journal of Drug and Alcohol Abuse* 13, 281–91.

Hasin, D.S. (1991) Diagnostic interviews for assessment: background, reliability, validity. *Alcohol Health and Research World* 15, 293–302.

Heather, N., Booth, P. and Luce, A. (1998) Impaired control scale: cross validation and relationships with treatment outcome. *Addiction* 93, 765–75.

Hesselbrock, M., Babor, T.F., Hesselbrock, V., Meyer, R.E. and Workman, K. (1983) 'Never believe an Alcoholic?' On the validity of self report measures of alcohol dependence and related constructs. *International Journal of Addiction* 18, 593–609.

Hyams, G., Cartwright, A. and Spratley, T. (1996) Engagement in alcohol treatment: the client's experience of, and satisfaction with, the assessment interview. *Addiction Research* 4, 105–23.

Kranzler, H.R., Kadden, R.M., Babor, T.F., Tenner, H. and Rounsaville, B.J. (1996) Validity of the SCID in substance abuse patients. *Addiction* 91, 859–64.

Love, A., James, D. and Willner, P. (1998) A comparison of two alcohol craving questionnaires. *Addiction* 93, 1091–102.

McCrady, R.G., Rogler, L.H. and Tryon, W.W. (1992) Issues of validity in the Diagnostic Interview Schedule. *Journal of Psychiatric Research* 26, 59–67.

Månsson, M., Hansson, M., Hoberg, A-L. and Berglund, M. (1993) Severity of alcohol dependence, rating by patient records. *Alcohol and Alcoholism* 28, 347–51.

Miller, W.R., Heather, N. and Hall, W. (1991) Calculating standard drink units: international comparisons. *British Journal of Addiction* 86, 43–7.

Novey, S. (1968) *The Second Look*. Baltimore: Johns Hopkins Press.

Orford, J. and Edwards, G. (1977) *Alcoholism: a Comparison of Treatment and Advice, with a Study of the Influence of Marriage*. Maudsley Monograph No. 26. Oxford: Oxford University Press.

Orford, J., Natera, G., Davies, J. et al. (1998) Tolerate, engage or withdraw: a study of the structure of families coping with alcohol and drug problems in South West England and Mexico City. *Addiction* 93, 14–15.

Orford, J., Natera, G., Velleman, R. et al. (2001) Ways of coping and the health of relatives facing drug and alcohol problems in Mexico and England. *Addiction* 96, 761–74.

Prochaska, J.O. and DiClimente, C.C. (1984) *The Transtheoretical Approach: Crossing Traditional Boundaries of Therapy*. New York: Daw-Jones Ireven.

Rollnick, S., Heather, N., Gold, R. and Hall, W. (1992) Development of a short 'readiness to change questionnaire' for use in brief, opportunistic interventions among excessive drinkers. *Addiction* 87, 743–54.

Segal, D.C., Hersen, M. and Van Hasselt, V.B. (1994) Reliability of the Structured Clinical Interview for DSM-III-R; an evaluative review. *Comprehensive Psychiatry* 35, 316–27.

Skinner, H.A. (1981) Primary syndromes of alcohol abuse: their measurement and correlates. *British Journal of Addiction* 76, 63–76.

Skinner, H.A. and Allen, B.A. (1982) Alcohol dependence syndrome: measurement and validation. *Journal of Abnormal Psychology* 91, 199–209.

Stockwell, T., Hodgson, R., Edwards, G., Taylor, C. and Rankin, H. (1979) The development of a questionnaire to measure severity of alcohol dependence. *British Journal of Addiction* 74, 79–87.

Thom, B., Brown, D., Drummond, C., Edwards, G., Mullan, M. and Taylor, C. (1992) Engaging patients with alcohol problems in treatment: the first consultation. *British Journal of Addiction* 87, 601–11.

Turner, C. (1990) How much alcohol in a 'standard drink'? An analysis of 125 studies. *British Journal of Addiction* 85, 1171–5.

Vaillant, G.E. (1983) *The Natural History of Alcoholism.* Cambridge, MA: Harvard University Press.

Witte, J.S. and Haile, R.W. (1996) Agreement in alcohol consumption levels as measured by two different questionnaires. *Journal of Studies on Alcohol* 56, 406–9.

World Health Organization (1992) *The ICD-10 Classification of Mental and Behavioural Disorders: Clinical Descriptions and Diagnostic Guidelines.* Geneva: World Health Organization.

16

Withdrawal states and treatment of withdrawal

Withdrawal in perspective

Different needs of differing patients

Many patients who have sustained serious problems as a result of their drinking have not contracted the dependence syndrome and will experience no significant physiological disturbance on withdrawal. A further important group of patients will be showing dependence to slight or moderate degree, but will not suffer from withdrawal symptoms which are to any major extent debilitating. However, there are patients who will feel wretched on withdrawal, and a small group for whom withdrawal will precipitate life-threatening disturbance.

Given diversity in possible withdrawal experience, it makes no sense to approach the treatment of withdrawal in terms of a fixed regime for all-comers. A spectrum of likely withdrawal experiences suggests the need for a spectrum of treatment approaches as corollary. Many patients will need no medication at all to help them come off alcohol, and for many others withdrawal can be safely managed on an out-patient basis with minimum drug cover. In only the minority will withdrawal require admission to hospital, but for some of those patients the effective use of medication will be vital. The clinical significance of withdrawal is firstly, therefore, the demand it makes on the clinician to see the different needs of different patients and to manage minor withdrawal states without unnecessary fuss, while at the same time learning to recognize the necessity for very great care in treating the potentially dangerous situation. This chapter discusses treatment in terms of different regimes for different intensities of need.

Significance of withdrawal as barrier to 'coming off'

Some patients will present themselves as unable to come off alcohol because of their incapacity to cope with the withdrawal symptoms. This plea may be entirely genuine. A patient who has previously experienced an attack of delirium tremens may know full well that when they are in a state of severe relapse there is a grave risk of precipitating a further attack of delirium if they attempt abruptly to stop drinking. Their pleas for admission should be heeded. But there are patients with less severe degrees of dependence whose belief that they cannot stop drinking without coming into hospital should be kindly resisted. It is important for such patients to learn that they can cope with withdrawal at home, with minimal ado, and without repeated admissions which reinforce the idea of incapacity to deal with relapse themselves. Unnecessary admissions which mean invalidism and time off work must be avoided.

Withdrawal and team work

Given that drugs may have to be prescribed for out-patient withdrawal, and given also the potential seriousness of the major withdrawal experience which demands in-patient admission, it is evident that the medical practitioner has an important role to play in the treatment of these conditions. If the case is primarily being handled by non-medical staff, this implies the need for good medical liaison. The counsellor in a voluntary agency must, for instance, know when to make the quick out-patient referral, or call on the advice of the general practitioner with whom there is a working relationship.

Detoxification in context

Mere drying out is not by itself an effective way of helping a patient, and whatever is done about withdrawal only has its meaning within the context of other strategies for aiding the patient. When plans for withdrawal are being made at the same time as initial assessment and goal setting, the withdrawal phase is easily placed within the wider frame. When, however, withdrawal is being dealt with in response to relapse and in an atmosphere of crisis, it is easy to react precipitously and forget the context within which decisions about withdrawal treatment ought to be made. Questions which should be asked in such circumstances centre on what *use* the patient is to make of this help (either as out-patient or in-patient), and what the patient's expectations are of this particular aspect of the contract to help. What plans has the patient got for the far side of withdrawal? Treatment of relapse is discussed further in Chapters 17 and 19.

A checklist for detoxification in the community

It should be possible safely and effectively to detoxify the majority of patients in the community (Collins et al., 1990; Stockwell et al., 1991). This section considers the ways in which community or out-patient detoxification of the not too severely dependent patient can be managed.

Does the patient want to come off alcohol?

To put this item first in the checklist may seem an over-emphasis of the obvious, but it is not uncommon to see medical prescribing which suggests a confusion of logic. The doctor has given the patient drugs to treat withdrawal because the doctor believes that the patient ought to come off alcohol, rather than because the patient seriously intends to come off alcohol. The patient leaves the interview with a prescription for a bottle of tranquillizers which they will use to supplement their continued alcohol intake.

Is it safe to conduct withdrawal in an out-patient setting?

This decision is made without difficulty when, as commonly happens, it is obvious that the patient has not got a severe dependence syndrome. They are, for instance, suffering from morning shakes of only moderate intensity which have been present for not much longer than 6 months, and they came off alcohol for 2 weeks on their own initiative and without any untoward happenings only a month ago. A brief review with the patient of such points as these will usually settle the question of whether out-patient withdrawal is appropriate. A similarly quick answer can be reached in the other direction if there is a previous history of major withdrawal experience and the patient has now reinstated dependence of serious degree. It is decisions in the middle ground which set difficulty and which call for the most experienced skill. Handling this problem will, as ever, depend on a relationship with the patient which allows open discussion of the issues involved. Such a patient may come into hospital for an admission of only 2 or 3 days 'to see how things go', or alternatively may opt initially to try detoxification at home provided there is good support.

In addition to severity of dependence, a number of other specific pointers may offer further guidance regarding the safety of a community 'detox'. Has out-patient detoxification failed previously and, if so, why? Is there any specific medical reason why community detoxification may be hazardous – for example, a history of delirium tremens or withdrawal seizures? Is the home environment sufficiently supportive, both in terms of family or friends who may summon help if needed and in terms of support for treatment of the drinking problem? This is discussed further below.

A summary of the indicators which might suggest that detoxification is more safely and effectively conducted on an in-patient basis is given in Box 16.1.

> **BOX 16.1 Contra-indications to a community detoxification**
> - Severe dependence
> - History of delirium tremens or withdrawal seizures
> - Previous failed community detoxification
> - Unsupportive home environment

Is there likely to be a withdrawal experience which requires treatment?

If it is necessary to make sure that the patient is not so dependent as to preclude the out-patient approach, it is also necessary to ensure that they are indeed suffering from a dependence syndrome, or from dependence of more than minimal degree. Otherwise, one may fairly talk about treatment of their drinking problem and the strategies they may apply for abstinence or ameliorated drinking, but there is no sense in setting up a withdrawal regime when there is no significant withdrawal disturbance to be treated. This might again seem a too obvious point if it were not common to find patients routinely medicated with minor tranquillizers without any enquiry being made into their true needs.

What is the best time?

It may be asking too much for a man or woman with a busy job to try to achieve successful withdrawal in the midst of engagements and in the full setting of usual drinking pressures. Discussion may suggest that the patient should set aside a long weekend or take a holiday specially for this purpose. To suggest this degree of forward planning may usefully help to focus commitment.

Is there adequate support?

Although there are plenty of people who at some time in their lives have been so determined to deal with their drinking that they have come off alcohol in such adverse surroundings as a drink-laden doss house, it is always useful to think through with the patient how environmental supports may be deployed to maximize the chances of success. If there is a husband or wife to give support, that person should be brought into the discussion and the active engagement of the spouse may have benefit for both partners. This may also be the moment when a patient will be particularly able to accept the usefulness of Alcoholics Anonymous (AA): getting out, perhaps, to an AA meeting and hearing how others dealt with this problem, or a phone call from an AA member giving a feeling of contact and fellowship, with a follow-through to more continuing involvement. The hospital doctor must also ensure that the general practitioner is kept in the picture. Support from the hospital may imply the offer of daily appointments over the period of a few days, and staff should be prepared to make a home visit if necessary. If there is no other social support available, day-patient facilities for a short period may be helpful.

Use of drugs

Some practical aspects for the use of drugs in out-patient withdrawal are briefly discussed in this section, both to provide background information for the person other than the doctor who wants to understand this aspect of the patient's treatment, and to emphasize points of immediate medical concern.

Given that assessment suggests that a major withdrawal state is not a risk but that there is reason to believe that some degree of withdrawal symptoms is going to be experienced, most patients within this band of the dependence spectrum are going to require prescription of a minor tranquillizer. The same drug may be used for daytime and night-time sedation. Within this spectrum there will, however, be a range of severities, so therapy may involve a range of drug doses, with the emphasis always on avoiding needless over-medication.

There is a number of different drugs which are effective for this purpose. A drug of the benzodiazepine group should be considered as the first choice. It is best for the individual doctor to become familiar with one drug, so as to develop a sense of the likely dosages needed in particular circumstances, rather than switching from drug to drug. Among the benzodiazepines, chlordiazepoxide (trade name Librium) may be prescribed in a dose of, say, 5–10 mg three or four times per day.

Although chlormethiazole (trade name Heminevrin) has been popular in the UK in the past, and may still have a role for in-patient detoxification, it is contra-indicated in the out-patient context. This is because of the potentially fatal inter-action with alcohol in the case of the patient who continues drinking (McInnes, 1987). Chlormethiazole is not licensed for prescription in the USA.

The dose and frequency of medication should be discussed with the patient and spouse, and instructions written down explicitly. A prescription should not be given for more than 3–7 days, and prescribing should not be allowed to trail on unnecessarily once the patient has withdrawn. A community detoxification regime does not need to be longer than 1 week. The patient should be cautioned against the risks of driving when under the influence of drugs.

Prescription of vitamins is not an absolute requirement of withdrawal treatment within this severity range, but oral supplements may be offered, and may sometimes be specifically indicated on other grounds such as clinical evidence of malnutrition. Similarly, electrolyte disturbance is unlikely to be a major concern in this group. However, it should be remembered that serum potassium levels can fall, and oral potassium supplementation may be required, even in the relatively mild cases of alcohol withdrawal which are treated in the community (Burin and Cook, 2000).

A checklist for in-patient treatment of withdrawal (other than delirium tremens or withdrawal seizures)

In this section, the treatment of the greater part of the spectrum of withdrawal states seen in the in-patient setting is discussed, but treatment of delirium tremens and of alcohol withdrawal seizures is held over for discussion in the next section. The checklist here bears on medical and nursing practice.

Remember that in the in-patient setting (as with out-patients), a wide range of withdrawal states will be encountered

It is inappropriate for a ward to operate in terms of any fixed drug regime. At the time of admission, a patient-specific withdrawal regime has to be set up for each case, and this regime must be flexible in response to unfolding events.

Monitoring is very important

Competent routine ward monitoring provides the basis for treatment which is alert, flexible and able rapidly to be escalated in case of need. There is much to be said for the use of standardized scales to facilitate this process, and several suitable instruments are available. For example, the Selective Severity Assessment scale (SSA: Gross et al., 1973) provides precise instructions for rating 11 variables: eating disturbance, sleep disturbance, agitation, hallucinations, tremor, sweats, clouding of consciousness, quality of contact, temperature, pulse and convulsions. The revised Clinical Institute Withdrawal Assessment for Alcohol scale (CIWA-Ar: Sullivan et al., 1989) is a more recent, ten-item, derivation of the SSA, which has been refined and modified in various ways. An example of a briefer, eight-item, scale (Mainz Alcohol Withdrawal Scale: Banger et al., 1992) is given in Table 16.1. Careful monitoring, combined with supportive care can reduce the need for medication (Shaw et al., 1981).

A sensible ward procedure may be for the nurses to make at least 8-hourly observations on all withdrawing patients for the first 3 days, but this may need to be more frequent during the first 24 hours. Observations may be discontinued with the senior nurse's approval if all areas are normal. Every now and then, a patient who has given an incomplete history and who is expected to show only mild withdrawal will unexpectedly develop more severe symptoms. Routine observations over the first few days are therefore essential.

In addition to rating withdrawal symptoms, breath alcohol should be measured when the patient arrives on the ward, and again an hour or so later. This allows an estimation of the actual blood alcohol concentration and also confirms the rate of fall of blood alcohol. This is important for several reasons. Firstly, if estimated blood or breath alcohol is high, there may be a danger of interaction with prescribed

Table 16.1 Mainz Alcohol Withdrawal Scale (MAWS)

Item	Rating			
	0 None	1 Mild	2 Marked	3 Severe
Disorientation		Full orientation but sluggish answers	Blurred orientation in at least one quality	Disorientation in at least one quality
Hallucinations		Occasional, distancing possible	Frequent, sometimes distancing still possible	Nearly permanently, no distancing at all
Inattentiveness		Slip of the tongue, misunderstanding	High suggestibility: string catching, reading	Spontaneous illusions
Disturbance of contact		Good contact with investigator, but not with environment	Sometimes poor contact with investigator	No contact with investigator
Agitation		Feeling nervous	Physical restlessness	Absolute psychomotor agitation
Tremor		Extended fingers	Extended hands	Tremor of hands or body when resting
Hyperhidrosis		Palpable on hands and forehead	Visible on hands and forehead	Visible on total body
Anxiety		Reported on questioning only	Expressed by behaviour	Panic

From Banger et al. (1992).

medication during the first few hours of admission, and particular care must be taken with prescribing during this period. Secondly, if the patient has consumed a significant amount of alcohol immediately before admission, their blood alcohol levels may still be rising. This should generate even greater caution in the prescribing and administration of medication immediately after admission.

Environment

That the environment should be properly supportive is as important here as when the patient is detoxifying at home. General and psychiatric nursing skills have to be employed to help the patient through what may be a few unpleasant days, and the ability of the patient to tolerate this experience will depend in part on the sort of friendliness which they are being offered. Mobilizing support from other patients and from visiting relatives can also be valuable.

Drug treatments

Prescription of a number of different types of drugs may be appropriate. They are each considered here in turn.

Minor tranquillizers

The same types of drugs can be prescribed here as for ambulatory treatment, but in a setting which allows close monitoring and where the severer grades of withdrawal are sometimes being dealt with, considerably larger doses may on occasion be employed. There is an old saying that the proper dose of any drug is *enough*, and that certainly applies in these circumstances. The skilled use of a drug with the intention of ameliorating severe withdrawal distress or aborting risk of delirium is a matter of titrating the drug dose against the symptoms. The withdrawal symptoms occur because the level of alcohol in the brain is falling, and these symptoms will be ameliorated when the level of prescribed drug is high enough to compensate for the fall in alcohol. What one is in fact doing is substituting a monitored drug intoxication for an alcohol intoxication, and it is in those terms necessary and rational in the severe case to press the drug dose boldly.

With a benzodiazepine, in severe withdrawal, one may have to give quite large doses. For example a dose of 40–60 mg chlordiazepoxide, three or four times a day, or even more than this, may be required. If there is immediate need to bring severe symptoms under control, then lorazepam may be given by intramuscular injection, with an initial dose of, say, 25–30 mg/kg. Alternatively, diazepam may be given by slow intravenous injection or per rectum (as a suppository or enema).

If chlormethiazole is given, the dose may be pressed up to, say, 600 mg of chlormethiazole base, four times daily by mouth. Note that chlormethiazole syrup contains chlormethiazole edisylate, and that 250 mg chlormethiazole edisylate in syrup is therapeutically equivalent to approximately 192 mg chlormethiazole base as a capsule. If in doubt about dosage, current information should be obtained from the manufacturer or the relevant national formulary. In the in-patient setting, this drug can be safely and effectively employed in the treatment of alcohol withdrawal. However, there is no particular advantage over the benzodiazepines. In that in-patient practices are often seen as a model to copy in primary care, it may indeed be best avoided.

It should again be stressed that what is 'enough' is determined by clinical observation of response, rather than by any rule book. If the patient becomes excessively drowsy or if there is a large fall in blood pressure, drugs should be cut back or temporarily withheld. Such an approach is far more in the patient's interests than a blind reliance on heavy mixed drug schedules, which will be unnecessarily extreme in many instances and yet insufficient in other cases.

If it has been necessary in the acute phase to load the patient with a drug, one is then in effect subsequently carrying out a drug withdrawal rather than an alcohol withdrawal procedure. This implies gradually tailing off the drug dose at a rate which will not produce significant drug withdrawal symptoms. The rate of reduction must once more be patient specific and in accord with monitored symptoms. Problems may in particular arise if withdrawal from a large dose of chlormethiazole is carried out too quickly, resulting in confusion or symptoms of delirium. There is evidence that few, if any, patients actually require medication with a benzodiazepine for more than 2 days (Saitz et al., 1994), and regimes of longer than 7–10 days are rarely, if ever, necessary for uncomplicated alcohol withdrawal.

Vitamins

With patients who have had a heavy alcohol intake, there is the risk of an acute Wernicke's encephalopathy developing with disastrous suddenness (see Chapter 7), and it is therefore a wise prophylactic measure to give thiamine (vitamin B_1) supplements. These may be given orally, for example in a dose of 100 mg daily, but there is evidence that absorption is particularly poor in this group of patients (Thomson et al., 1970). Parenteral administration (either intramuscular or slow intravenous) is therefore essential where there is any specific cause for concern (Cook and Thomson, 1997). For example, in cases of malnutrition, peripheral neuropathy or signs and symptoms of a Wernicke–Korsakoff syndrome, it is particularly important to employ this approach. Because the diagnosis of Wernicke's encephalopathy is easily missed, a presumptive diagnosis should be made, and treatment instituted, with a low threshold of suspicion (Cook et al., 1998). A presumptive diagnosis should be made in any patient undergoing alcohol withdrawal who shows signs of acute confusion, ataxia, ophthalmoplegia, memory disturbance, hypothermia or hypotension.

The correct dose of thiamine is a subject of debate, but one pair of ampoules of high-potency parenteral B vitamins, once or twice daily for 3–5 days, is probably effective in preventing the onset of Wernicke–Korsakoff syndrome. A higher dose may well be required in established cases and treatment should not be considered ineffective unless at least two pairs of ampoules of high-potency parenteral B vitamins have been given three times daily for at least 2 days (Cook et al., 1998).

Administration of parenteral vitamins has become much less popular following reports of very rare, but sometimes severe, adverse reactions (O'Brien, 1995). However, it must not be forgotten that Wernicke's encephalopathy is potentially fatal, and that the sequelae can be severely disabling. In a properly supervised in-patient setting, where some patients may be at particular risk of Wernicke–Korsakoff syndrome, the balance of risks and benefits will usually be in favour of parenteral vitamin supplementation. However, parenteral administration of B complex vitamins should only be used in circumstances which will allow emergency cardiopulmonary resuscitation to be offered if necessary.

Major tranquillizers

Phenothiazines and other major tranquillizers have no part to play in the treatment of this spectrum of withdrawal, and only add to the risks.

Specific treatment to avert withdrawal seizures

The effective use of minor tranquillizers should be sufficient to minimize the development of withdrawal convulsions, and it is usually neither necessary nor useful to give additional medication for this purpose. (See below for further discussion of this matter.)

The treatment of delirium tremens

This section deals with technical issues which are mainly the concern of medical and nursing staff, but it may again be of interest to other professionals to acquaint themselves with at least the outlines of how such problems are handled. (See Chapter 7 for a full discussion of the causes and clinical features of delirium tremens.)

The best hope here is, in fact, that the condition will not arise and not have to be treated. If severe withdrawal is adequately managed with appropriate drug doses, the risk of delirium tremens will in many instances be aborted. However, despite best efforts, ward admission and alcohol withdrawal will sometimes precipitate delirium tremens, and cases of already established delirium will also sometimes present directly for admission. Once a fully developed attack of delirium tremens is under way, it is uncertain whether any treatment will actually shorten the course of the disorder, but there is persuasive evidence that the difference between competent and less competent treatment may be the survival as opposed to the death of the patient. The dangers of death from delirium tremens should not be exaggerated, but they exist.

Here is the list of matters to be kept in mind when treating this condition (see also Box 16.2).

What setting for treatment?

Given the risks to life, patients suffering from this condition should have the benefit of being treated in a setting where the medical and nursing staff are as experienced

---

BOX 16.2 Important requirements in the treatment of delirium tremens
- In-patient environment, preferably with experienced staff
- Careful assessment and monitoring for co-morbid physical and psychiatric disorders – especially head injury, intercurrent infection, liver disease and hepatic coma, gastrointestinal bleeding and acute Wernicke–Korsakoff syndrome
- Chlordiazepoxide is the preferred drug treatment
- Careful monitoring of body temperature, fluids, electrolytes and blood sugar
- Parenteral vitamin supplementation
- Availability of emergency medical facilities

---

as possible. When a case occurs on a psychiatric ward, there may be uncertainty as to whether the patient should remain on that ward or be transferred to a general medical unit. The decision can only be made in the light of an appraisal of the skills and resources available in either setting.

Whatever the ward on which the patient is to be treated, the basic elements which the setting must provide are much the same. First-rate nursing is required, both for observation and for care. The situation must be one in which a potentially disturbed patient can be cared for without staff becoming flustered, and there must be precaution against a patient sustaining accidental injury whilst in a state of confusion. A safe nursing environment must be established, with no possibility of the patient falling out of the window or wandering off the ward. A patient who is only uncertainly in contact with reality is going to be helped by friendliness, reassurance and by good room lighting rather than a side room with shadowy corners.

Depending upon the mental health legislation of the country concerned, it may be necessary to consider formal admission if the patient refuses to stay in hospital. The risks to such patients, should they be allowed to take their own discharge, would be considerable and there should be no hesitation to arrange an assessment for compulsory detention. In the UK, this would be under a section of the Mental Health Act (1983). Note that it is the delirium tremens, not alcohol dependence, which would justify detention against the patient's will.

What underlying or complicating conditions may be missed?

Those patients who die in delirium tremens perhaps most often do so as a result of a medical complication which has been overlooked. Such oversight, unless actively guarded against, can easily come about when all energies are being concentrated on dealing with the immediate and acutely worrying presentation. The patient is probably in no condition to give an accurate history or an account of other symptoms.

The conditions which may have to be recognized are many, and no checklist can substitute for full initial examination and subsequent continued watchfulness. However, the conditions specially to be borne in mind include the possibility of head injury, intercurrent infection (particularly chest infection), liver disease and hepatic coma, gastrointestinal bleeding, and the acute onset of the Wernicke–Korsakoff syndrome. The picture may also be complicated if the patient has been taking barbiturates or another depressant.

What drug to use for specific treatment?

Much the same considerations apply here as with the choice of drugs for treatment of less severe withdrawal symptoms. A great deal of research has been aimed at determining which drug is likely to be most useful in treating delirium tremens, and the evidence is still conflicting. On the whole, it seems best to employ a drug with cross-tolerance to alcohol, and hence one which effectively *substitutes* for alcohol. Chlordiazepoxide may be given in a dose up to 400 mg daily by mouth in divided doses. When a rapid response is required, it may be necessary to supplement this with intramuscular, intravenous or rectal medication, as described above. As ever, an intravenous drug should not be used if avoidable. The dose of chlormethiazole will usually be in the region of 600 mg by mouth, four times daily (but see the note above regarding the dosage of chlormethiazole syrup, which is slightly different), with higher doses employed with care if indicated. Phenothiazines and other major tranquillizers may increase the risk to life, although some clinicians do prescribe them in delirium tremens, to control acutely disturbed behaviour (Chick, 1989) or hallucinations (Fish, 1991).

The use of an intravenous chlormethiazole infusion is worthy of especial mention, because of the particular dangers associated with its use. It is rarely, and in our experience virtually never, necessary to resort to such treatment if oral chlordiazepoxide has been employed boldly in conjunction with good nursing care. Where chlordiazepoxide is employed, we would urge that it should only be when high doses of oral chlordiazepoxide have failed to control the delirium, and when the uncontrolled withdrawal state itself poses a serious risk to the safety of the patient. The correct protocol is for 24–60 mg/min (as a 0.8% solution of chlormethiazole edisylate) until shallow sleep is induced. This should then be reduced to the lowest possible rate to maintain shallow sleep with spontaneous respiration. Such treatment should never be employed unless adequate resuscitation facilities are available, and then only with constant monitoring of cardiorespiratory function and consciousness level. Sudden changes in cardiorespiratory function or consciousness are a notorious and unpredictable complication of such treatment, and may have fatal consequences in the absence of unceasing vigilance. Prolonged treatment should be avoided as it may be associated with accumulation of the drug, electrolyte imbalance and delayed recovery. At intervals, the flow of the infusion should therefore be reduced, in order to check that consciousness lightens rapidly. Especial care must be taken when drug clearance is reduced by hepatic impairment or when cerebral, pulmonary or cardiac function is compromised, and in the elderly. Drug interactions (especially with other depressants such as chlordiazepoxide) are also a potentially fatal concern. If these warnings have not discouraged the reader from ever using this treatment, then the manufacturer's data sheet, and an appropriate formulary (for instance the British National Formulary) should be consulted for further advice before prescribing or administering intravenous chlormethiazole.

Fluids and electrolytes

Patients who are over-active, sweating and feverish (and perhaps also suffering from gastrointestinal disturbance) are candidates for serious disturbances in fluid and electrolyte balance, which must therefore be monitored. A dangerous fall in potassium level must be averted, and there have been suggestions that decreased magnesium levels are a particular likelihood in delirium tremens (Turner et al., 1989). Blood sugar levels should also be watched. Although a drip may have to be set up, fluid and electrolyte correction should be managed as far as possible by oral administration: keeping a drip in position with a delirious patient can lead to problems.

Vitamins

Given the dangers of a Wernicke–Korsakoff syndrome, there can be no doubt that the patient with delirium tremens should receive heavy intravenous or intramuscular doses of thiamine for several days. With the virtual impossibility at an early stage of distinguishing the signs and symptoms of delirium tremens from those of Wernicke's encephalopathy, a presumptive diagnosis of the latter condition should be made, and treatment instituted accordingly (see above).

Life support

Emergency facilities must be available in the event of acute circulatory failure. A rare complication is hyperthermia with the temperature suddenly rising to 40.5 °C or more. Hepatic coma is sometimes precipitated when the previously malnourished patient begins to take protein.

Alcohol withdrawal seizures

Seizures usually occur within the first 24 hours of admission (Turner et al., 1989), but they may also happen during the course of delirium (see Chapter 7). They are less likely to develop if the patient has been adequately sedated, and the same basic drug treatment as for withdrawal symptoms is in general the correct prophylaxis for withdrawal seizures, rather than additional anti-convulsant medication being given. However, opinions differ on this matter and there may be an argument for prescribing anti-convulsant medication for patients whose past history suggests a particular risk of withdrawal seizures (Turner et al., 1989). If a sequence of seizures occurs or status epilepticus develops (a run of seizures in continuous succession), intravenous medication will have to be given to bring the situation rapidly under control, and the usual measures deployed as for any patient suffering from convulsions.

A case history

A 33-year-old man, living alone, asked his social worker for help with 'coming off' alcohol. A previous episode of withdrawal, a year earlier, had failed because he recommenced drinking whilst still taking medication prescribed for his withdrawal symptoms. He therefore reluctantly agreed that on this occasion he would go into hospital for detoxification. On arrival on the ward, he was intoxicated, with a blood alcohol concentration of 350 mg/100 ml. An hour later, a repeat measurement indicated a decrease to 335 mg/100 ml, at which point the patient was starting to sweat and suffering from a coarse tremor. Regular observations of withdrawal symptoms were commenced using the CIWA-Ar and chlordiazepoxide was prescribed, commencing with a cautious dose of 25 mg in view of the high breath alcohol.

In view of the evidence of poor nutritional status, a high-dose B-complex vitamin preparation was prescribed, for intramuscular administration once daily for 5 days.

Over the first 24 hours, a total of 250 mg chlordiazepoxide was administered to the patient orally and this was effective in keeping him reasonably comfortable, albeit he was rather sleepless for the first night on the ward. Gradually lower doses of chlordiazepoxide were prescribed over succeeding days, and the drug was discontinued completely after 5 days on the ward.

The patient was discharged after 10 days. By this time, after encouragement and advice from the ward staff, he had made his own arrangements to be admitted to a residential rehabilitation facility in another part of the country. Arrangements had also been made by the medical staff for him to receive investigation and treatment for a suspected peptic ulcer. The ward occupational therapist had taught him some basic anxiety management techniques, as he had indicated that he often drank in response to symptoms of anxiety, due to various life stresses.

Withdrawal from drugs other than alcohol

Some patients may be dependent upon other drugs, in addition to their dependence on or misuse of alcohol (see Chapter 9). Some patients who are experiencing drinking problems but who are not dependent upon alcohol may nevertheless be dependent upon a drug or drugs other than alcohol. In all of these circumstances, appropriate medical management of withdrawal from drugs other than alcohol must be provided. It is not possible to describe here in detail the clinical management of withdrawal from all other types of drugs. However, a few comments may be in order in relation to dependence upon benzodiazepines and opioids, and the interested reader is referred to more detailed sources for further information in relation to these and other drugs (e.g. Frank and Pead, 1995).

Benzodiazepine dependence is usually best managed in the community, with gradual dose reduction being undertaken over a period of weeks or months (Higgitt et al., 1985; Schweizer and Rickels, 1998). However, where concomitant alcohol withdrawal is involved, admission may be required in order to ensure appropriate monitoring and prescribing during the acute phase of alcohol and early benzodiazepine withdrawal. It is usually best to convert other benzodiazepines into the equivalent dosage of diazepam or chlordiazepoxide and then to adjust the dose of this single drug in accordance with alcohol withdrawal symptoms. Managing the doses of several benzodiazepines prescribed concomitantly can be confusing at best, and dangerous at worst. Whereas benzodiazepines are usually discontinued after 7–10 days in cases of acute alcohol withdrawal alone, concomitant benzodiazepine dependence will usually require that the patient be discharged to the community on a lower dose, which is then gradually tailed off over a period of weeks or months. More rapid withdrawal can lead to prolonged symptoms of anxiety, and a risk of benzodiazepine withdrawal seizures.

Opioid dependence may be managed either by gradual dose reduction of the drug in question (e.g. methadone or codeine) or by substitution with methadone and then gradual methadone reduction over a period of weeks or months. Alternatively, other drugs may be prescribed in order to ameliorate the symptoms of acute opioid withdrawal. Amongst the drugs used in this way are drugs such as lofexidine (Bearn et al., 1996; Sheridan et al., 1999) which also have a reported benefit in the management of mild alcohol withdrawal (see, for example, Cushman and Sowers, 1989).

Withdrawal symptoms in summary

From what has been said in this chapter, it must be evident that the clinical skills required effectively to respond to the range of alcohol withdrawal pictures that will be encountered involve the ability to deploy a range of techniques apposite to varied presentations. The proper use of drugs can sometimes be very important, but this should not lead to any neglect of the importance of support and encouragement. The trust and the relationships established during the treatment of the crisis can be valuably carried through to the next phase of treatment.

REFERENCES

Banger, M., Philipp, M., Herth, T., Hebenstreit, M. and Aldenhoff, J. (1992) Development of a rating scale for quantitative measurement of the alcohol withdrawal syndrome. *European Archives of Psychiatry and Clinical Neuroscience* 241, 241–6.

Bearn, J., Gossop, M. and Strang, J. (1996) Randomised double-blind comparison of lofexidine and methadone in the in-patient treatment of opiate withdrawal. *Drug and Alcohol Dependence* 43, 87–91.

Burin, M.R.M.J. and Cook, C.C.H. (2000) Alcohol withdrawal and hypokalaemia: a case report. *Alcohol and Alcoholism* 35, 188–9.

Chick, J. (1989) Delirium tremens. *British Medical Journal* 298, 3–4.

Collins, M.N., Burns, T., Van den Berk, P.A.H. and Tubman, G.F. (1990) A structured programme for out-patient alcohol detoxification. *British Journal of Psychiatry* 156, 871–4.

Cook, C.C.H., Hallwood, P.M. and Thomson, A.D. (1998) B vitamin deficiency and neuropsychiatric syndromes in alcohol misuse. *Alcohol and Alcoholism* 33, 317–36.

Cook, C.C.H. and Thomson, A.D. (1997) B-complex vitamins in the prevention and treatment of Wernicke–Korsakoff syndrome. *British Journal of Hospital Medicine* 57, 461–5.

Cushman, P. and Sowers, J.R. (1989) Alcohol withdrawal syndrome: clinical and hormonal responses to α2-adrenergic agonist treatment. *Alcoholism: Clinical and Experimental Research* 13, 361–3.

Fish, D.N. (1991) Treatment of delirium in the critically ill patient. *Clinical Pharmacology and Therapeutics* 10, 456–66.

Frank, L. and Pead, J. (1995) *New Concepts in Drug Withdrawal*. Monograph Series, No. 4. Melbourne: The University of Melbourne.

Gross, M.M., Lewis, E. and Nagarajan, M. (1973) An improved quantitative system for assessing the acute alcoholic psychoses and related states (TSA and SSA). In *Alcohol Intoxication and Withdrawal: Experimental Studies*, Vol. 35, ed. Gross, M.M. New York: Plenum Press, 365–76.

Higgitt, A.C., Lader, M.H. and Fonagy, P. (1985) Clinical management of benzodiazepine dependence. *British Medical Journal* 291, 688–90.

McInnes, G. (1987) Chlormethiazole and alcohol: a lethal cocktail. *British Medical Journal* 294, 592.

O'Brien, P. (1995) Parenteral vitamin therapy in alcoholism. *Psychiatric Bulletin* 19, 788.

Saitz, R., Mayo-Smith, M.F., Roberts, M.S., Redmond, H.A., Bernard, D.R. and Calkins, D.R. (1994) Individualized treatment for alcohol withdrawal. A randomized double-blind controlled trial. *Journal of the American Medical Association* 272, 519–23.

Schweizer, E. and Rickels, K. (1998) Benzodiazepine dependence and withdrawal: a review of the syndrome and its clinical management. *Acta Psychiatrica Scandinavica* 98 (Suppl. 393), 95–101.

Shaw, J.M., Kolesar, G.S., Sellers, E.M., Kaplan, H.L. and Sandor, P. (1981) Development of optimal treatment tactics for alcohol withdrawal. I. Assesment and effectiveness of supportive care. *Journal of Clinical Psychopharmacology* 1, 382–8.

Sheridan, J., Cook, C. and Strang, J. (1999) Audit of the in-patient management of opioid withdrawal using lofexidine hydrochloride. *Journal of Substance Use* 4, 29–34.

Stockwell, T., Bolt, L., Milner, I., Russell, G., Bolderston, H. and Pugh, P. (1991) Home detoxification from alcohol: its safety and efficacy in comparison with in-patient care. *Alcohol and Alcoholism* 26, 645–50.

Sullivan, J.T., Sykora, K., Schneiderman, J., Naranjo, C.A. and Sellers, E.M. (1989) Assessment of alcohol withdrawal: the revised Clinical Institute Withdrawal Assessment for Alcohol scale (CIWA-Ar). *British Journal of Addiction* 84, 1353–7.

Thomson, A.D., Baker, H. and Leevy, C.H. (1970) Patterns of ^{35}S-thiamine hydrochloride absorption in the malnourished alcoholic patient. *Journal of Laboratory and Clinical Medicine* 76, 34–45.

Turner, R.C., Lichstein, P.R., Peden, J.G., Busher, J.T. and Waivers, L.E. (1989) Alcohol withdrawal syndromes: a review of pathophysiology, clinical presentation, and treatment. *Journal of General Internal Medicine* 4, 432–44.

17

The basic work of treatment

The structure of this chapter is as follows. The meaning given to the term 'basic work' is first defined and the significance of the therapeutic relationship discussed. Some guiding principles to provide a frame within which the therapy will be conducted are outlined, and the likely content of the basic therapeutic work is considered, with emphasis on a person-specific approach. Attention is then given to such issues as how the effort to achieve sobriety is to be made worthwhile, for the patient, how to deal positively with relapse, basic work with the family, and matters relating to the duration and termination of treatment. A note is given on basic approaches in the generalist setting. The chapter is rounded off with a summary which identifies 12 core elements fundamental to the treatment process.

What is meant by 'basic work'?

Special techniques, such as various psychotherapies, cognitive and behavioural therapy or the use of drugs, can all make contributions to an individual's treatment programme (see Chapter 19). It is these approaches which offer the conventional headings for discussion, while the undramatic basics of the helping process tend to be passed by, or dismissed as the background to the application of specialized techniques. It is, however, vital that attention should be given to the subtle and important range of happenings which occur whenever patient and therapist interact – the what, when and how of what is felt and said and done between them. Otherwise, we are at risk of throwing out as packaging the essential content of the parcel. Here is how a patient saw what happened between him and a doctor.

I remember when I first met that doctor. She seemed friendly, but when I tried to con her, she laughed and told me to get my priorities right. Typical alcoholic thinking – just told myself that she didn't understand, and I didn't bother to turn up for the next appointment. What happened next? I get a letter, not one of those form-letters that hospitals send out, but a personal letter from this doctor saying something like, 'I know it's difficult. I don't want to push you into anything, but I'll be in the clinic on Friday afternoon if you want to talk about things further.' So I went back to tell her she didn't understand!

Concern for the impression made at the first encounter (Thom et al., 1992), the ability to combine being 'friendly' with confrontation, finding a phrase like 'priorities' to sort out complexity, the way a letter is written (Batel et al., 1995) – these are examples which point to what is meant by 'basic work'.

Interventions are only likely to produce movement when in alignment with the real possibilities for change within the individual, the family and the social setting (Vaillant, 1983, 1993). The basic work of therapy is largely concerned with nudging and supporting movement along these 'natural' pathways of recovery. We need a more developed sense of people's innate capacity for recovery and the possible dimensions of recovery, rather than a belief that we can impose therapies on people who are to be marched along at our dictate. The clumsy therapist is like someone who tries to carve a piece of wood without respect for the grain. The basic work of treatment requires immense respect for that grain, and therapy must always be matched to individual needs.

This chapter is written largely in terms of the patient or client who is aiming at abstinence rather than at modification of drinking. That latter question is dealt with in Chapter 20. Much of what is said in this chapter is, however, generally applicable, whatever the chosen goal.

The relationship

The relationship between patient and therapist is fundamental, both to what can be achieved in any one therapeutic session and to what changes can be won over time (Carroll and Rounsaville, 1993; Luborsky et al., 1985). It begins to be built at the first moment of contact, is developed during the assessment interview (or interviews), is vital to the effectiveness of the initial counselling and goal-setting, and continues thereafter as an important component of therapy (Edwards, 1996). 'What is said' matters, but it cannot be abstracted from the feelings between the two people who are doing the saying and the listening. Take, for instance, the following remarks by a therapist, which might be necessary at a certain point in an individual's treatment.

You know that I believe you can stop drinking and make sense of your life, but things can't usefully just drag on. You've been coming up here regularly to talk about your problems for the last 6 months, and we are both aware that you're now becoming badly caught up in this business of 'I'll start tomorrow...the day after'. Here's a challenge. I'm not giving you an appointment for next week but instead am going to propose that you come back in 6 weeks and show me that by then you have stopped these binges and started instead to do some of those things with your family that you have been talking about. I want you to show yourself that you can succeed, and that will be a great feeling. It's time to make a start. You *can* make a start.

That same form of words may have three different types of impact. The impact may be negative, with the patient reinforced in their sense of hopelessness. The second alternative is for the patient in effect not to hear what is said, because no words spoken within a meaningless relationship can matter: if they bother to come back in 6 weeks' time, it will be with nothing having changed, and with what was said in that previous session blandly neutralized. Lastly, there is the possibility that the challenge is taken and used as a turning point, but this outcome can only be expected when the relationship positively matters. At worst, the word 'relationship' is devalued into a catch-phrase of professional jargon, and yet every now and then one senses again the intensely important reality of what is being talked about.

Work with drinking problems requires awareness of how relationships are made and used, but there is little which is unique to alcohol problems in this regard. The same basic skills are needed in any area of therapy and the general nature of a therapeutic relationship will not be discussed here in detail. It may, however, be useful to list a number of considerations which derive from psychotherapeutic principles (Luborsky and Crits-Christoph, 1990; Malan and Osimu, 1992), but which have to be thought through when working with drinking problems (Levin and Weiss, 1994). These issues are summarized in Box 17.1

> **BOX 17.1 The therapeutic relationship**
> *The quality of the relationship between therapist and client is fundamental to what can be achieved:*
> - The ability to show empathy
> - Avoiding possessiveness and the lure of directiveness
> - Conferring worth and giving hope

Showing warmth and empathy

Warmth cannot be invented, and a show of pretended warmth will be transparent. When warmth is genuinely experienced, it still has to be conveyed, and there are skills in the use of voice and gesture as well as in learning how to convey warmth in words which are not cloying.

Possessiveness and directiveness

The seeming helplessness of the patient who is caught up in drinking and their pleas for rescue, if not guarded against, may set up a relationship in which the patient is invited to slip into the regressed role of a child. The therapist takes the position of the perplexed and guilt-ridden parent, loaded with responsibility to save the child from its wilful destructiveness. Such a relationship is the antithesis of one which encourages growth towards autonomy. Directiveness may work in the short term as the patient is carried along by the therapist's will and demand, but progress of that kind is unlikely to be sustained. The patient will sooner or later rebel and drinking is the likely act of rebellion.

Conferring worth and giving hope

The way in which the patient's bad feelings about themselves are to be handled within the relationship is another important question. Feelings of worthlessness, helplessness, pessimism and unresolved guilt are common in the person who has experienced years of excessive drinking, and can handicap the attempt at recovery. The therapist's job is not to give cheery and false comfort which will carry no conviction, but to attempt by many small strategies to help towards better feelings.

To predict at baseline which patient will form an effective therapeutic alliance with a particular patient is, however, difficult, and research reveals few strong statistical pointers. The patient's depression may handicap the process, while a strong initial motivation for change may help towards a positive relationship (Project MATCH, 1998; Gerdner and Holmberg, 2000; Connors et al., 2000; Carroll, 2001).

Work with the patient: some guiding principles

What actually happens when, after the initial assessment, formulation and goal-setting, the client and therapist, on a series of later occasions, sit down together and talk? Here are some principles which can guide the work and they are summarized in Box 17.2.

BOX 17.2 **Working with the patient: guiding principles**
- Seek to maintain continuity of purpose. Use the initial formulation and goal-setting, check on what has been achieved, set further goals in concrete terms.
- Be flexible, listen to what the patient brings to the session, but identify leading issues for the session.
- Be aware of what is happening in the therapeutic relationship.
- Hold on to the family perspective.
- Monitor progress and engage the patient in self-monitoring.
- Keep a balance between dynamics and realities.
- Maintain a balance of emphasis between drinking and other areas for work.

Maintain continuity of purpose

Both patient and therapist have to maintain a sense of progress and purpose, and avoid confusion and drift. Recovery needs a maintained sense of direction. This is achieved in a number of ways.

1. *Make use of the initial formulation and goal-setting.* The initial exercise in clarification of understanding and purpose should be referred to as the continued basis for action (see Chapter 15).

2. *Emphasize what has been achieved.* At each session, it is useful for the therapist to help the patient identify what has been achieved since the last meeting and thus reinforce the patient's own sense of achievement: for instance, a day or so many days or weeks of abstinence, a difficult situation dealt with successfully, a new job started, an outing with the family, or new aspects of self-understanding.

3. *Set the next task for the short term.* The meeting also has to identify what are to be the next steps, with the patient making a commitment to attempt these steps. The work plan is of no value if it is only in terms of generalities, such as 'getting some other interests going' or 'trying to be more understanding of the wife's point of view'.

4. *An eye on the slightly longer term.* Although it is useful to concentrate on the short term (Alcoholics Anonymous's 'day at a time'), patients will also, to varying extents, want to see further ahead, and be helped forward by thoughts of what things may look like in 6 months or a year hence. The person who thinks concretely will be happier to plan their steps in such visible terms as new possessions, whereas someone else may chart their progress in terms of personal changes and changes in relationships.

Be aware of the relationship

The importance of the therapeutic relationship has already been noted, and continuing thought has to be given to what is occurring in this regard. Is the therapist, for instance, being edged into a too authoritarian role, or being moved towards argument or sterile intellectual debate?

Hold on to the family perspective

Despite intentions, it is easy to become too focused on the individual and to discover after some months that the needs of the family and the relevance of the home situation have been allowed to slip from sight, with adverse consequences. If the patient has a family, what is happening within the family and within other close relationships has to be discussed and plans made for continuing work with the people involved.

Monitor progress

Implicit in the idea of commitment is the expectation that commitment will be met, but the process only works if the therapist checks on what is agreed. It is helpful for the patient to feel that their progress is being monitored, and periodic reporting to the therapist can be supported by an element of self-monitoring. The patient may, for instance, be asked to keep a daily diary, with headings to deal with such issues as drinking, craving, 'tricky situations' and the use of leisure time.

Maintain a balance between dynamics and realities

The treatment approach which is outlined in this chapter embraces a concern with psychodynamics, cognitive–behavioural aspects and external realities. There is danger in putting too heavy an emphasis on one area while others are neglected.

Keep a balance between drinking and other issues

Each interview is likely to reinforce the agreed drinking goal and monitor progress along the drinking dimension. Work towards recovery also has to be planned, pursued and monitored along other dimensions, often bearing on enhancement of the quality of sobriety. It is when the therapist or patient focuses too much on one sector to the cost of any other that things go wrong (see Chapter 21).

The therapeutic work

So much for a discussion of the general framework. With those headings in mind, we can now go on to look at some likely detailed content of the therapeutic work.

Working on the drinking problem

According to the phase of recovery to which the patient has progressed, this heading will have different meanings. It should again be emphasized that this discussion is worded in terms of the patient who is aiming at abstinence, although with due modification the same principles apply to work towards a controlled drinking goal. For instance, at the earliest stage the immediate question is how the patient who is aiming at abstinence is to come off drink and be helped where necessary with detoxification (see Chapter 16), whereas for the patient who has chosen the goal of controlled drinking, the immediate task is to get the drinking under control (Chapter 20). Whichever the chosen goal, the patient has to be presented with the unambiguous message that dealing with the drinking problem is a high priority. In terms of Prochaska and DiClimente's 'Stages of Change' model (Prochaska et al., 1994), much of the initial work under this heading may be concerned with helping patients to move from 'precontemplation' to 'contemplation', 'preparation' and then on to 'action' and 'maintenance'. Many therapists find that this model provides them with a useful map for charting individual progress, although at the theoretical level there is debate as to the validity of this segmentation (Davidson, 1996; Sutton, 1996). A further psychological approach relevant to this phase of work is that of *motivational interviewing* (Rollnick and Miller, 1995). Some patients may find a self-help manual useful (Heather et al., 1990).

When the patient is off alcohol – focusing again primarily on the present discussion on the abstinence goal – there is important work to be done on consolidation. The patient's basic understanding of the nature of their drinking problem (and the nature of dependence) has to be rehearsed and reinforced. This is not accomplished by the therapist giving a lecture, but by them pointing up a discussion: 'Just how do you *understand* this drinking problem? How would you explain to another person what's different between your relationship with alcohol and their drinking?' Work on ambivalence is also a continuing task, rather than something ever settled once and for all: 'What would you lose now if you went back to drinking? What so far looks like the best thing that's coming out of sobriety?'

Discussion will usefully focus on questions such as the degree to which the patient is thinking about or craving for alcohol, the cues and circumstances which trigger these subjective experiences, and the ways in which the patient copes with such feelings (Gossop, 1996). Personal coping mechanisms must be identified and it is important to teach patients to think in these terms and rehearse the strategies which are going to be employed in difficult situations. Much of the psychological underpinning of this phase of the work will come from a relapse prevention approach.

Mental health

A patient will often bring up problems related to their 'nerves' – anxiety, phobic symptoms, irritability, jealousy, depression or difficulty in sleeping. During the initial weeks (or even months) of sobriety, these symptoms may still be related to withdrawal, and can therefore be expected gradually to clear. What at first appear to be handicapping phobic symptoms may, for instance, fade out with 2–3 months of sobriety. In practice, the contribution made to the patient's 'nerves' by the biological processes of withdrawal will, over the initial period of sobriety, be inseparable from symptoms which may stem from their rediscovery of what it is like to be their real self, unshielded by alcohol. Their real self may be anxious and irritable, but for years alcohol has blotted out, exacerbated or confused these underlying propensities.

No matter which of the above factors may explain the patient's psychological discomfort, the best immediate response is not heedlessly to offer drugs, but to employ a commonsense and supportive approach. A reflex assumption which has been reinforced over many years' drinking has to be overcome: psychic distress may be part of the human condition and not something which has to be immediately and chemically ablated. The patient is, as it were, too anxious about being anxious.

The patient is then likely to be helped if, together with these basic messages, some ideas are offered as to how distress is to be ameliorated more constructively than by resort to tranquillizers. They may be helped by learning a relaxation technique, or by developing a variety of simple coping strategies such as listening to music, going for a walk or telephoning a friend. While the basic approach to many psychological problems is best made in this low-key fashion, the therapist must also keep an eye open for the presence of more serious disturbances (see Chapters 7 and 8) which may require very active attention.

Social and family adjustment

A wide range of problems may need to be discussed and monitored under this heading, as the patient works towards agreed goals. It may be wise for the therapist on each occasion to make at least a general enquiry as to what is happening within the family, how things are going at work (or as regards looking for a job), and how leisure is being spent. Financial problems, housing or any court proceedings may also need to be checked on. Basic work with the family is discussed later in this chapter.

Physical health

Particularly in the early stages of sobriety, there may be problems in the patient's physical health which require attention or referral, and which must not be lost from sight because of everything else that is on the agenda. A feeling of rediscovered physical well-being may be one of the prime rewards of sobriety.

Slotting in more specific treatments

The use of the more specific treatment approaches which are discussed in Chapter 19 requires discretion and timing. Every session, besides its immediate contact, is also potentially a routing point.

Making the effort worthwhile

No-one is likely to achieve long-term success in dealing with a drinking problem unless sobriety (or ameliorated drinking) proves to be a personally rewarding experience (Vaillant, 1983; Edwards et al., 1992). If all that is won by the effort to stop drinking is a grey and empty existence, it will not be long before there is a relapse.

When sobriety is unrewarding, there is also the danger that alcohol will be substituted by uncontrolled gambling or by excessive use of tranquillizers or sedatives. Many patients move spontaneously towards discovery of rewards, and two general patterns of development can often then be seen – either a wide new engagement in life or, alternatively, a much narrower substitute activity. The first of these two pathways – the wide new engagement – is, in fact, often a re-engagement in life rather than an entirely new series of moves, and is characteristic of the person who had a positive involvement in life before the emergence of the drinking problem overwhelmed these enjoyments. The second pathway – that of narrower substitute activity – more often characterizes the recovery of the person who never, at any previous period, achieved any great base of enjoyment. In this instance, it is not that a happy pattern of living was overwhelmed by drinking, but, on the contrary, that the drinking problem initially developed in the setting of unrewarding relationships and activities. Recovery may be marked by an almost frenetic commitment to one particular interest.

When no rewarding pattern of new involvement develops in the wake of sobriety and as the months go by there is instead a continued complaint that 'it was better when I was drinking', thought has to be given to what can be done to obtain constructive movement. The therapist's role is firstly that of identifying the problem and encouraging the patient to identify small, real steps towards a solution and to take those steps. This is often a stage in which the family again needs to be involved. Beyond commonsense advice, there are various other lines of approach. For instance, the passivity and pessimism which stand in the way of a determined attempt to find rewards seem often to have the characteristics of a learnt expectation of failure – 'I just can't get on with people, I'm no good at anything'. Even one small, limited success may begin to offer a new sense of possibilities – success generalizes.

On other occasions, the rewards of sobriety take a turn for the better after a major life change which is more or less accidental or very purposely brought about, such as a shift to a new locality, a new job, the break-up of a marriage, or a new relationship. These are the kind of solutions which tend traditionally to be looked on with suspicion as 'geographical escape', with the problems in no way resolved but taken along to be acted out again in the new personal setting. Such strategies are, admittedly, in some instances no more than unprofitable escapism, but it is wrong automatically to take a negative view of what is likely to be achieved by these large shifts. At times the patient is precisely right in taking the bold and simple view that 'what is wrong is living in this street'. The move to the new house, with the decorating, furniture buying and pride in ownership, the shared family involvement, the escape from the old social environment and all the drinking friends who used to knock on the door, can then mark the start of a new epoch.

The therapeutic use of the concept of alcoholism as a disease

A proportion of patients may find the concept of alcoholism as a disease (Jellinek, 1960; Edwards, 2000) helpful to recovery. Such a formulation can serve as an idea around which that patient organizes understanding of his or her condition and a personal programme of recovery. This concept is central to the philosophy of Alcoholics Anonymous (see Chapter 18).

The advantages inherent in such a simple definition of the problem can, for many patients, be considerable. There is comfort in the view that they are suffering from a condition which can be understood within much the same model as diabetes: guilt is relieved and acceptance of the inexorable fact that the only remedy for this disease is to stop drinking offers a clear personal goal. Seen in these terms, the disease is 'incurable', and recovery is a lifetime programme centred around vigilant avoidance of the first drink.

The disease concept is sometimes seized on as a revelation by a patient who has previously been thrashing around chaotically, with self-defeating attempts to 'control' their drinking. There are, however, therapists who are unhappy with this formulation or unwilling to work within its constraints. They see the disease concept as inviting the patient to avoid self-responsibility – 'It's a disease, I can't help it'. They may also see it as a formulation which detracts attention from the wider spectrum of drinking behaviours and alcohol-related problems and over-emphasizes the dependence element.

From the therapeutic angle, the reasonable position to take must be that there are different ways of formulating problems which will be more or less helpful to different patients, and with which different therapists will be more or less comfortable. The patient can be rendered a disservice if the therapist insists on a dogmatic view of either kind. In reality, the risk of damage is usually obviated by the patient shopping around until a model of understanding is found which suits that person best.

How to deal positively with relapse

Relapse is a common event. This statement will be interpreted pessimistically if one has misread the treatment of drinking problems as being only about rapid and maintained 'success'. More often, real success involves trial and error along the way. Dealing with and learning from relapse are part of the process of recovery, but such a view is not to be read as favouring a *laissez-faire* attitude. Relapse has to be taken seriously by patient and therapist alike, but in another sense it has also to be demystified. It is a piece of behaviour to be objectively understood rather than a fall from grace.

Relapse can take many different forms. It may be precipitate and explosive, or it may be a matter of a slow slide; the pace of relapse is often directly related to the degree of dependence. The patient may then stay relapsed for months or years, and the Alcoholics Anonymous member of 20 years' standing may seem tragically to have lost all their gains. However, relapse may be short lived, with the patient pulling back after a day or two. Beyond the surface description of these different patterns, there is then the question of the cause and meaning of the occurrence, and it is these inner significances which, in the individual case, have to be examined if there is to be profit from the experience and recovery is to move forward.

Some of the commoner circumstances of relapse are set out below, but in reality the determinants are often likely to be multiple and will require varied responses (Carroll, 1996).

An initial and ambivalent sobriety overthrown

Here, one is dealing with patients who relapse in the early days of treatment because they have not as yet satisfactorily sorted out the balance of their motivations. They are in two minds as to whether or not they want to stop drinking, and the relapse indicates that there is still important initial work to be done in sorting out these ambivalences. Motivation has got to be strengthened.

Insufficiency in coping mechanisms

Here, the same surface picture has a different inner meaning and different therapeutic implications. These patients have, to a greater extent, overcome their ambivalence, but they are unskilled in defending their sobriety. They know what they want to do, but are caught out and fail in their intentions. Effort has to be directed at better learning of coping mechanisms.

Failure to find sobriety rewarding

Sobriety has not been consolidated and no satisfactory substitutes have been found for drinking. This is the type of relapse which occurs after perhaps 6–12 months of uneasy sobriety. The need is to work again on the rewards of sobriety.

Disturbance of mood

Relapse is, in such instances, an indication that the patient has been unable to cope with an upset in mood. Patients may have experienced a transient patch of gloom, anxiety, or irritability, which has overwhelmed their defences, or they may be prone to cyclical mood swings. Depressive illness is a not uncommon cause of relapse, and the possibility of hypomanic illness may also have to be considered.

Overcome by events

In such instances, an event or series of events proves too much for the individual's defences. Rather than drinking being a response to catastrophic happenings, the more usual story is of an event which, to the outsider, might seem trivial, or a cluster of seemingly minor troubles. For instance, the patient has had a row with her husband and, that same morning, the water tank in the roof has leaked, and the desire to bring back a bottle of gin from the supermarket is irresistible. To dismiss such a story as 'just a bundle of excuses' is unhelpful. Its analysis tells us that, for this woman, ordinary marital discord gives rise to feelings of insecurity which are hard to bear, and that when subjected then to a little extra stress, she will be without any means of coping other than resort to drink.

Failure in vigilance

Sometimes it seems that the patient has been careless. They were half aware that it would be dangerous to go to that party, but such considerations were less important than the prospect of fun. They knew that it would be risky to start drinking in such a setting, but by the time the party was in full swing, they 'thought they could get away with it'. This lack of vigilance is often related to a fading of memory; the pains previously experienced with drinking are now rather distant, while the pleasure of a glass of wine is immediate.

Whether relapse is insidious or abrupt, it is a happening to be *used* in treatment. The usefulness of the experience is, however, lost if the incident is met inappropriately: for instance, if it is passed by as trivial and unimportant, interpreted as a reason for pessimism and surrender of therapeutic effort, or taken as an occasion for abandonment of the patient's and family's active responsibility with an unnecessary retreat to hospital. Relapse is best met with no retreat from expectations of the patient's self-responsibility. That responsibility now includes getting out of the relapse, working out its meaning, and setting things up so that further relapse is less likely.

Many relapses are short lived, with the patient regaining sobriety before harm is done. It is potentially misleading to use the same word to describe the happenings when a patient takes a few drinks one evening and then stops drinking again completely, as opposed to sliding into a rapid reinstatement of dependence and being once more in the grip of very threatening drinking. Some therapists therefore prefer to distinguish between 'lapse' (transient or minor) and 'relapse' (major and perhaps with reinstatement of dependence). A lapse may lead on to the relapse, but this is not the inevitable march of events, and what the therapist at first views as 'lapse' may be the patient's tentative move towards the re-establishment of normal drinking.

As well as therapy seeking to enable patients and their families to learn from the incident, there may be immediate actions needed to minimize the harm done by any such occurrence. The patient may, for instance, need to avoid losing their job and to get back to work as soon as possible. Where there are particular dangers to physical health, such as may be present if the patient is suffering from pancreatitis or liver disease, then the sooner drinking is stopped the better. Relapse may sometimes pose dangers of suicide if the patient believes that 'the last chance has gone'.

Basic work with the family

The importance of the family dimension in the initial assessment and goal-setting and the value of the initial interview with the spouse have already been discussed (see Chapter 15).

Work with the spouse

The spouse's behaviour patterns may have become stuck in a rut, and be producing no benefit, and sometimes just trying a change of tack can help. Constructive help-seeking and constructive management seem on the whole to be more effective than continued attack or manipulation (Orford and Edwards, 1977). It may generally be beneficial if the spouse can reach a decision as to what they definitely will not do, and what are their limits. For instance, they may decide as an act of definite policy that they will abandon arguing and nagging, or that they will not give their partner money or go out and buy them drink. It is the open identification of a set of intentions, the sense of something to do, the drawing up of a personal programme which is useful in such a situation.

It is often helpful to hold a few joint sessions to try to ensure that mutual goals are understood and that there is shared commitment to constructive change. This can be used to give the sense of a new start, with an emphasis on the positive, on identifying what is good in the marriage, what each in practical terms wants from the other and what each will give to the other partner. There is no evidence that a routine, major therapeutic intervention with the spouse is of benefit.

Help for the children

The best help for the child is restoration of the happiness of the home. The fact of a previously alcohol dependent parent ceasing to drink, of rowing and violence no longer being the continuing experience, can be dramatically beneficial to the child's happiness and well-being (Lynskey et al., 1994). Sometimes the changes are evident within a week. The teacher notices that the child is concentrating at school, the mother knows that a child has stopped bed-wetting or will say, 'It's lovely, they're talking to their dad again.' More often, the changes are going to be seen over a longer period, and the restoration of confidence will take many months, with the previously drinking parent hurt and discouraged because their children have not sooner come towards them.

Given that help for the problem drinking parent (and the partner) may be of indirect benefit to the children, other ways of aiding the children have also to be considered, especially where there is no immediate treatment response from the adult (Zeitlin, 1994). There can be instances in which urgent thought has to be given to removal of the child from the home as an immediate measure of physical protection, or in which high priority has to be given to social work supervision of an intensity which can monitor the child's safety (in Chapter 12 we give a case example of such a situation).

As regards individual help for the child remaining in the disturbed home, much the same range of approaches is applicable as with a child or young person facing any other disturbing home influence. The offer of a good and confident relationship is itself valuable, but with a child who is of an age to verbalize problems, it is helpful to discuss directly the parent's drinking – to listen to and offer understanding of the child's distress, to find some more satisfactory way of looking at the parents and of coping with the anger and hurt, to offer straightforward information, to discuss the child's role within the family, what the child 'can do to help' and the limits of those possibilities, and to aid towards good friendships outside the home. Children, too, have their coping mechanisms, which can be adaptive or maladaptive.

There may be occasions when older children should be involved in family therapy in a formal sense, but the skills necessary to handle the interactions of children and parents in such a forum should not be underestimated. More often, what is useful is the home visit or series of home visits during which children can experience a family discussion in a natural setting and family members drop in and out as they feel like it. The role of Al-Ateen (a self-help group deriving from Alcoholics Anonymous and Al-Anon) is discussed in Chapter 18.

The use of therapeutic groups

The place of group therapy as a special technique to be deployed at the stage when patients are consolidating their recovery, is discussed in Chapter 19. Alcoholics Anonymous and Al-Anon also provide group experience. However, groups can also have their place in the basic work of treatment, and many therapists would see involvement in groups at an early stage of the treatment process as being useful for information giving, shared solution of problems, and support. There is no evidence that more intensive group work at these earlier stages brings special benefit.

Spacing of appointments

There is no one rule for the spacing of appointments, and some patients will need to be seen more frequently than others. In general, the emphasis on autonomy and self-determination is best supported by giving more spaced rather than more frequent appointments, with escalation into a modal routine of intensive intervention resisted. Much must depend on the thoroughness and purposiveness of the initial assessment and exercise in goal-setting. It is better to put investment in that direction, with similarly purposeful but spaced follow-up, than to start from an incomplete assessment with a follow-through which lacks direction despite frequency of contact.

As for how long a session should last, this again must be individually determined. On many occasions, a 20-minute interview can give sufficient time for a focused monitoring of progress, while in other instances it may be necessary to find 45–60 minutes for listening and detailed discussion.

The treatment organization should also have the capacity to respond to emergency and be able to see the patient who experiences a crisis between the fixed appointments. It will, however, be unhelpful to see a patient on a free-demand basis if their demands are witness to their over-dependence on other people. It will be better to encourage them to meet their own crises and keep to the schedule of appointments.

When a patient fails to keep an appointment, there should be an administrative mechanism which ensures that they are not then lost from sight. A personal letter offering a further appointment should be written or a phone call made and, if contact is not re-established, a home visit should perhaps be arranged. When all else fails, the patient should still be left with the indication that the door remains readily open.

Duration and termination of treatment

The duration of treatment may be proposed by the therapist, but it is effectively determined by the patient. There are patients who appear to have benefited from one or two sessions and who decide this is all they need, whereas at the other extreme there are those who want to maintain at least intermittent contact over years.

A fixed course of so many sessions over so many months cannot in reality meet the needs of an enormously varied patient population. Judgement needs to be made in terms of the patient's progress along a number of dimensions of recovery, the likelihood of further useful work, the timeliness of a move which further emphasizes the patient's ability to handle their own responsibilities, and negotiation on timing between therapist and patient. Rather than there then being a 'this is the end of your treatment' type of announcement, what is said might often be something like this.

We've been meeting each month for the last 8 months, and you've achieved a great deal. If you agree, what I would now suggest is that we meet again just before Christmas – that's 5 months hence. But if for any reason you wanted to see me earlier, 'phone and let me know.

The question arises in a different form when making this decision not in relation to the patient who has made substantial progress, but in a case in which after 6 months of work the drinking is continuing unabated. Does one 'terminate treatment' on the grounds that the patient is failing to benefit or show commitment to change? In general, rather than such a situation being an indication for the termination of treatment, it more often suggests the need for reassessment of what is being done.

Basic work in the generalist setting

This chapter and the book as a whole for the most part focus on how to respond to drinking problems of significant severity and dealt with by professionals with more than a few minutes of time to deploy. Help given in the primary care, general hospital ward or other generalist frontlines is, however, of such importance as to make it mandatory to enter a note on this matter within a chapter which discusses 'basic work' (Anderson, 1995; Heather, 2001). These issues are taken up again within the service planning context in Chapter 22.

Here, what needs to be underlined is that within the generalist setting the basic skills which are required relate firstly to case identification (Chapter 14). Professionals working in a specialist clinic are likely to have the task of case recognition already accomplished for them, in that the referral letter will tell them that this is a patient with a drinking problem. Not so the general practitioner or other generalist working in settings in which the patients come unsorted and unlabelled, and the challenge is to recognize heterogeneous drinking problems which can exist in all shades of degree.

The majority of cases dealt with in these types of generalist setting will be of lesser severity than those encountered by the specialist. In most instances, the appropriate treatment will be brief intervention, directed at milder or earlier alcohol-related pathologies, or at excessive alcohol intake where there is as yet no evidence of adverse consequences. With the case identified, the necessary skills include the ability to give succinct and intelligible advice to encourage explicit and targeted change (for instance bringing down weekly intake to 21 units or, say, 170 g absolute alcohol per week for men and 14 units or 110 g for women, with concomitant lowering of liver enzymes). Along with the advice should go monitoring and feedback to the patient. The generalist will also on occasion be identifying and dealing with more severe drinking problems or alcohol dependence, and decisions will have to be made as to when and from what direction specialist support should be sought.

Basic work: bringing the ideas together

It would be misleading to present a carefully ordered flow chart or series of ordered steps to describe the basic work of treatment, for this would contradict the message that what is most required is the flexibility to meet the needs of the individual patient as their recovery evolves. However, with that caution in mind, it may be useful to have a checklist.

1. Assessment with patient and spouse is the initiation of therapy, and a shared experience.
2. The case formulation orders the material obtained in the assessment, and is again shared with patient and spouse.
3. Goal-setting must be negotiated in similar terms. Goals must be specific and cover non-drinking as well as drinking issues. There must be an invitation to a tangible commitment to working towards those goals.
4. The therapeutic relationship is important and must be skilfully fostered. The therapist must learn how to show warmth and give hope, but should not be lured into over-directiveness, either with the patient or their spouse. Self-responsibility should be fostered.
5. Some basic therapeutic principles should be borne in mind: continuity of purpose and sense of movement must be maintained; salient questions must be identified at each interview, with the patient allowed to define what is of importance; and the family perspective must be maintained. Therapy requires continuous monitoring, and the patient may usefully engage in self-monitoring. Balances have to be struck, both between a focus on reality and dynamics and between drinking and other topics. Commitment may at various points need to be re-examined. An eye has constantly to be kept on the development of the relationship.
6. The actual content of the interview includes work on the drinking problem and attention to problems in the areas of mental and physical health and social adjustment.
7. Each interview, as well as being concerned with the continuing basics of treatment, is also an occasion for deciding whether it is timely to signpost the patient towards any more specialized type of help.

8. The effort towards recovery by the patient and spouse has to be worthwhile. They must be helped to anticipate the gains, and a sobriety which is only negative will not be maintained. The *quality* of sobriety is important. Strengthening of the patient's motivation is basic to therapy.

9. Relapse is not to be considered a taboo subject. If relapse does occur, it should be possible to learn from the event. The many different patterns, causes and meanings of relapse must be understood.

10. Basic work with the family may also be needed. This includes meeting the immediate needs of the spouse and children, as well as work which facilitates conjoint efforts towards the patient's recovery.

11. The pacing and intensity of help must be kept under review and ultimately tailed off, perhaps with the offer of an 'open door' rather than formal closure of the case. What must be guarded against is an automatic escalation into heavy intervention. Once there has been full assessment and careful and agreed goal-setting, much may then often be left to the patient and family, with monitoring and encouragement and a little talking through.

12. Basic treatment is an alliance with the natural processes of recovery; it is a matter of discovering rather than imposing possibilities for change, a matter of teaching map-reading skills rather than pushing people along a path which we dictate.

REFERENCES

Anderson, P. (1995) *Alcohol and Primary Health Care.* European Series No. 64. Copenhagen: WHO Regional Office for Europe.

Batel, P., Pessione, F., Bouvier, A-M. and Rueff, B. (1995) Prompting alcoholics to be referred to an alcohol clinic: the effectiveness of a simple letter. *Addiction* 90, 811–14.

Carroll, K.M. and Rounsaville, B.J. (1993) Implications of recent research on psychotherapy for drug abuse. In *Drugs, Alcohol and Tobacco: Making the Science and Policy Connections,* ed. Edwards, G., Strang, J. and Jaffe, J. Oxford: Oxford University Press, 210–21.

Carroll, K.M. (1996) Relapse prevention as a psychosocial treatment: a review of controlled clinical trials. *Experimental and Clinical Psychopharmacology* 4, 46–54.

Carroll, K.M. (2001) Constrained, confounded and confused: why we really know so little about therapists in treatment outcome research. *Addiction* 96, 203–6.

Connors, G.J., DiClimente, C.C., Dermen, K.H., Kadden, R., Carroll, K.M. and Frone, M.R. (2000) Predicting the therapeutic alliance in alcoholism treatment. *Journal of Studies on Alcohol* 61, 139–49.

Davidson, R. (1996) Motivational issues in the treatment of addictive behaviour. In *Psychotherapy, Psychological Treatments and the Addictions,* ed. Edwards, G. and Dare, C. Cambridge: Cambridge University Press, 173–88.

Edwards, G. (1996) Addictive behaviours: the next clinic appointment. In *Psychotherapy, Psychological Treatments and the Addictions*, ed. Edwards, G. and Dare, C. Cambridge: Cambridge University Press, 94–109.

Edwards, G. (2000) The mysterious essences of treatment. In *Alcohol, the Ambiguous Molecule*. London: Penguin, 136–47.

Edwards, G., Oppenheimer, E. and Taylor, C. (1992) Hearing the noise in the system. Exploration of textual analysis as a method for studying change in drinking behaviour. *British Journal of Addiction* 87, 73–81.

Gerdner, A. and Holmberg, A. (2000) Factors affecting motivation to treatment in severely dependent alcoholics. *Journal of Studies on Alcohol* 61, 548–560.

Gossop, M. (1996) Cognitive and behavioural treatments for substance abuse. In *Psychotherapy, Psychological Treatments and the Addictions*, ed. Edwards, G. and Dare, C. Cambridge: Cambridge University Press, 158–72.

Heather, N. (2001) Brief interventions. In *International Handbook of Alcohol Dependence and Problems*, ed. Heather, N., Peters, T.J. and Stockwell, S. Chichester: John Wiley and Sons, 605–26.

Heather, N., Kisson-Singh, J. and Fenton, W. (1990) Assisted natural recovery from alcohol problems: effects of a self-help manual with and without telephone contacts. *British Journal of Addiction* 85, 1177–85.

Jellinek, E.M. (1960) *The Disease Concept of Alcoholism*. New Brunswick, NJ: Hillhouse Press.

Levin, J.D. and Weiss, R.H. (eds) (1994) *The Dynamics and Treatment of Alcoholism: Essential Papers*. Northvale, NJ: Jason Aronson.

Luborsky, L. and Crits-Christoph, P. (1990) *Understanding the Transference*. New York: Basic Books.

Luborsky, L., McLellan, A.J., Woody, G.E., O'Brien, C.P. and Anerback, A. (1985) Therapist success and its determinants. *Archives of General Psychiatry* 42, 602–11.

Lynskey, M.T., Fergusson, D.M. and Horwood, J. (1994) The effect of parental alcohol problems on rates of adolescent psychiatric disorder. *Addiction* 89, 1277–86.

Malan, D.H. and Osimu, F. (1992) *Psychodynamics Training and Outcome*. New York: Basic Books.

Orford, J. and Edwards, G. (1977) *Alcoholism. A Comparison of Treatment and Advice, with a Study of the Influence of Marriage*. Maudsley Hospital Monograph No. 26. Oxford: Oxford University Press.

Prochaska, J.O., Nacross, J.C. and DiClimente, C.C. (1994) Stages and processes of self-change of smoking: toward an integrative model of change. *Psychotherapy: Theory, Research and Practice* 19, 276–88.

Project MATCH (1998) Matching alcoholism treatments to client heterogeneity: Project MATCH three-year drinking outcomes. *Alcoholism: Clinical and Experimental Research* 22, 1300–11.

Rollnick, S. and Miller, W.R. (1995) What is motivational interviewing? *Behavioural and Cognitive Psychotherapy* 23, 325–34.

Sutton, S. (1996) Can 'stages of change' provide guidance in the treatment of addictions? A critical examination of Prochaska and DiClimente's model. In *Psychotherapy, Psychological Treatments and the Addictions*, ed. Edwards, G. and Dare, C. Cambridge: Cambridge University Press, 184–205.

Thom, B., Brown, D., Drummond, C., Edwards, G., Mullan, M. and Taylor, C. (1992) Engaging patients with alcohol problems in treatment: the first consultation. *British Journal of Addiction* 87, 601–11.

Vaillant, G.E. (1983) *The Natural History of Alcoholism*. Cambridge, MA: Harvard University Press.

Vaillant, G.E. (1993) *Wisdom of the Ego*. Cambridge, MA: Harvard University Press.

Zeitlin, H. (1994) Children with alcohol misusing parents. In *Alcohol and Alcohol Problems*, ed. Edwards, G. and Peters, T.J. British Medical Bulletin No. 50. Edinburgh: Churchill Livingstone, 139–51.

18

Alcoholics Anonymous

Alcoholics Anonymous (AA) was founded in the USA in 1935 by two alcoholics (Wilson, 1994). Its growth since then has been dramatic. There are now more than 51 000 groups and over 1.1 million members in the USA alone, and there are more than 100 000 groups in total in almost 170 countries worldwide. The estimated world membership is over 2 million. AA first began to establish itself in the UK in the late 1940s and there are now 3000 groups in Great Britain.

AA has helped countless individuals (often when professional intervention has failed), is a repository of astonishing experience and subtle and often humorous wisdom, and has had a profound influence in humanizing social attitudes towards people with drinking problems. It is thus an enormous potential resource, and it is a dereliction of duty if patients go through treatment without AA ever being mentioned or, worse still, if they are deflected from AA involvement by some negative statement born of ignorance and misunderstanding – 'I think you would find it all too religious.'

The therapist must be willing to find out how AA operates and what its beliefs are, and the best way of doing so is to pay a personal visit to an open meeting of AA – a meeting open to all-comers, as opposed to closed meetings which are restricted to AA membership.

AA meetings

The AA meeting is of central importance to AA's functioning. It has a unique atmosphere, marked by a seeming informality but with an underlying and purposeful method of working. The number of people at a meeting will vary from group to group, but is typically around 10 to 20. Some of those present will have been attending AA for years, whereas the man or woman sitting in the back row may have just walked hesitantly through the door for the first time. A chairman will have been elected for that evening and will probably be sitting at a table with one or two members who have been asked 'to give their stories'. The newcomer will notice a lot of friendly greeting and talking.

The meeting will start with the chairman saying 'My name is...' (only first names are used), 'I am an alcoholic'. These words carry immense implications: the speaker is not ashamed of their alcoholism, but without reservation acknowledges their condition as an inalienable fact. The starting point of the evening is thus one individual's reaffirmation, for all present, of what in AA terms must be the starting point of recovery for every individual, namely the admission that he or she is suffering from 'alcoholism'.

The chairman will then read the AA preamble.

Alcoholics Anonymous is a fellowship of men and women who share their experience, strength, and hope with each other that they may solve their common problem and help others to recover from alcoholism. The only requirement for membership is a desire to stop drinking. There are no dues or fees for AA membership; we are self-supporting through our own contributions. AA is not allied with any sect, denomination, politics, organization or institution; does not wish to engage in any controversy, neither endorses nor opposes any causes. Our primary purpose is to stay sober and help other alcoholics to achieve sobriety. (Leach and Norris, 1977).

With these preliminaries out of the way, the first speaker of the evening will then be called. Their introduction will again be in terms of 'My name's..., and I'm an alcoholic'. He or she will speak for 20–30 minutes, giving an account of their personal background and then going on to describe the development of their drinking problem, the sufferings they endured or inflicted on others, the deceptions and prevarications of their drinking days, and then often some final turning-point or 'rock bottom' experience. They will go on to describe their introduction to AA and their recovery within the programme of that fellowship, and their evolving understanding of the meaning of AA as a way of life. Within this biographical format, different speakers develop their own approach, and the ability of the person who has never given a public speech in any other setting to make a personal statement which is both moving and convincing is no doubt related to the unwritten guidelines which propose that a personal *story* should be given, rather than an abstract lecture. The story which is told in unadorned manner by the person with fairly recent experience of recovery seems often to be better received than the highly polished performance by the person who has told their story many times, but who is by now rather distanced from the acuteness of their experience. Also, stories which deal with recovery, and which offer practical hints on how to work at recovery, are likely to be better received than long-drawn-out accounts of drinking days.

These life stories are followed by comments and personal statements from the floor. Themes are caught up and explored by the listeners, who often stress their identification with the speaker's story – 'That happened to me too . . .'. No-one is forced to speak and it is realized that for weeks the new member may want to do no more than sit and listen.

Reference is often made during the meeting to 'The Twelve Steps', which enshrine the basic ideology of AA. These steps are as follows.

1. We admitted we were powerless over alcohol – that our lives had become unmanageable.
2. Came to believe that a Power greater than ourselves could restore us to sanity.
3. Made a decision to turn our will and our lives over to the care of God *as we understood Him*.
4. Made a searching and fearless moral inventory of ourselves.
5. Admitted to God, to ourselves and to another human being the exact nature of our wrongs.
6. Were entirely ready to have God remove all these defects of character.
7. Humbly asked Him to remove our shortcomings.
8. Made a list of all persons we had harmed, and became willing to make amends to them all.
9. Made direct amends to such people wherever possible, except when to do so would injure them or others.
10. Continued to take personal inventory, and when we were wrong, promptly admitted it.
11. Sought through prayer and meditation to improve our conscious contact with God *as we understood Him* praying only for knowledge of His will for us and the power to carry that out.
12. Having had a spiritual awakening as the result of these steps we tried to carry this message to alcoholics and to practice these principles in all our affairs. (Alcoholics Anonymous, 1977)

A speaker may comment on the meaning which any one of these steps has had for them personally and describe their efforts to achieve this step. For instance, the meaning to be given to step 2 with its idea of 'a Power greater than ourselves' (usually referred to as a 'Higher Power') often attracts discussion. The Higher Power is usually interpreted in terms of an open and individually determined concept of God – the 'God *as we understood Him*', of steps 3 and 11. This seemingly theistic formulation does not in practice debar an atheist from finding help in AA.

The formal proceedings end with the meeting saying together what is known as the Serenity Prayer:

> God grant me the serenity
> To accept the things I cannot change
> The courage to change the things I can
> And the wisdom to know the difference.

The members then chat and exchange news over tea or coffee, and subtle but positive effort is likely to be made to put the new attender at their ease and draw them into contact. Frequently, the new member will, after some weeks, find a 'sponsor' who will offer personal advice and a special degree of availability – a phone number to contact, an arrangement to meet in the evening to attend an AA meeting, and so on. The sponsor is also a role model.

Besides the meetings themselves, much else is potentially on offer. Members may start to visit each other at home, go out to meals together or share other social activities. Old drinking friends are dropped, and new friends found who think and talk AA. In some localities, routine meetings will be supplemented by study groups, and AA literature shared and passed around. Regional and national AA conventions may be attended, and the more experienced member may give time to 'twelfth-stepping' (acting as sponsor and working with new members); they may help with prison or hospital groups, or offer availability as a speaker at meetings of community organizations.

The 'Minnesota Model'

AA itself is a worldwide network of self-help groups, with no allegiance to any other institution. However, it has been extremely influential upon the working of many individuals and organizations, particularly in North America, where its principles have been applied to institutional forms of treatment now known commonly as the 'Minnesota Model' (Cook, 1988a; see Chapter 22).

In some countries, entry into this form of treatment may begin with an 'intervention' in the client's home. This strategy, directed mainly at the drinker who denies having any problem with alcohol, requires the gathering of family, friends, colleagues and significant others under the direction of a trained therapist. The unsuspecting 'alcoholic' then arrives home to be confronted by the assembled gathering. The aim of the confrontation, in which each person presents examples of the drink-related harm that they have witnessed, is to challenge the drinker's denial that they have a problem, and to encourage them to enter a suitable programme of treatment. Such interventions may be very effective when expertly managed, but could easily be destructive and counter-therapeutic if ill-considered or attempted by the inexperienced. However, they illustrate the principle that, in the first instance, treatment may have to be taken to the problem drinker, rather than expecting the drinker to seek help themselves in the clinic or treatment centre.

Whether or not an 'intervention' has been employed as the starting point, the typical Minnesota Model treatment package commences with a residential phase, typically lasting 1–2 months, with a packed programme of group therapy, lectures, work assignments, daily reading groups and other activities, notably attendance at AA meetings. The staff are mainly, or even entirely, comprised of recovering 'alcoholics' and drug 'addicts' who have themselves worked through the Twelve Steps and demonstrated a commitment to abstinence for a period of some years.

Such individuals, even in recovery, would consider themselves to be suffering from 'alcoholism' or 'chemical dependency' and the terms 'problem drinker' or 'drug misuser' would be quite alien in these settings.

In addition to 'alcoholics', residents in such centres usually also include addicts to other drugs, who will work through the programme of Narcotics Anonymous (NA; Peyrot, 1985). A range of 'behavioural' addictions is also treated in many such centres, including eating disorders, relationship or sexual addictions, and a diverse group of other problems.

Following the residential phase of treatment, the 'alcoholic' may be encouraged to participate in a programme of aftercare offered by the same institution. One of the great strengths of this approach, however, is its ability to link people in to their local AA groups for long-term or lifelong support. No other approach to the treatment of drinking problems can boast an international network of support groups on such a scale as this.

The Minnesota Model has been criticized in some quarters as being expensive and ineffective. In fact, it need not be any more expensive than other residential approaches to treatment, and is potentially cheaper than in-patient units which provide expensive medical and nursing care. Reliance on self-help groups rather than professional therapy offered after discharge may actually result in cost savings (Humphreys and Moos, 2001). Such evidence as has been published suggests also that the Minnesota Model is no less effective than many other treatment programmes (Cook, 1988b; Kownacki and Shadish, 1999; Humphreys and Moos, 2001).

Essential processes

What are the essential processes through which AA operates? There have been many attempts to answer this question, and in summary the following dimensions can probably be identified.

Coherent, flexible ideas

A coherent but flexible set of ideas is offered (an ideology), which can relieve the individual's sense of hopelessness and explain the nature of their problem. They are suffering from 'the disease of alcoholism', which is pictured as metaphorically akin to an 'allergy to alcohol'. Their constitution is such that they will react to this drug differently from other people. They can never be 'cured', but the disease will be 'arrested' if they do not drink again. Lifetime abstinence must be their only goal. It is the first drink that they cannot risk.

It is likely that the hopeless and despondent drinker who has finally realized their need for help will be more receptive to the explanation and meaning of their experience which the ideology of AA offers. Affiliation with AA, and engagement in its programme of recovery, may then offer a reduction in the form of anxiety known as cognitive dissonance. The resolution of this anxiety by means of adoption of the AA philosophy is not dissimilar to religious conversion, and is often understood as being a profoundly spiritual experience (Tiebout, 1944; Galanter, 1999).

Action programme

AA offers an action programme, and 'The Twelve Steps' outline the actions which have to be taken. The 'alcoholic' must join AA and stay close to AA. They will be advised to take things 'one day at a time' and to work for short-term goals. The stories and discussions they listen to at AA meetings and the guidance from their sponsor will provide them with many hints on coping and problem solving. Their first priority is to deal with their drinking, but the programme will also require them to examine psychological problems – their guilt, their 'resentment', their tendency to blame others, their 'stinking thinking'. The 'personal inventory' which is a key part of this process of self-examination may also be a key to the efficacy of the Twelve Step programme (Khantzian and Mack, 1994; Kownacki and Shadish, 1999).

AA is 'a selfish programme' and each individual is working for sobriety for their own sake and not to please anyone else, and they thus give no hostages to fortune. If they relapse, they are not rejected but may return any number of times to try again. The programme will finally include 'twelfth-stepping', but by then members should have learnt that in the process of helping other people they will help themselves and confirm their own strength; it is not, however, their job to proselytize, 'pull people down lamp-posts', or put their own sobriety at risk.

Rewards of sobriety

AA carries the message that sobriety is rewarding, and helps the individual to discover these rewards. It gives people new friends, introduces them to a new social network, relieves their loneliness, helps them to structure and employ their time, removes a stigma and confers on them a sense of personal worth. If they have been sober for 1 day, they have been a success. Through AA, they may ultimately achieve serenity, with sobriety a way of life.

Possibility of recovery

AA's ideology is persuasive and an approach to recovery is made to appear possible. This last heading bears on each of the previous headings. AA does not 'work' through an abstract set of ideas, but through those ideas being found persuasive by the individual. The most apt theoretical definition of the disorder and the pathways to recovery would remain useless if AA did not have the ability to persuade the new member that AA is about him or her as an individual, can meet their problems, and show them personally the way ahead. AA can carry this conviction because its members so evidently know what they are talking about; they, too, have been through it all and know every stratagem of deceit and denial, while at the same time bearing tangible witness to the possibility of success.

AA as a spiritual programme

It is often said that the AA programme is 'spiritual rather than religious' (Kurtz, 1991). We have already noted that the Twelve Steps unambiguously talk about God as a Higher Power essential to recovery, and yet that this is not seen as incompatible with membership of the atheist or agnostic. Similarly, the adoption of the ideology of AA has been seen as a spiritual process not dissimilar to religious conversion. The twelfth step specifically refers to a 'spiritual awakening'. What, then, is spirituality? And what is its place within the Twelve Step programme?

There is no agreed answer to the first of these questions, and thus it is difficult to answer the second. However, a number of themes appear to emerge from the literature (see Box 18.1). Spirituality is seen as being concerned with a transcendent dimension of life, which is as clearly identified with the divine for some people as it is not for others. It is concerned also with what it means to be 'human', and there is frequent reference to an inner 'core' or force within people. It is often understood as being concerned with finding meaning or fulfilment in life. Perhaps most frequently, it is understood as concerning relationships – with others, with the world around, and with God. It is sometimes seen as opposed to the material world. For some, it is closely involved with religion, and for others it is to be contrasted with religion.

BOX 18.1 **Themes in the definition of spirituality**
- Relationship
- The transcendent/divine/absolute
- Being human/being a 'person'
- Inner 'core' or force
- Search for meaning or fulfilment
- Spirit versus material
- Religion

AA is also concerned with a transcendent dimension to human experience. It is concerned with human relationships – both within its meetings and also with those that have been damaged as a result of alcoholism (see, for instance, steps 8 and 9). For some, it reveals the characteristics of a religious sect (Jones, 1970), whereas for others it is to be contrasted with religion. For some, meaning and fulfilment are encountered in a new way in the course of working through the Twelve Step programme. It would thus appear that AA and spirituality have much in common. More important is the testimony of many members of AA who have found the spiritual dimension of this programme of recovery to be central to their own understanding of its strength and efficacy.

Spirituality has been described as the 'silent dimension in addiction research' (Miller, 1990). New research instruments are being developed and applied to this field, which make it likely that it will become a much greater focus of future research attention (Miller, 1998).

Who will affiliate with AA?

Like other approaches to treatment, AA is not a panacea. Its membership is almost exclusively composed of people who have suffered from moderate or severe alcohol dependence, and group cohesion is therefore built around total acceptance of the abstinence goal. The person who is not dependent and who does not wish to aim for abstinence is unlikely to find AA compatible.

Drinkers who go to a meeting where everyone is of another social background are also unlikely to feel at home, although this problem can be met by individuals shopping around until they find a group of people with whom they can identify. Different AA meetings vary in composition; some operate with a wide mix of social backgrounds, whereas others seem tacitly to have recruited their membership with a bias towards a particular socio-economic stratum. Also, some groups will emphasize the spiritual aspect of AA ideology much more than others. It may therefore take some time and perseverance for the new member to find the group which most suits their needs. Some groups may have a particular reputation for being helpful to the newcomer, who may be guided in their direction.

It is always difficult to predict who will and who will not find AA helpful, and patients should be advised to go along to meetings and see for themselves whether AA offers an answer.

The therapist and co-operation with AA

As was stated earlier, the therapist should, whenever appropriate, signpost the way to AA. This not only implies being able to provide the appropriate phone number (which is available in the local telephone directory), and perhaps being able to effect a direct introduction to an AA sponsor with whom the patient is likely to identify, but also means having the knowledge and sympathy which will enable them to convey to the patient that attending some AA meetings is likely to be eminently worthwhile. The therapist who, on occasion, is able to attend AA open meetings will enhance his or her credibility as informant and build up valuable contacts with local groups.

The therapist will know that only a minority of their patients (perhaps no more than 5–10%) will enter into a full and prolonged relationship with AA, but even a lesser exposure can be beneficial. AA attendance should always be voluntary, and any attempt at coercion is only likely to be counterproductive (Kownacki and Shadish, 1999).

Co-operation is, of course, a two-way business, and AA needs to understand the workings of the local services and be able to make a direct referral for professional advice if assistance is thought necessary. Many centres have established a fruitful two-way relationship of this sort, and at the national level AA has set up mechanisms for liaison with hospitals and prisons. A centre which is offering a normal drinking goal for some of its patients will, however, need to talk through this aspect of its work with AA if misunderstanding is to be avoided. Another difficulty can stem from the anti-drug attitude of some AA members, which may result in advice to a new member that they should stop taking antidepressant drugs, or disulfiram, against their own best interests. At the extreme, some AA members may be so convinced that AA offers the only true pathway to recovery as to make co-operation with other agencies difficult. However, such difficulties are rare and, with open communication and mutual respect, problems can usually be sorted out.

The relationship of AA to the in-patient unit is discussed in Chapter 22.

Research on AA

Although there is a considerable research literature on AA, definitive studies proving (or disproving) its efficacy are lacking. This is a result of the methodological problems that are inherent in the study of a voluntary programme of self-help with which people may affiliate, or from which they may disaffiliate, at will (Glaser and Ogborne, 1982) as well as of the heterogeneity of members' experiences and outcomes, and the poor design of many studies (Tonigan et al., 1996). The evidence of efficacy is therefore largely suggestive, being based upon popularity, personal testimony and perceived benefit rather than scientific proof (Edwards, 1995). Surprisingly, there is somewhat more evidence (although still far from being definitive) to support the contention that there is an aggregate level effect of AA in reducing alcohol-related problems in the population as a whole (Babor, 1995).

A recent large, multi-centre study in the USA, known as Project MATCH, has shown that 'Twelve Step Facilitation' (TSF) is equally effective as cognitive–behavioural therapy and motivational enhancement therapy. For patients without severe psychiatric problems, TSF was actually superior to the other two treatments after 12 months (Project MATCH Research Group, 1997). After 3 years, TSF was superior to motivational enhancement for patients whose previous social networks had been supportive of their drinking (Longabaugh et al., 1998). This benefit was partly mediated by AA attendance: i.e. those with networks supportive of drinking were more likely to attend AA, and AA attendance was associated with better outcome.

TSF is not to be equated with either AA attendance or the Minnesota Model. However, TSF includes amongst its objectives a fostering of commitment to attend AA and to begin working through the Twelve Steps. In terms of findings that are supportive of the benefits of these objectives, Project MATCH is therefore certainly the most important research project ever to have been undertaken.

A detailed analysis of research on AA is beyond the scope of this book, but the interested reader should consult the review by McCrady and Miller (1993).

One member of AA speaking

Here is the account given by one member of AA, in his own words.

I crawled into AA, physically, mentally and spiritually bankrupt, to find an amazing bunch of men and women who had suffered the same physical and mental agony as myself.

At last there were people who thought like me. Dear God – I was no longer alone. And, slowly, slowly, the fog has started to clear. Today, nearly 4 years later, I have not had a drink and am happy and contented for the first time in nearly 50 years of existing. Now I am really starting to Live with a capital 'L' – and it's just great. I never knew that life could be such fun without booze.

Learning from AA

Claims for the success and universality of AA can easily be exaggerated, and its emphasis on the disease concept may be out of tune with the model employed by some therapists. But there can be no doubt that, as well as the direct benefit which AA offers to individual drinkers, it also has much to teach the therapist about the processes which aid and influence recovery. There is wisdom to be borrowed from AA.

Al-Anon

Al-Anon is an organization which is independent of, but allied with, AA (Al-Anon Family Groups UK and Eire, 1980). It is a self-help group which caters for the families of 'alcoholics' – for 'anyone who loves an alcoholic'. It has its own 'Twelve Steps', which mirror AA thinking. Quite often, an AA meeting will be going on in one room and an Al-Anon meeting in the next room, with everyone getting together afterwards over the tea and biscuits.

The functioning of Al-Anon will not be discussed here in detail, because its principles and methods of working have much in common with AA. That Al-Anon can fulfil an extremely important function does, however, need to be emphasized, and the therapist should again be able knowledgeably to point the way. Al-Anon may give immediate relief to the wife who has been struggling by every stratagem to stop her husband from drinking, and who has in the process been experiencing stress and frustration. Al-Anon will teach her to 'let go' and to give up the hope of trying to control her husband's behaviour or solve his problem for him. He must find his own answers to *his* own problem and, similarly, she must examine *her* own behaviour: the only behaviour which she is directly able to control or alter is, indeed, her own.

Al-Ateen

Al-Ateen is a self-help group operating along AA lines which aims to help the teenage children of families in which there is an alcoholic parent. To date, this organization has become more widely established in North America than in the UK or other parts of Europe. That children living in such families are often experiencing distress and conflict cannot be doubted (see Chapter 5), and Al-Ateen potentially meets the needs of a group which the professional services involved with the parents may all too easily pass by.

Other self-help groups

Although AA is the largest and best-known self-help group for people with drinking problems, on a local basis other self-help groups may be available. In the UK, for example, there is a special group for doctors and dentists (the 'British Doctors and Dentists Group'; Anonymous, 1995). This profession-specific self-help group is often more approachable for a practitioner who may have fears of traditional AA groups, not least that they may meet their patients at the meetings. However, the group does have a close affinity to AA.

Other groups have deliberately set out to take a different approach from AA. For example, in the USA, Secular Organizations for Sobriety (SOS) and Rational Recovery (RR) have taken a non-religious stance (Connors and Dermen, 1996); Women for Sobriety (WFS) has taken a holistic and feminist approach; and Moderation Management® has provided group support for moderation of drinking rather than total abstinence (Emrick, 2001).

No other mutual help movement for people with drinking problems has become as international as AA, but, within their countries of origin, some of these other organizations have attracted large memberships, which in some cases far exceed the national membership of AA itself (Mäkelä et al., 1996).

REFERENCES

Al-Anon Family Groups UK and Eire (1980) Help for families of problem drinkers. *Health Trends* 12, 8.

Alcoholics Anonymous (1977) *Twelve Steps and Twelve Traditions.* New York: Alcoholics Anonymous World Services.

Anonymous (1995) The British Doctors' and Dentists' Groups: over two decades of successful work. *Addiction Counselling World* 6, 26–7.

Babor, T. (1995) The social and public health significance of individually directed interventions. In *Alcohol and Public Policy: Evidence and Issues*, ed. Holder, H.D. and Edwards, G. Oxford: Oxford University Press, 164–89.

Connors, G.J. and Dermen, K.H. (1996) Characteristics of participants in Secular Organizations for Sobriety (SOS). *American Journal of Drug and Alcohol Abuse* 22, 281–95.

Cook, C.C.H. (1988a) The Minnesota model in the management of drug and alcohol dependency: miracle method or myth? Part I. The philosophy and the programme. *British Journal of Addiction* 83, 625–34.

Cook, C.C.H. (1988b) The Minnesota model in the management of drug and alcohol dependency: miracle method or myth? Part II. Evidence and conclusions. *British Journal of Addiction* 83, 735–48.

Edwards, G. (1995) Alcoholics Anonymous as mirror held up to nature. In *Psychotherapy, Psychological Treatments, and the Addictions*, ed. Edwards, G. and Dare, C. Cambridge: Cambridge University Press, 220–39.

Emrick, C. (2001) Alcoholics Anonymous and other mutual aid groups. In *International Handbook of Alcohol Dependence and Problems*, ed. Heather, N., Peters, T.J. and Stockwell, T. Chichester: John Wiley and Sons, 663–78.

Galanter, M. (1999) Research on spirituality and Alcoholics Anonymous. *Alcoholism: Clinical and Experimental Research* 23, 716–19.

Glaser, F.B. and Ogborne, A.C. (1982) Does AA really work? *British Journal of Addiction* 77, 123–9.

Humphreys, K. and Moos, R. (2001) Can encouraging substance abuse patients to participate in self-help groups reduce demand for health care? A quasi-experimental study. *Alcoholism: Clinical and Experimental Research* 25, 711–16.

Jones, R.K. (1970) Sectarian characteristics of Alcoholics Anonymous. *Sociology* 4, 181–95.

Khantzian, E.J. and Mack, J.E. (1994) How AA works and why it's important for clinicians to understand. *Journal of Substance Abuse Treatment* 11, 77–92.

Kownacki, R.J. and Shadish, W.R. (1999) Does Alcoholics Anonymous work? The results from a meta-analysis of controlled experiments. *Substance Use and Misuse* 34, 1897–916.

Kurtz, E. (1991) *Not-God: a History of Alcoholics Anonymous.* Center City, MN: Hazelden.

Leach, B. and Norris, J.L. (1977) Factors in the development of Alcoholics Anonymous (AA). In *Treatment and Rehabilitation of the Chronic Alcoholic*, ed. Kissin, B. and Begleiter, H. *The Biology of Alcoholism*, Vol. 5. New York: Plenum Press, 441–543.

Longabaugh, R., Wirtz, P.W., Zweben, A. and Stout, R.L. (1998) Network support for drinking, Alcoholics Anonymous and long-term matching effects. *Addiction* 93, 1313–33.

Mäkelä, K., Arminen, I., Bloomfield, K. et al. (1996) *Alcoholics Anonymous as a Mutual-help Movement: a Study in Eight Societies.* Wisconsin: University of Wisconsin Press.

McCrady, B.S. and Miller, W.R. (eds) (1993) *Research on Alcoholics Anonymous. Opportunities and Alternatives.* Brunswick, NJ: Rutgers Center of Alcohol Studies.

Miller, W.R. (1990) Spirituality: the silent dimension in addiction research. *Drug and Alcohol Review* 9, 259–66.

Miller, W.R. (1998) Researching the spiritual dimensions of alcohol and other drug problems. *Addiction* 93, 979–90.

Peyrot, M. (1985) Narcotics Anonymous: its history, structure, and approach. *International Journal of the Addictions* 20, 1509–22.

Project MATCH Research Group (1997) Matching alcoholism treatments to client heterogeneity: Project MATCH post treatment drinking outcomes. *Journal of Studies on Alcohol* 58, 7–29.

Tiebout, H.M. (1944) Therapeutic mechanisms of Alcoholics Anonymous. *American Journal of Psychiatry* 100, 468–73.

Tonigan, J.S., Toscova, R. and Miller, W.R. (1996) Meta-analysis of the literature on Alcoholics Anonymous: sample and study characteristics moderate findings. *Journal of Studies on Alcohol* 57, 67–72.

Wilson, W. (1994) The society of Alcoholics Anonymous. *American Journal of Psychiatry* 151, 259–62.

Special techniques

Introduction

No single treatment approach is effective for all individuals with alcohol problems (Institute of Medicine, 1990). There is now evidence that some treatments are more effective than others for certain patients, but which treatments work? In very general terms, about one-third of individuals entering treatment will do very well during the first year after the treatment episode. Here, improvement means abstinence, moderation of drinking and freedom from or a reduction in alcohol-related problems (Miller et al., 2001). The remaining two-thirds will continue to have periods of heavy drinking, but they drink less frequently and when they drink they consume less. This certainly results in a reduction in alcohol-related health and social problems. A narrow focus on drinking outcomes misses the fact that treatment confers substantial benefits on patients. It is also likely that factors outside the treatment setting have a differential impact on the behavioural change process. Another issue, not always considered, is that treatment outcomes are likely to be different in different countries. For instance, European outcomes are not as favourable as those from the USA (see Miller et al., 2001). It must be remembered, however, that there will always be a proportion of dependent drinkers who go on to kill or wreck themselves, despite treatment.

Our basic plea is that treatment choices should, wherever possible, be research based while at the same time a spurious scientism should not be allowed to inhibit the efforts of the individual therapist who is trying to help the individual patient in difficult and unique circumstances. Box 19.1 summarizes in round terms our judgement as to the extent of current research underpinning for different treatments.

In this chapter, four broad approaches to the treatment of drinking problems are discussed: motivational interviewing, cognitive–behavioural therapy, psychotherapy and pharmacotherapy. These are prefaced by an account of the stages of

> BOX 19.1 **Special treatments for drinking problems: an appraisal of their research underpinning**
>
> - *Psychosocial treatments* including motivational interviewing, social skills training, the community reinforcement approach, behaviour contracting, self-monitoring. Well supported by research.
> - *Individual psychotherapies* other than cognitive–behavioural. Little or no research support. Deploy with discrimination.
> - *Group therapy.* Probably useful for basic support, but efficacy as a treatment of choice not supported.
> - *Behavioural marital therapy.* Well supported by research.
> - *Alcoholics Anonymous.* The impact of AA has not, as yet, been conclusively researched.
> - *Disulfiram.* Not without side effects, but useful in some circumstances.
> - *Anti-craving drugs* including naltrexone and acamprosate. Naltrexone and acamprosate supported by research.

change model which is relevant to most treatments. There will then be an account of Project MATCH and its implications for the 'real world' of treatment. Finally, the efficacy of different treatments is discussed and the future of alcohol treatment services considered (see also Chapter 22). The aim is to outline different techniques and discuss their value and limitation; no attempt is made to go into details about their application. Anyone wanting to acquire the necessary specialist clinical skills will do best to train under the guidance of someone familiar with such methods.

What are described as 'special techniques' may be considered routine by some practitioners, whereas others would place a lesser emphasis on these approaches from that given here. The adjective 'special' is still useful to differentiate these methods from the basic approaches discussed in Chapter 17, and most experienced therapists would agree that, whatever the special approach favoured, it is only valuable within the context of the general therapeutic work discussed in that chapter.

Stages of change

The 'stages of change' model, which acknowledges the pivotal role of the patient in the process of behavioural change, describes five discrete stages of change which can be applied both to an understanding of drinking behaviour and to the practical work of treatment (Prochaska and DiClemente, 1986; Prochaska et al., 1992, DiClemente and Prochaska, 1998). These stages are *Precontemplation, Contemplation, Preparation (originally called the Determination stage), Action and Maintenance* (see page 248). In the *precontemplation* stage, individuals are not considering a change in their drinking habits in the next 6 months. They may present to treatment services because they are under pressure from a partner, family, employer or general practitioner. Individuals in the *contemplation* stage recognize that they have a problem and begin to consider the implications for change. They have not yet made a commitment to take action and may remain at this stage for long periods if they do not resolve their ambivalence to change. Individuals in the *preparation* stage are intending to take action and may already have tried to cut down on their alcohol consumption. Having made a decision to change, individuals move forward into the *action* stage. They make a commitment to change and try to modify their drinking behaviour, often needing considerable support and encouragement. If successful action is sustained for a period of 3–6 months, the individuals move into the *maintenance* stage, in which they seek to integrate the changes into their lifestyle in order to prevent relapse.

The 'stages of change' model was first put forward as a linear schema and then as a circular or revolving-door model. Because individuals usually relapse, and re-enter the cycle, often moving through the stages several times before achieving long-term maintenance, Prochaska et al. (1992) have more recently presented a spiral model.

Prochaska and DiClemente's model provides a useful and practical framework in the treatment setting. It is helpful for the therapist to consider the degree to which the patient is prepared to change. Thus patients in the precontemplation stage are not impossible to treat, and patients in the action stage will not always succeed. The view that relapse is part of the process helps to avoid a sense of failure, and allows it to be seen as part of the natural process rather than as a catastrophe. This model has intuitive appeal and has been influential in guiding clinical practice (Davidson, 1992). However, the discrete categorization of the various stages is perhaps over-simplified and artificial. Although the stages tell us something about when people change, they do not explain how or why they change (Davidson, 1998). Self-efficacy, intention and motivation all appear to facilitate the change process. Despite its shortcomings, the 'stages of change' model is routinely used by clinicians in the alcohol and addictions field, perhaps because it helps to set motivational interviewing in context (Davidson, 1998). It continues to provide debate and is possibly best viewed as a model of ideal change that may be helpful in the design of interventions (Sutton, 1996).

Motivational interviewing

Since its original description as a therapeutic technique for use with problem drinkers, motivational interviewing has emerged as a practical and acceptable treatment approach for individuals who are reluctant to change and who are ambivalent about changing. It draws on strategies from client-centred counselling, cognitive therapy, systems theory and the social psychology of persuasion (Miller and Rollnick, 1991, 2002). The therapist does not assume an authoritarian or confrontational role, but seeks to create a positive atmosphere conducive to change. The overall goal is to increase the intrinsic motivation of patients, leaving them with the responsibility to effect their own change. It is helpful to view motivational interviewing in the context of the 'stages of change' model. In the early stages, patients are helped to explore their ambivalence to address reasons for change, using strategies derived from client-centred counselling, such as open-ended questions, reflective listening, affirmation and summarizing. Self-motivational statements are elicited from patients in order to help them to develop a perceived discrepancy or dissonance between their present behaviour and their stated goals. Motivational interviewing develops and amplifies this discrepancy, ultimately allowing the patient to present the reasons for change without feeling coerced. It has been shown to be effective in reducing alcohol consumption in problem drinkers from a variety of health settings, including primary care and general hospitals (Bien et al., 1993). Project MATCH found no difference in outcomes between Motivational Enhancement Therapy (MET), Cognitive–Behavioural Therapy (CBT) and Twelve Step Facilitation (TSF) after a 12-week treatment period. The improvements that occurred during treatment were still evident at 1-year and at 3-year follow-up (Project Match Research Group, 1997a, 1997b, 1998a). Angry clients did particularly well after MET.

Cognitive–behavioural therapy

The cognitive–behavioural approach to treatment is based on the assumption that it is the problem drinking which is to be treated, as opposed to the psychoanalytic view that the drinking is a symptom or symbol of an underlying psychodynamic conflict or neurosis. Implicit in this approach is the belief that problem drinking is mainly a learned behaviour and that treatment involves replacing the maladaptive pattern of drinking behaviour with more appropriate drinking, or abstinence. Cognitive–behavioural psychology also highlights the role of expectations about alcohol in the development of drinking and its consequences.

Broad-spectrum approaches

A further development of the cognitive–behavioural approach has been the inclusion of training in skills thought to be lacking in patients with drinking problems. Drinkers may, for instance, use alcohol to cope with anxiety or anger or as a result of negative cognitions associated with low self-esteem and depression. Such individuals may benefit from specific techniques including relaxation training, anger management and cognitive restructuring. These approaches are not specific to alcohol problems, but find their application as treatments aimed at dealing with postulated psychological causes of excessive drinking. Within this spectrum, at least the following kinds of intervention can be listed.

Social skills training

Some patients with drinking problems are handicapped by an underlying inability to function confidently in social situations. Social skills training concentrates on developing assertion and communication skills. Social skills deficits are assessed and patients are then taught how to initiate social interactions and express their thoughts and feelings. This is typically done in a group setting where role play, desensitization and other behavioural methods can be used. For instance, the patient who is unassertive may find it difficult to say 'no' to an offered drink; one element in therapy may involve teaching them to rehearse saying 'no'. Social skills training which includes assertiveness training is an extremely effective method of treatment for alcohol problems (Holder et al., 1991; Miller et al., 1998). It can be delivered on an individual or group basis and is particularly suited to individuals with severe alcohol dependence. However, it requires a certain level of cognitive functioning, and patients with neuropsychological impairment/alcohol-related brain damage will not benefit from this approach.

Problem-solving skills

Individuals with drinking difficulties frequently have handicaps in solving problems and will then cope by denial or by further drinking. Training in problem-solving skills is similar to social skills training and aims to help the patient to develop alternative coping strategies for use in high-risk situations (Parks et al., 2001b). In Project MATCH, the coping skills model of CBT used was associated with better outcomes in less dependent clients.

Relaxation training

Many patients report that they initially began to drink in order to relieve feelings of anxiety. Anxiety disorders are not uncommon among such individuals (see Chapter 8). Teaching of relaxation by simple psychological techniques may be useful for a tense patient who drinks to relax, and can offer an alternative method of coping with cravings (Monti et al., 1989).

Anger management

Without alcohol, many patients experience difficulties coping with and expressing their anger. Training in anger management can be of benefit, particularly if carried out in conjunction with assertiveness training (Heather, 1995).

Cognitive restructuring

Often, patients will attribute their alcohol use to extrinsic factors such as stress and are not aware that their own negative thoughts are implicated (Beck et al., 1993). Cognitive restructuring helps the individual to interrupt the series of thoughts that would usually lead to drinking and to replace them with positive thoughts. This is an effective treatment, which should be used routinely as part of a cognitive–behavioural programme. It is particularly successful when used in combination with social skills training (Oei and Jackson, 1982).

Behavioural self-control

Behavioural self-control training is particularly effective in helping individuals at the less severe end of the dependence spectrum to reduce their alcohol consumption. Initially, the therapist and client negotiate sensible limits of alcohol consumption and the client keeps a drinking diary or fills out a self-monitoring card to record all drinks taken. A craving diary or daily activity diary can also be helpful. Clients are then taught techniques for reducing the rate of drinking and are helped to identify triggers to drinking, in particular negative moods (boredom, anxiety, depression), positive moods (excitement, happiness) and external cues (meeting with friends, particular time of day, a particular place). Behavioural self-control training can be used in the individual or group setting and self-help manuals are available (Heather, 1995).

Cue exposure

This approach is based on the principles of classical conditioning and borrows from a treatment strategy which was developed for phobias, obsessive–compulsive disorder and other anxiety disorders. The patient is exposed to conditioned stimuli or cues which have previously precipitated craving or excessive drinking, and encouraged either not to drink or not to drink excessively. For instance, they may be asked to carry around with them a bottle of whisky and sniff at it without drinking, or a therapist may accompany them on outings to a bar, or they may be asked to take sufficient alcohol to activate craving and then desist from further drinking. Cue exposure reduces the likelihood that the stimulus will trigger a response in the future and improves the individual's self-efficacy. It can be combined with coping skills (Monti et al., 1989; Marlatt, 1990) or incorporated into a relapse prevention programme (Drummond and Glautier, 1994; Drummond et al., 1995).

Aversion therapies

Aversion therapies based on the principles of classical conditioning came to the fore in the 1930s and are of historical importance because they fostered an optimistic interest in 'alcoholism' treatment at a time when little else appeared to be promising. The act of drinking alcohol is paired with a variety of unpleasant experiences, and the individual should show an automatic negative response when later exposed to alcohol. Such counter-conditioning techniques have included chemically induced nausea (using emetine and apomorphine), apnoea (using intravenous succinylcholine), electric shock and covert sensitization (Miller et al., 1995).

Nausea aversion therapy has shown positive outcomes in a number of studies. However, the favourable results reported in the literature are more likely to be due to the artefact of patient selection, rather than to any special effect: a patient would need to be highly motivated to volunteer for such an unpleasant experience in the name of treatment. As the dangers and unpleasantness of nausea aversion therapy outweigh any supposed advantages, we recommend that this treatment should no longer be used. Succinylcholine-induced apnoea (cessation of breathing) as a treatment should be discarded completely. It is also questionable whether electric shock treatment, which is associated with considerable pain, is an ethical mode of treatment.

Covert sensitization is the form of aversion therapy most commonly used. Here, patients are taught to associate the sight or taste of alcohol with unpleasant images which they learn actively to conjure up (conditioned aversion). Covert sensitization is suited to an abstinence goal, and is recommended for use on an individual basis, as the best results are thought to be achieved when the images are specific to the individual. Covert sensitization is an effective treatment (Holder et al., 1991) and its success can be predicted from the degree of conditioning established during treatment (Elkins, 1980).

The community reinforcement approach (CRA)

This approach is based on the principles of instrumental learning and the emphasis is on manipulation of real-life rewards in the patient's environment. The community reinforcement approach (CRA) focuses on altering reinforcement contingencies in the home environment, involves significant others and uses positive reinforcement. The family's positive reactions, aid with job-finding, membership of a social club and other social rewards are presented to the patient as contingent on treatment success, and the therapeutic team accepts responsibility to ensure that such rewards are, in fact, on offer (Hunt and Azrin, 1973; Azrin, 1976; Meyers and Miller, 2001). This technique has evolved over time. Components of earlier interventions have been dropped and new treatment components added, such as motivational counselling, drink-referral training, and immediate on-site disulfiram administration. It has, however, retained its focus on drinking behaviours, family and job-related problems. Although initially used with in-patients, it has been employed with out-patients and with supervised disulfiram. Married patients with family support do well using the stand-alone disulfiram component, whereas unmarried, unsupported patients benefit from the whole package (Azrin et al., 1982). Recent research shows that CRA-based strategies are also effective when disulfiram is not used (Meyers and Miller, 2001). Although CRA is an effective treatment, particularly for drinkers with serious problems, it has never been widely adopted in clinical practice. This is surprising, because the procedures are well specified and can be learned and applied successfully, even by novice therapists. The full package need not be time consuming or expensive, and positive outcomes have been reported even after five to eight sessions. It is more likely that CRA has not been disseminated distinctively or attractively enough to facilitate its transfer to routine clinical practice (Meyers and Miller, 2001).

Relapse prevention therapy

Some aspects of relapse have already been discussed in Chapter 17 (page 289–90) in relation to the basic work of treatment. The term relapse prevention refers to a wide range of techniques, many or all of which are cognitive or behavioural in their thrust. This approach has its origins within a theoretical model of relapse proposed by Marlatt and Gordon (1985). Within this perspective, relapse is not viewed as an inexplicable catastrophe, but as an event that takes place through a series of cognitive, behavioural and affective processes. One of the main objectives of the relapse prevention programme is preventing a lapse from becoming a relapse. Relapse is viewed as an untoward event which is to be avoided by careful forward planning and by the design of an individual relapse prevention programme. Patients themselves are active partners in identifying high-risk situations which are associated with a potential for relapse. Intrapersonal factors such as negative and positive emotional states, interpersonal conflict and social pressure can all be determinants of relapse. The patient then has to learn more effective coping mechanisms including cognitive strategies, or personally planned substitute activities and rewarding use of leisure. Strategies will thus involve learning both how to avoid unnecessary risks and how to deal positively and confidently with inevitable risks. Relapse prevention essentially addresses itself not just to changing a self-destructive habit, but beyond that to the maintenance of change, and to the development of self-efficacy and coping skills. The approach is applicable both to abstinence and the normal drinking goal.

Marlatt and Gordon also addressed lifestyle imbalance in their relapse prevention model. The individual experiencing feelings of self-deprivation may be particularly likely to relapse in high-risk situations. Cognitive factors such as rationalization or denial come into play when individuals are craving and are used to legitimize the drinking behaviour and to reduce feelings of guilt and anxiety. Covert planning of relapse through a series of seemingly irrelevant decisions is also described in this model. Beyond Marlatt and Gordon's pioneering formulation, several other authors have now contributed to elaboration of the relapse prevention model (Wanigaratne et al., 1990; Annis et al., 1996). Treatment outcome studies of relapse prevention have shown mixed results (Miller et al., 1995). Successful components include teaching individuals to recover quickly from lapses (Weingardt and Marlatt, 1998) and interventions to improve aftercare participation. Relapse prevention seems to be most effective when applied to alcohol dependent individuals at the more severe end of the spectrum. Treatment effects are maintained long term (Parks et al., 2001a).

Marital and family therapy

Alcohol problems have a far-reaching influence on family life, and are in turn affected by family dynamics. Many different types and intensities of family approach have been employed in the treatment of drinking problems, varying from informal chats with husband and wife to sophisticated therapeutic interventions based on a specific theory. The needs of the women partners of heavy drinking men have largely been ignored. In situations where it proves difficult to engage problem-drinking men in treatment, stress management sessions may help to ease the stresses and burden experienced by their women partners (Halford et al., 2001). Other family members besides the husband and wife may be involved in therapeutic sessions. Over recent years, there have been many advances in family therapy techniques and in the application of those techniques to this specialized sector of practice, and there is evidence that marital or family therapy improves the short-term outcomes. It is therefore important that anyone working with drinking problems should have some familiarity with family therapies. Two types of treatment, behavioural marital therapy (BMT) and spouse therapy, have been shown to be effective.

Behavioural marital therapy

This effective treatment approach focuses on the patient's drinking behaviour and the quality of the marital relationship (O'Farrell et al., 1993). Behavioural and disulfiram contracts are used to address the drinking behaviour. The marital interventions focus on improving the relationship and resolving conflicts and problems. A stable relationship is clearly a prerequisite. Some programmes incorporate a disulfiram contract in which the problem drinker takes disulfiram every day, observed by the spouse. BMT has been shown to improve drinking outcomes at 18 months, and to maintain marital stability and satisfaction (O'Farrell et al., 1993). Interactive couples' group therapy is another technique which shows promise (Bowers and Al-Rehda, 1990).

Spouse therapy

Here, the spouse is helped to encourage the problem drinker to seek help and is taught behavioural reinforcement strategies to support abstinence or reduced drinking. Spouse therapy is effective in improving treatment retention (Heather, 1995).

Cognitive–behavioural 'packages'

Anyone working with people who have drinking problems will recognize that they are a very heterogeneous population and that different approaches are needed for different patients. It is best to carry out an individual assessment, and on the basis of this assessment to identify the type of treatment best suited to that person. Thus a treatment 'package' may usefully incorporate several cognitive–behavioural techniques tailored to the individual's need.

Psychotherapy

Drinking and its psychodynamic meanings

In the past, some psychoanalytic writing has suggested that the dynamic meaning of drinking can be pronounced upon in universal terms – excessive drinking as always being a suicidal equivalent, for instance. Such a dogmatic view of the psycho-dynamics of drinking is as unhelpful to work in this field as are any fixed formulae for dynamic interpretations in the general field of psychotherapy.

Drinking and excessive drinking will, in fact, have different meanings for different patients, and often multiple meanings for any one patient. Without seeking to pre-empt the need to explore the individual, there are some recurrent themes with which it is useful to become familiar. Some of these themes are set out briefly below, but this list is not exhaustive.

1. Drinking may be an indicator of identification with a heavy-drinking parent or other key figure in the patient's childhood. The patient is, as it were, destined to act out someone else's life rather than their own. Other people in their present surroundings are also being set up as actors in the old play, for instance the wife is being forced into the same role as the patient once saw his mother play in relation to his own alcoholic father. The acutely traumatic early experiences of the child in an 'alcoholic' family, with the many unresolved conflicts of love, hate, rage, and pity, are particularly likely to result in a patient continuing to define relationships in terms of the play which they still desperately hope to resolve.

2. Related to the general framework proposed above, one may identify a variety of common sub-plots. A man with a drinking problem may, for instance, seek defeat, punishment or even destruction through drink, because they see themselves

(their father) as deserving such fate. They may be seeking to inflict punishment on others, believing that at some level their mother destroyed their father and that she (and now the patient's own wife) is in a sense, a dreaded enemy. He may see drinking as giving power, because his father was only powerful when drunk. However, drinking may also point directly to interpersonal dependency conflicts: the patient wants to be powerful and independent but also wants to be a dependent child who is sick, erring and repeatedly forgiven.

3. Patients sometimes seem to use alcohol as a way of entering a blissful state of reverie where they can engage in fantasy and wish fulfilment. The real world is too difficult. Alcohol is valued for its subjective effect, and it becomes symbolized as all-warm, mother-like or milk-like. The drink is then an indicator of the patient's general difficulty in consistently maintaining an engagement with the real adult world.

The meanings given to alcohol are not only individually determined and shaped by early personal experience, but are also often coloured by culture. The need to be sensitive to the special meanings that a woman may give to her drinking also needs to be noted, for symbolic meanings may differ between the sexes.

Psychotherapy is not a panacea and its deployment may pose particular difficulties for those with alcohol and other addiction problems (Davison, 1996). Insight-oriented psychotherapy has not been shown to be an effective treatment for drinking problems in controlled trials. Yet, it has something to offer the carefully selected patient, and may on occasion be essential to that improvement in the quality of sobriety which is such an important adjunct to recovery. The therapist who, with modesty, open-mindedness and guidance, engages in such work is also personally going to benefit and will round out their understanding of the extraordinarily complex human processes which often lie behind a drinking story.

Indications for psychotherapy

The position which is taken in this section on the place of psychotherapy is in tune with the overall emphasis which is being given to the importance of approaching each patient in terms of their unique needs. This is the way in which an experienced nurse therapist described her use of psychotherapeutic insights.

Most of the time I am not 'doing psychotherapy', at least overtly. I doubt whether most of my patients would regard themselves as 'being in psychotherapy'. I am in fact making use of psychotherapeutic principles in every interview – I am working through and with a relationship, and dealing with defence mechanisms. But all this work goes on in a setting which emphasizes the need to keep one's feet on the ground, deal with drinking, pay the bills, get the children to school.

Such deployment of dynamic skills in the everyday clinical setting merges with more formal and intensive psychotherapeutic strategies. We do not favour the routine and intensive deployment of formal psychotherapy as a treatment for drinking problems. The psychotherapeutic intervention, which is always put into top gear for every patient and family from the earliest stages, not only represents an un-economic and undiscriminating deployment of resources, but may damage the individual's and family's capacity to generate their natural and spontaneous ways of working for and consolidating recovery. Such a perspective must not be mis-interpreted as antipathetic to psychotherapy. On the contrary, the position which is being taken is both that an understanding of dynamic principles must underpin basic work in this area, and that formal psychotherapy can on occasion have an important part to play. The argument is, however, that formal psychotherapy is not universally applicable and that its deployment requires timing and discrimination.

Different therapists will have their own views as to whether suitability for psycho-therapy is determined restrictively or more freely. What should particularly be cautioned against is the danger of forgetting that suitability for psychotherapy does indeed have to be determined by careful assessment. The enthusiasm of those not specially trained in general psychotherapeutic work may lead to the prescription of psychotherapy for a patient whom no experienced psychotherapist would regard as a suitable patient for such engagement. Many psychotherapists will make the offer of psychotherapy actually conditional on the patient achieving a stable period of sobriety or other life changes.

Here is an example of a referral to psychotherapy which was timely and proved useful.

A woman aged 45 had presented 3 years previously with heavy, non-dependent drinking in the setting of a painful marital breakdown. After a year's total abstinence from alcohol, she had for 2 years been drinking in a moderate and controlled fashion. She was now contem-plating remarriage, but was worried that she might in this new relationship re-enact what she sensed as being life-long problems in close relationships with men. Her father had been a strong but distant figure whom she had been taught greatly to admire, but towards whom her feelings had been very ambivalent. After two assessment interviews by a psycho-therapist, she was offered a contract in terms of relatively short-term psychotherapy (6 months with weekly sessions), which was to focus on her problems with key relation-ships and her conflicting needs to be dominated together with her resentful and destructive responses to the people whom she manoeuvred into this role.

The alcohol team may have appropriate psychotherapeutic skills within its own resources, or it may be necessary to make referrals to psychotherapy specialists. This type of problem may, however, also be ideal for training staff in techniques for brief psychotherapy techniques, with the time of the experienced psychotherapist then devoted to case supervision rather than to the treatment of referred cases.

Group therapy

Group therapy has been widely employed in the treatment of drinking problems, even to the extent of sometimes being viewed as the treatment of choice (Falkowski, 1996). Despite this, there is little evidence that classical group psychotherapy has a lasting impact on drinking behaviour. In the alcohol field, a diversity of activities is likely to be operating under the broad label of 'group work', and relapse prevention and cognitive–behavioural treatment are commonly delivered in this way.

At their simplest, such groups would be of the kind described in Chapter 22 as often having a place within the therapeutic structure of a treatment centre. Such groups tend to have an open rather than a closed membership, as patients are admitted and discharged. At the other extreme, one may find practitioners who will work with closed groups of, say, eight to ten patients selected for their homogeneity (all women, for instance, or all of the same social background), and who will run these groups in terms of orthodox group therapy principles.

One can identify variations on some general themes as to the type of the work which is likely to be accomplished in group sessions. There may first be value simply in group *education*: for instance patients learn about the nature of dependence. A second important and general theme is *problem solving*: this may relate to such reality issues as how to find a job or deal with debts, or may focus on interpersonal and dynamic issues. Rehearsal of *relapse prevention strategies* is often a useful part of group work, as patients share ideas with each other on how sobriety is to be consolidated and relapse avoided. Cohesion of group sentiment can assist in *definition of goals*, in overcoming *resistance* and in *strengthening of motivation*. Lastly, the fellowship of the group and the opportunity to share problems may very generally contribute to support and help to overcome feelings of isolation.

The therapist should be willing to take responsibility for excluding any patient who comes to a group when intoxicated. Having anyone who has been drinking participate in a group usually causes such anxiety and anger as to rule out the possibility of constructive work.

Psychodrama

The use of psychodrama in the treatment of drinking problems has its advocates. Although special training is required for the skilled application of this approach, less complex role-playing techniques are more easily learnt. Patients may benefit greatly from group exploration of how they would, for instance, say 'no' to a drink, deal with anger or provocation, or manage a job interview.

Therapies for sexual problems

The sexual problems which may underlie or result from excessive drinking are too often overlooked, and insufficient help is therefore given with these problems. Specialized techniques exist for assisting with such difficulties. Although it is unlikely that the therapist who was working on drinking problems will be able to become fully trained in the application of sex therapies, he or she should be conversant with what such approaches have to offer and should be able to make appropriate referrals.

Pharmacotherapy

Over recent years, there have been major advances in understanding the neuro-pharmacological basis of alcohol dependence (see Chapter 3), and this has been paralleled by the introduction of newer pharmacotherapeutic agents, in particular drugs with anti-craving properties. Pharmacotherapy, however, is not a panacea, and should not be used in isolation, but in conjunction with psychosocial treatments. This chapter summarizes current knowledge on the older (disulfiram) and newer drugs in the field. Alcohol withdrawal is discussed in Chapter 16. This section of the present chapter discusses in turn: disulfiram (an alcohol-sensitizing agent); drugs that attenuate drinking behaviour (anti-craving drugs); drugs used to treat psychiatric disorders associated with alcohol dependence; and finally amethystic agents. A number of recent reviews will be of interest to readers seeking a more detailed account (Hughes and Cook, 1997; Moncrieff and Drummond, 1997; Garbutt et al., 1999; Kranzler, 2000).

Disulfiram

Since its introduction in the late 1940s, disulfiram (trade name Antabuse) has been used very widely in the treatment of alcohol problems. Disulfiram blocks the breakdown of alcohol at the acetaldehyde stage by inhibiting the hepatic enzyme aldehyde dehydrogenase (ALDH). This leads to an accumulation of acetaldehyde in the body and to the disulfiram–ethanol reaction, characterized by flushing of the face and upper trunk, throbbing headache, palpitations, tachycardia, nausea, vomiting and general distress. With large doses of alcohol, arrhythmias, hypotension and collapse may occur. The reaction usually starts within 10–30 minutes of drinking and can last several hours. The severity varies greatly: it may be so slight that the patient 'drinks through it', or so severe as to be life threatening. Patients with cardiac failure, coronary artery disease, hypertension, hepatic or renal impairment, respiratory disease, diabetes or epilepsy should not be given disulfiram. In the event of a severe reaction and cardiovascular collapse, the patient should lie down and the foot of the bed should be elevated. A vasopressor (blood pressure-raising drug) may be needed. Intravenous vitamin C or an antihistamine has also been recommended as an antidote. Patients prescribed disulfiram should carry a medical card with emergency instructions. The practice of exposing patients to a challenge dose of alcohol as a therapeutic test is not routinely justified.

The rationale of this treatment is that patients cannot drink while under the protective cover of the drug, and they will thus only have to take a daily decision to take the medication rather than have to resist the sudden temptation to drink of any moment. Disulfiram is thus not primarily a conditioning treatment, though a variety of secondary learning processes may be involved.

Although disulfiram is used for its deterrent action, it also has effects on the central nervous system, inhibiting dopamine β-hydroxylase and increasing concentrations of dopamine in the mesolimbic system. Patients taking disulfiram have reported a reduction in desire for alcohol.

Disulfiram is usually given in a daily dose of 100–200 mg. It is absorbed slowly, and therefore must be taken for a few days so as to build up a satisfactory blood level. Side effects include initial lethargy and fatigue, vomiting, an unpleasant taste in the mouth and halitosis, impotence and unexplained breathlessness. Other less usual side effects include psychosis (usually accompanied by delirium), allergic dermatitis, peripheral neuritis and hepatic cell damage. Disulfiram also interacts with other drugs, enhancing the effect of warfarin and inhibiting the metabolism of tricyclic antidepressants, phenytoin and benzodiazepines such as diazepam and chlordiazepoxide. It is therefore a drug which should only be used with discretion and its dangers should not be discounted.

Despite the many years during which disulfiram has been in use, it is still difficult to form a view as to its place in treatment. Most studies of disulfiram have been of short duration, used small numbers of 'severe alcoholics', were not methodologically sound and were associated with some form of coercion – from the courts, clinics or doctors (Hughes and Cook, 1997). Results have been equivocal, but Fuller et al.'s (1986) multi-centre trial suggested that unsupervised oral disulfiram may help to reduce the frequency of drinking in men who are not abstinent but who are reasonably motivated. It has been argued that this 'harm reduction' effect is a clinically important one (Heather, 1993). Supervised oral disulfiram appears to be effective when incorporated into a comprehensive treatment programme, when used in association with a contingency management plan, a community reinforcement approach (Azrin et al., 1982) or counselling (Chick et al., 1992). Garbutt et al. (1999) concluded that the evidence supporting the efficacy of disulfiram was 'fair'.

The disadvantages of disulfiram include the potential dangers of the drug–ethanol reaction, side effects of the drug and a covert message that more basic therapeutic work is not needed. However, some patients find disulfiram helpful, especially in the early stages of abstinence. Others may prefer to take a low maintenance dose over many years and others will use it intermittently to cover high-risk periods, for instance the executive going to a conference where they know they will be exposed to much entertaining.

In the light of present evidence, the best results with disulfiram are probably likely to be seen when one or both of the following conditions are fulfilled. Firstly, the use of the drug should be explained to, and negotiated with, the patient, so that the taking of these tablets becomes not only acceptable but wanted; the patient is not being muzzled, or surrendering autonomy, but making a free decision to engage in this type of treatment. Secondly, an acceptable degree of supervision should be set up (the tablet taken in the doctors office, for instance, or in the medical room at work, or under the eyes of the wife or partner), or a contingency management plan or therapeutic contract established. Disulfiram has been used in this way within industrial treatment programmes and, in the USA, within court probation programmes.

Disulfiram is also available in a long-acting implant form, but research evidence in favour of this route of administration is negative. The technique involves implantation of disulfiram pellets beneath the skin by means of a surgical operation conducted under local anaesthetic. The preparation is not officially approved in all countries. The pellets sometimes work their way to the surface and are scratched out, and unpleasant septic complications can occur. Pharmacologically effective blood levels of the drug are not obtained, and any success which results must depend more on expectancy than on chemistry. The occasional patient may, however, be found who has great faith in this treatment and who will regularly attend for a 3-monthly implant – a patient who, for example, has experienced frequent imprisonment for drink-related crime, and who believes that only with this seeming extreme of external control can further trouble be avoided.

Drugs that attenuate drinking behaviour

The emergence of naltrexone and acamprosate as substances targeted at the treatment of drinking problems has occurred only over the last few years. Controlled research results to date are promising (Garbutt et al., 1999, Miller and Wilbourne, 2002). Both drugs are discussed below, together with other drugs that have been evaluated in alcohol dependence over recent years. These include serotonergic agents, such as selective serotonin reuptake inhibitors (SSRIs), buspirone hydrochloride and ondansetron hydrochloride.

Naltrexone

The opioid receptor antagonist naltrexone, in a dose of 50 mg daily, has been shown to reduce relapse rates in alcohol dependent patients, in combination with out-patient psychosocial treatment (O'Malley et al., 1992; Volpicelli et al., 1992; Anton et al., 1999; Morris et al., 2001). It seems to be less effective in promoting abstinence, and the treatment effect is dependent on patient compliance (Volpicelli et al., 1997; Anton et al., 1999). In one study, compliance was greater in those with a higher urge to drink in response to alcohol stimuli in a laboratory situation (Rohsenow et al., 2000). Naltrexone may reduce the euphoria associated with alcohol intake and an action on craving has been suggested (Volpicelli et al., 1995; Monti et al., 1999). When social drinkers take naltrexone, they experience less stimulation and a less positive effect after consuming alcohol (Davidson et al., 1999).

Two large multi-centre trials (one American and one carried out in the UK) failed to replicate the above findings with respect to abstinence and relapse. The American study used veterans with chronic, severe alcohol dependence, almost all of whom were men (Krystal et al., 2001). It is therefore possible that these results cannot be generalized to patients with less chronic and less severe alcohol dependence, and to women. The UK study found that total consumption, liver enzymes and alcohol craving were significantly reduced in compliant patients treated with naltrexone as compared to placebo (Chick et al., 2000a). It also demonstrated that naltrexone was effective when used in association with a range of psychosocial treatments which were less intensive than those applied in the American studies.

Studies to date have involved a 12-week trial of naltrexone with a 12-week follow-up. Further research is needed to assess the longer term efficacy of naltrexone.

Naltrexone is a reasonably safe drug. Side effects include nausea, vomiting, abdominal pain, headache, reduced energy, joint and muscle pain, and sleeping difficulty. Loss of appetite, diarrhoea, constipation, increased thirst, chest pain, increased sweating, increased energy, irritability, chills, delayed ejaculation and decreased potency are less frequent side effects. Liver function abnormalities and reversible thrombocytopaenia (reduction in platelet count) have been reported but are rare.

Most people tolerate the daily 50 mg dose, though in some instances the 25 mg dose will be better. It may be helpful to take the lower dose for the first 3–4 days of treatment to minimize side effects. Individuals who are troubled with persistent craving may need a dose of 100 mg daily. Treatment is usually for 3–6 months in the first instance. However, the effect may fall off after 6 months and some patients may need longer term prescribing, up to 1 year (O'Malley et al., 1996). Naltrexone appears to be safe when used with antidepressants, but more studies are needed to evaluate its role in depression and alcohol dependence (Croop et al., 1997).

Naltrexone should only be used in alcohol dependent patients who are medically and socially stable, have no active liver disease and are not taking opioids. Patients should have an abstinence goal, should be engaged in a psychosocial treatment programme and should want to take naltrexone. Abstinence for 3–7 days before starting treatment is recommended. Liver toxicity tests should be carried out before starting treatment, and at regular intervals while patients are taking the drug. The use of opiates and opioid-containing medications is contra-indicated and patients should be careful about using other drugs with potential liver toxicity, e.g. paracetamol and disulfiram. In special instances, naltrexone can be used alongside disulfiram as long as great care is taken to ensure that liver toxicity tests are done at regular intervals.

In individuals taking naltrexone, pain should be treated with aspirin, paracetamol (bearing in mind the potential complication mentioned above) or ibuprofen. When opioid analgesia is needed, naltrexone should be discontinued for 2–3 days. People taking naltrexone should carry a naltrexone card providing information that they are on this drug and regarding emergency analgesia. Naltrexone is licensed for use in alcohol dependence in the USA and a number of European countries. It is not licensed for use in alcohol dependence in the UK, but is available at specialist clinics, where its use is authorized on a named patient basis.

Nalmefene, another opoid antagonist, appears to have a similar action to naltrexone (Mason et al., 1994, 1999) and may be more effective.

How does naltrexone work? Alcohol is thought to be reinforcing because it stimulates brain opioid activity (see Chapter 3). Opioid antagonists such as naltrexone should theoretically block or reduce the effect of alcohol on opioid receptor activity, and decrease the pleasure or 'high' experienced by drinkers. This mechanism would explain the lower rates of drinking or relapse in the naltrexone groups in the American studies. Naltrexone may also reduce cravings or urges to drink. Another potential mechanism relates to what happens when someone drinks while taking naltrexone. Here, naltrexone is thought to increase the aversive effects of alcohol (e.g. nausea) and/or to increase intoxication for a given dose of alcohol.

Acamprosate

Acamprosate (calcium bis acetyl homotaurinate) has been used in the treatment of alcohol dependence in France for several years. Clinical trials suggest that it may help to prevent relapse in alcohol dependent patients when used as part of a therapeutic programme (Paille et al., 1995; Whitworth et al., 1996; Sass et al., 1996; Pelc et al., 1997; Poldrugo, 1997; Besson et al., 1998; Tempesta et al., 2000). The German study showed that the effects lasted for 1 year after stopping the medication (Sass et al., 1996). However, the UK study was negative, probably because of (i) a higher dropout rate and relapse into drinking before starting the drug; (ii) a higher proportion of episodic drinkers in the sample; and (iii) a background of less intensive treatment than in the other European studies (Chick et al., 2000b).

Acamprosate is a safe drug which does not interact with alcohol or diazepam and appears to have no addictive potential itself. It has been used safely with antidepressants. The recommended treatment dose is 1998 mg daily for body weight over 60 kg and 1332 mg daily for body weight under 60 kg. Acamprosate should not be prescribed to individuals with renal insufficiency or severe hepatic failure, or to women who are pregnant or breast-feeding. About 10% of patients experience diarrhoea and abdominal discomfort. Acamprosate is licensed for use in most European countries, several Latin American countries and Australia.

The mechanism of action of acamprosate is uncertain (Littleton, 1995). It has been reported to block presynaptic $GABA_B$ receptors and to antagonize NMDA receptor activation in the hippocampus and nucleus accumbens. Its effectiveness may be related to its ability to restore glutamatergic transmission reduced by alcohol (Berton et al., 1998; see Chapter 3).

Selective serotonin reuptake inhibitors (SSRIs)

SSRIs are amongst the newer antidepressants which have relatively few side effects. A variety of SSRIs, including fluoxetine and citalopram, have been shown to reduce alcohol consumption temporarily by about 20% in social drinkers and early problem drinkers. The results with alcohol dependence are less clear cut. A recent Italian study suggested that fluvoxamine and citalopram, in combination with cognitive–behavioural therapy, decreased relapse rates in non-depressed, alcohol dependent patients compared with placebo (Angelone et al., 1998). Patients treated with citalopram reported a significant reduction in craving.

'Alcoholic' subtypes may respond differentially to serotonergic medication. One study showed that Type B 'alcoholics' (higher risk/severity: Babor et al., 1992) had poorer drinking outcomes with fluoxetine 60 mg daily than with placebo (Kranzler et al., 1996). However, in a more recent study, sertraline 200 mg/day was associated with better drinking outcomes than placebo in Type A alcohol dependent subjects (Pettinati et al., 2000).

SSRIs may prove to be a useful addition to psychosocial treatment in a proportion of non-depressed, alcohol dependent patients. This effect appears to occur independently of their action on mood. However, the evidence to date does not support the routine use of SSRIs in clinical practice. Their use in depressed, alcohol dependent patients is discussed on page 332.

Buspirone

Buspirone, a 5-hydroxytryptamine ($5\text{-}HT_{1A}$) partial agonist, has been shown to reduce alcohol consumption in anxious, alcohol dependent patients and to improve treatment retention (Kranzler et al., 1994). Its action on drinking is thought to be mediated through a reduction in anxiety, and alcohol dependent individuals with anxiety might benefit (Malec et al., 1996). Buspirone appears to have little effect in non-anxious, alcohol dependent patients (George et al., 1999).

Ondansetron

Ondansetron, a specific 5-HT$_3$ antagonist, may have a role in early onset 'alco-holism' (onset in individuals under the age of 25 years), decreasing drinking and increasing abstinence rates (Johnson et al., 2000; see page 39). This sub-type is characterized by greater serotonergic abnormality and greater antisocial behaviour.

Drugs used to treat psychiatric co-morbidity

As mentioned in Chapter 8, alcohol dependence is commonly associated with psy-chiatric co-morbidity and the combination tends to lead to poorer outcomes. Judicious treatment of co-morbid depressive, anxiety and psychotic disorders should help to ameliorate psychological symptoms and improve drinking out-comes.

Antidepressants

Depressive symptoms commonly occur in patients with drinking problems, par-ticularly during the alcohol withdrawal phase. Treatment with antidepressants (tri-cyclics, SSRIs) should be delayed until the 'depressed' patient has been abstinent for at least 10–14 days. The tricyclic antidepressants imipramine and desipramine have been shown to improve depression and reduce the risk of relapse in alcohol dependent individuals with co-morbid depression (McGrath et al., 1996; Mason et al., 1996). Fluoxetine has been shown to reduce depressive symptoms and alcohol consumption in patients with alcohol dependence and co-morbid major depressive disorder (Kranzler et al., 1995; Cornelius et al., 1997).

Carbamazepine

Carbamazepine, an anticonvulsant agent with mood-stabilizing properties has been shown to increase the time to first drink in a small placebo-controlled study (Mueller et al., 1997). The use of carbamazepine as a mood stabilizer in patients with bipolar affective disorder (manic–depressive disorder) is well established.

Lithium

Despite early promise, lithium therapy does not appear to be of direct benefit in the treatment of alcohol dependence (Dorus et al., 1989). However, it is widely used for the treatment and prophylaxis of bipolar affective disorder.

Dopamine antagonists

Tiapride, a selective D$_2$ antagonist, has been used in a clinical sample where it was shown to improve abstinence in anxious or depressed 'alcoholics' (Shaw et al., 1987). However, its side-effects profile limits its widespread use.

Amethystic agents

The search for a drug to reverse alcohol intoxication dates back to the time of Greek mythology. However, no effective and safe alcohol antagonist has been found to date.

Project MATCH and the 'real world' of treatment

Project MATCH, a multi-site study carried out in nine centres in the United States involved a total of 1726 individuals with a diagnosis of alcohol dependence/abuse who were randomly assigned to one of three distinct, individually delivered treatments: (1) a TSF therapy designed to enable engagement in Alcoholics Anonymous (12 sessions); (2) CBT designed to teach coping skills to prevent relapse to drinking (12 sessions); and (3) MET designed to increase motivation for and commitment to change (four sessions) (Project MATCH Research Group, 1997a, 1997b, 1998a, 1998b). There was no control group and treatment was for 12 weeks. Clients were followed up over a 1-year period and a proportion at 3 years after completion of treatment. Two groups were recruited to the study, an aftercare group and an out-patient group. The more severely dependent aftercare sample ($n = 774$; 80% male) was recruited immediately following a period of in-patient or intensive day-hospital treatment. The out-patient sample ($n = 952$; 72% male) had not received any prior treatment.

Inclusion criteria were stringent. Essentially, subjects were alcohol dependent and had no other drug-use disorder. The average ages in the sample were 41.9 years for the aftercare sample and 38.9 years for the out-patient sample. About one-third were married; half were in employment and just over three-quarters were white. Compliance with treatment was excellent, with clients attending over two-thirds of scheduled treatment sessions.

The study set out to assess the benefits of matching clients to the three treatment modalities on a number of client characteristics, hence the acronym MATCH (Matching Alcoholism Treatments to Client Heterogeneity). It was hypothesized that certain clients would do better if matched to specific treatments.

At 1-year follow-up, 35% of the aftercare clients had remained completely abstinent, compared with 20% of the out-patient sample. It was thought that the period of abstinence during in-patient treatment may have conferred a beneficial effect on the aftercare group. However, many other factors were thought to be involved, precluding the conclusion that aftercare was superior to out-patient treatment. There were no real differences in the efficacy of CBT, MET and TSF during the year following treatment. The TSF-treated out-patients did better at 1-year and 3-year follow-up than the other two groups (Project MATCH Research Group, 1998a). Analysis of the treatment effect in the out-patient group over time showed that the

MET group initially did less well in terms of abstinence than the other two groups, but had 'caught up' by the time of the 3-year follow-up.

Therapist effects on drinking outcome were minimal (Project MATCH Research Group, 1998c), probably reflecting the fact that the therapists were carefully selected and trained, used manual-guided treatment and were closely supervised (Carroll, 2001). The study design therefore reduced variability among therapists and excluded the possibility of examining their impact on treatment.

Project MATCH was a huge, methodologically rigorous and highly technical study. The conclusions were complex and it is possible that some important messages are still buried in the sheer complexity and detail of the data. The sample was highly selected and not very heterogeneous. The drinking outcome measures were perhaps too simple, given the overall complexity of the study. The extensive research assessments may well have conferred some therapeutic benefit on the clients, thus reducing possible differences among the treatment modalities. The three treatments were all delivered in a similar way, again reducing variability. It could be argued that the use of manuals does not reflect a 'real-world' setting. If anything, the commonalities across the treatments modalities were highlighted. TSF was slightly unusual in that it was delivered by therapists in individual sessions. It must be remembered that TSF is not Alcoholics Anonymous and it is not the same as the treatment delivered in Twelve Step programmes.

It might be argued that the four-session MET was more 'value for money' than the other treatments. Closer scrutiny of the data on treatment intensity suggests that the TSF and CBT groups did not get three times as much treatment as the MET clients, particularly when these sessions were combined with the extensive assessment and research contacts. The average number of sessions for aftercare and out-patient clients for the three treatments was as follows: MET – an average of 3.1 and 3.3 sessions respectively; CBT – an average of 8.0 and 8.3 sessions respectively; and TSF – an average of 7.3 and 7.5 sessions respectively.

Project MATCH has been complemented by a naturalistic long-term treatment outcome study, carried out at 15 substance misuse programmes attached to Veterans Affairs (VA) hospitals in the USA (Ouimette et al., 1997). This study was carried out in a 'real-world' setting in the sense that it was an evaluation of treatment programmes already running at these centres. The effectiveness of Twelve Step, Cognitive Behavioural (CB) and an eclectic mix of both treatments was compared in a treatment sample of 3698 male clients who had been in residential substance abuse programmes for an average of 25 days.

Overall, subjects showed substantial declines in substance use at 1-year follow-up, with clients treated in Twelve Step programmes doing better (more likely to be abstinent) than those in CB or eclectic programmes (Moos et al., 1999). The

Twelve Step group was also more likely to be free of substance abuse problems and employed at 1-year follow-up. This 'real-world' study also failed to find consistent patient–treatment matching effects for Twelve Step and CB treatments.

The efficacy of treatments for alcohol use disorders

In an influential review, Miller and Hester (1986) highlighted the fact that the effectiveness of treatment methods being widely used in alcohol treatment programmes, particularly in the USA, was not supported by controlled research. In fact, treatment methods with proven efficacy were not, at that time, commonly used in treatment settings.

Over recent years, the number of treatment outcome studies in the alcohol literature has burgeoned and many attempts have been made to rate the efficacy of these treatments. Miller and colleagues have attempted to review and rate controlled outcome studies according to rigorous predefined criteria, thus facilitating a rank ordering of treatment efficacy (Miller et al., 1998; Miller and Wilbourne, 2002). The psychosocial treatments with the strongest evidence for efficacy were brief interventions, social skills training, the community reinforcement approach, behaviour contracting, BMT and care management. The opiate antagonists (naltrexone and nalmefene) and acamprosate also performed well (see Box 19.2).

BOX 19.2 The top-ten list of treatment methods supported by controlled trials

1. Brief intervention
2. Motivational enhancement
3. GABA agonist acamprosate
4. Opiate antagonist (naltrexone, nalmefene)
5. Social skills training
6. Community reinforcement
7. Behaviour contracting
8. Behavioural marital therapy
9. Case management
10. Self-monitoring

From Miller and Wilbourne (2002).

Essentially, behaviour techniques that build on the inner resources of the individual and their social support system and that facilitate motivation for change and self-efficacy appear to be effective. Here, or elsewhere, the qualities of empathy, non-possessive warmth and genuineness on the part of the therapist are likely to facilitate improvement (Rogers, 1957).

Treatments at the bottom of the table include educational methods, confrontational and general counselling, psychotherapy, relaxation training and standard treatment 'as usual'. All too often, these are the only treatments available in alcohol treatment programmes. Clinical services need to incorporate evidence-based treatment methods into their repertoire. This is a challenge, because the 'real world' of the community, out-patient or in-patient setting can be chaotic, fraught with day-to-day crises, staff shortages and poor morale. Delivery systems also need to be considered and patients offered more choice in terms of actual treatment, rapid treatment entry and 'meeting them where they are' (Humphreys and Tucker, 2002). Individuals with severe chronic alcohol dependence should have the option to be followed up for lengthy periods, in much the same way that diabetics are followed up in specialized clinics, i.e. treatment needs to be more 'extensive' (Humphreys and Tucker, 2002). Many alcohol dependent individuals live sad, isolated lives, with little in the way of positive features in their social environment. In these situations, the therapeutic intervention must become a positive, enduring feature of their environment. The therapist becomes someone they can rely upon and trust to act as an advocate with the rent arrears, to facilitate referral to a physician, someone to whom they can show their holiday photographs, share their grief about the death of a parent, sister, spouse. The therapist may be the only person who remembers their birthday, supports them when they get into trouble with the police (again), or takes the time to ensure that they are admitted to hospital when they are suicidal.

'Extensive' interventions can take the form of long-term out-patient treatment, peer-managed residential accommodation and extended care monitoring. These interventions can be combined with pharmacotherapy and other psychosocial treatments. Voluntary and self-help organizations are other 'extensive' resources, many of which engage with individuals indefinitely. A real culture shift, therefore, must take place within services, so that they are more appealing to users. Equally, patients should not be discharged just because they fail to attend three consecutive appointments, particularly if the therapist has failed to find out what has been happening to them. Effective treatments for alcohol dependence are only effective in the context of the individual strengths and social environment of the patient. Clinicians and therapists lose sight of this at their peril.

The present position

In this chapter we have attempted to outline the main special approaches available today in the treatment of drinking problems. We hope that this discussion will stimulate the reader to explore these treatments further and in actuality. The fundamental position taken in this chapter is that choosing the best treatment for the individual patient is a skilled and highly responsible undertaking which needs to be negotiated and later reviewed with the patient, guided by clinical experience, and illuminated by a critical understanding of what an evolving research base can tell.

REFERENCES

Angelone, S.M., Bellini, L., Di Bella, D. and Catalano, M. (1998) Effects of fluvoxamine and citalopram in maintaining abstinence in a sample of Italian detoxified alcoholics. *Alcohol and Alcoholism* 33, 151–6.

Annis, H.M., Herie, M.A. and Watkin-Merek, L. (1996) *Structured Relapse Prevention: an Outpatient Counselling Approach*. Toronto: Addiction Research Foundation of Ontario.

Anton, R.F., Moak, D.H., Waid, R., Latham, P.K., Malcolm, R.J. and Dias, J.K. (1999) Naltrexone and cognitive behavioral therapy for the treatment of out-patient alcoholics: results of a placebo-controlled trial. *American Journal of Psychiatry* 156, 1758–64.

Azrin, N.H. (1976) Improvements in the community-reinforcement approach to alcoholism. *Behaviour Research and Therapy* 14, 339–48.

Azrin, N.H., Sisson, R.W., Meyers, R. and Godley, M. (1982) Alcoholism treatment by disulfiram and community reinforcement therapy. *Journal of Behaviour Therapy and Experimental Psychiatry* 13, 105–12.

Babor, T., Dolinsky, Z., Meyer, R., Hesselbrock, M., Hoffman, M. and Tennen, H. (1992). Types of alcoholics: concurrent and predictive validity of some common classification schemes. *British Journal of Addiction* 87, 1415–31.

Beck, A.T., Wright, F.D., Newman, C.F. and Liese, B.S. (1993) *Cognitive Therapy of Substance Abuse*. New York: Guilford Press.

Berton, F., Francesconi, W.G., Madamba, S.G., Zieglgänsaerger, W. and Siggins, G.R. (1998) Acamprosate enhances N-methyl-D-aspartate receptor-medicated neurotransmission but inhibits presynaptic GABA$_B$ receptors in nucleus accumbens neurons. *Alcoholism: Clinical and Experimental Research* 22, 183–91.

Besson, J., Aeby, F., Kasas, A., Lehert, P. and Potgieter, A. (1998) Combined efficacy of acamprosate and disulfiram in the treatment of alcoholism: a controlled study. *Alcoholism: Clinical and Experimental Research* 22, 573–9.

Bien, T.H., Miller, W.R. and Tonigan, J.S. (1993) Brief interventions for alcohol problems: a review. *Addiction* 88, 315–36.

Bowers, T.G. and Al-Rehda, M.R. (1990) A comparison of outcome with group/martial and standard/individual therapies with alcoholics. *Journal of Studies on Alcohol* 151, 301–9.

Carroll, K.M. (2001) Constrained, confronted and confused: why we really know so little about therapists in treatment outcome research. *Addiction* 96, 203–6.

Chick, J., Anton, R., Checinski, K. et al. (2000a) A multicentre, randomised, double-blind, placebo controlled trial of naltrexone in the treatment of alcohol dependence or misuse. *Alcohol and Alcoholism* 35, 587–93.

Chick, J., Gough, K., Falkowski, W. et al. (1992) Disulfiram treatment of alcoholism. *British Journal of Psychiatry* 161, 84–9.

Chick, J., Howlett, H., Morgan, M.Y. and Ribon, B. (2000b) United Kingdom multicentre acamprosate study (UKMAS): a 6-month prospective study of acamprosate versus placebo in preventing relapse after withdrawal from alcohol. *Alcohol and Alcoholism* 35, 176–87.

Cornelius, J.R., Salloum, I.H., Ehler, J.G. et al. (1997) Fluoxetine in depressed alcoholics: a double-blind, placebo-controlled trial. *Archives of General Psychiatry* 54, 700–5.

Croop, R.S., Faulkner, E.B. and Labriola, D.F., for the Naltrexone Usage Study Group (1997) The safety profile of naltrexone in the treatment of alcoholism. *Archives of General Psychiatry* 54, 1130–5.

Davidson, D., Palfai, T., Bird, C. and Swift, R. (1999) Effects of naltrexone on alcohol self-administration in heavy drinkers. *Alcoholism: Clinical and Experimental Research* 23, 195–203.

Davidson, R. (1992) Prochaska and DiClemente's model of change: a case study? *British Journal of Addiction* 87, 821–2.

Davidson, R. (1998) The transtheoretical model: a critical overview. In *Treating Addictive Behaviours*, 2nd edn, ed. Miller, W.R. and Heather, N. New York: Plenum Press, 25–38.

Davison, S. (1996) Psychotherapy: why do some need more and some need less? In *Psychotherapy, Psychological Treatments and the Addictions*, ed. Edwards, G. and Dare, C. Cambridge: Cambridge University Press, 77–93.

DiClemente, C.C. and Prochaska, J.O. (1998) Towards a comprehensive, transtheoretical model of change. In *Treating Addictive Behaviours*, 2nd edn, ed. Miller, W.R. and Heather, N. New York: Plenum Press, 3–24.

Dorus, W., Ostrow, D.G., Anton, R. et al. (1989) Lithium treatment of depressed and non-depressed alcoholics. *Journal of the American Medical Association* 262, 1646–52.

Drummond, D.C. and Glautier, S. (1994) A controlled trial of cue exposure treatment in alcohol dependence. *Journal of Consulting and Clinical Psychology* 62, 802–17.

Drummond, D.C., Tiffany, S.T., Glautier, S. and Remington, B. (1995). *Addictive Behaviour: Cue Exposure, Theory and Practice.* Chichester: John Wiley and Sons.

Elkins, R.L. (1980) Covert sensitization and alcoholism: contributions of successful conditioning to subsequent abstinence maintenance. *Addictive Behaviours* 5, 67–89.

Falkowski, W. (1996) Group therapy and the addictions. In *Psychotherapy, Psychological Treatments and the Addictions*, ed. Edwards, G. and Dare, C. Cambridge: Cambridge University Press, 206–19.

Fuller, R.K., Branchey, L., Brightwell, D.R. et al. (1986) Disulfiram treatment of alcoholism: a Veterans Administration co-operative study. *Journal of the American Medical Association* 256, 1449–55.

Garbutt, J.C., West, S.L., Carey, T.S., Lohr, K.N. and Crew, F.T. (1999). Pharmacological treatment of alcohol dependence. *Journal of the American Medical Association* 281, 1318–25.

George, D.T., Rawlings, R., Eckardt, M.J., Phillips, M.J., Shoaf, S.E. and Linnoila, M. (1999) Buspirone treatment of alcoholism: age of onset, and cerebrospinal fluid 5-hydroxyindolacetic acid and homovanillic acid concentrations, but not medication treatment, predict return to drinking. *Alcoholism: Clinical and Experimental Research* 23, 272–8.

Halford, W.K., Price, J., Kelly, A.B., Bouma, R. and Young, R. McD. (2001) Helping the female partners of men abusing alcohol: a comparison of three treatments. *Addiction* 96, 1497–508.

Heather, N. (1993) Disulfiram treatment for alcohol problems: is it effective and, if so, why? In *Treatment Options in Addiction. Medical Management of Alcohol and Opiate Abuse*, ed. Brewer, C. London: Gaskell, 1–18.

Heather, N. (1995) *Treatment Approaches to Alcohol Problems*. Copenhagen: World Health Organization Regional Publications European Issues No. 65.

Holder, H., Longabaugh, Miller, W.R. and Rubonis, A.V. (1991) The cost effectiveness of treatment for alcoholism: a first approximation. *Journal of Studies on Alcohol* 52, 517–40.

Hughes, J.L. and Cook, C.C.H. (1997) The efficacy of disulfiram: a review of outcome studies. *Addiction* 92, 381–96.

Humphreys, K. and Tucker, J.A. (2002) Towards more responsive and effective intervention systems for alcohol-related problems. *Addiction* 97, 126–32.

Hunt, G.M. and Azrin, N.H. (1973) A community-reinforcement approach to alcoholism. *Behaviour Research and Therapy* 11, 91–104.

Institute of Medicine (1990) *Broadening the Base of Treatment for Alcohol Problems*. Washington, DC: National Academy Press.

Johnson, B.A., Roache, J.D., Javors, M.A. et al. (2000) Ondansetron for reduction of drinking among biologically predisposed alcoholic patients. A randomized controlled trial. *Journal of the American Medical Association* 284, 963–71.

Kranzler, H.R., Burleson, J.A., Del Boca, F.K. et al. (1994) Buspirone treatment of anxious alcoholics. *Archives of General Psychiatry* 51, 720–31.

Kranzler, H.R. (2000) Pharmacotherapy of alcoholism: gaps in knowledge and opportunity of research. *Alcohol and Alcoholism* 35, 537–47.

Kranzler, H.R., Burleson, J.A., Korner, P. et al. (1995) A placebo-controlled trial of fluoxetine as an adjunct to relapse prevention in alcoholics. *American Journal of Psychiatry* 152, 391–7.

Kranzler, H.R., Burleson, J.A., Brown, J. and Babor, T.F. (1996) Fluoxetine treatment seems to reduce the beneficial effects of cognitive–behavioural therapy in Type B alcoholics. *Alcoholism: Clinical and Experimental Research* 20, 1534–41.

Krystal, J.H., Cramer, J.A., Krol, W.F., Kirk, G.F. and Rosenheck, R.A. (2001) Naltrexone in the treatment of alcohol dependence. *New England Journal of Medicine* 345, 1734–9.

Littleton, J. (1995) Acamprosate in alcohol dependence: how does it work? *Addiction* 90, 1179–88.

McGrath, P.J., Nunes, E.V., Stewart, J.W. et al. (1996) Imipramine treatment of alcoholics with primary depression: a placebo-controlled clinical trial. *Archives of General Psychiatry* 53, 232–40.

Malec, T.S., Malec, E.A. and Dongier, M. (1996) Efficacy of buspirone in alcohol dependence: a review. *Alcoholism: Clinical and Experimental Research* 20, 853–8.

Marlatt, G.A. (1990) Cue exposure and relapse prevention in the treatment of addictive behaviours. *Addictive Behaviours* 15, 395–9.

Marlatt, G.A. and Gordon, J.R. (1985) *Relapse Prevention*. New York: Guilford Press.

Mason, B.J., Ritvo, E.C., Morgan, R.O. et al. (1994) A double-blind, placebo-controlled pilot study to evaluate the efficacy and safety of oral nalmefene HCl for alcohol dependence. *Alcoholism: Clinical and Experimental Research* 18, 1162–7.

Mason, B.J., Kocsis, J.H., Ritvo, E.C. and Cutler, R.B. (1996) A double-blind placebo-controlled trial of desipramine for primary alcohol dependence stratified on the presence or absence of major depression. *Journal of the American Medical Association* 275, 761–7.

Mason, B.J., Salvato, F.R., Williams, L.D., Ritvo, E.C. and Cutler, R.B. (1999) A double-blind placebo-controlled study of oral nalmefene for alcohol dependence. *Archives of General Psychiatry* 56, 719–24.

Meyers, R.J. and Miller, W.R. (2001) *A Community Reinforcement Approach to Addiction Treatment.* International Research Monographs in the Addictions. Cambridge: Cambridge University Press.

Miller, W.R., Andrews, N.R., Wilbourne, P. and Bennett, M.E. (1998) A wealth of alternatives: effective treatments for alcohol problems. In *Treating Addictive Behaviors*, 2nd edn, ed. Miller, W.R. and Heather, N. New York: Plenum Press, 203–16.

Miller, W.R., Brown, J.M., Simpson, T.L. et al. (1995) What works? A methodological analysis of the alcohol treatment outcome literature. In *Handbook of Alcoholism Treatment Approaches: Effective Alternatives*, 2nd edn, ed. Hester, R.K. and Miller, W.R. Needham Heights, MA: Allyn and Bacon, 12–44.

Miller, W.R. and Hester, R.K. (1986) The effectiveness of alcoholism treatment: what research reveals. In *Treating Addictive Behaviors: Processes of Change*, ed. Miller, W.R. and Heather, N. New York: Plenum Press, 121–74.

Miller, W.R. and Rollnick, S. (1991) *Motivational Interviewing: Preparing People to Change Addictive Behavior.* New York: Guilford Press.

Miller, W.R. and Sanchez, V.C. (1993) Motivating young adults for treatment and lifestyle change. In *Issues in Alcohol Use and Misuse by Young Adults*, ed. Howard, G.S. and Nathan, P.E. pp 55–81. Notre Dame: University of Notre Dame Press, 55–81.

Miller, W.R. and Rollnick, S. (2002) *Motivational Interviewing: Preparing People to Change Addictive Behaviour*, 2nd edn. New York: Guilford Press.

Miller, W.R., Walters, S.T. and Bennett, M.E. (2001) How effective is alcoholism treatment in the United States. *Journal of Studies on Alcohol* 62, 211–20.

Miller, W.R. and Wilbourne, P.L. (2002) Mesa Grande: a methodological analysis of clinical trials of treatments for alcohol use disorders. *Addiction* 97, 265–77.

Moncrieff, J. and Drummond, D.C. (1997) New drug treatments for alcohol problems: a critical appraisal. *Addiction* 92, 939–47.

Monti, P.M., Abrams, D.B., Kadden, R.M. and Cooney, N.L. (1989) *Treating Alcohol Dependence.* New York: Guilford Press.

Monti, P.M., Rohsenow, D.J., Hutchison, K.E. et al. (1999) Naltrexone's effect on cue-elicited craving among alcoholics in treatment. *Alcoholism: Clinical and Experimental Research* 24, 1542–9.

Moos, R.H., Finney, J.W., Ouimette, P.G. and Suchinsky, R.T. (1999). A comparative evaluation of substance abuse treatment orientation, amount of care, and 1-year outcomes. *Alcoholism: Clinical and Experimental Research* 23, 529–36.

Morris, P.L.P., Hopwood, M., Whelan, G., Gardiner, J. and Drummond, E. (2001) Naltrexone for alcohol dependence: a randomised controlled trial. *Addiction* 96, 1565–73.

Mueller, T.I., Stout, R.L., Rudden, S. et al. (1997) A double-blind placebo-controlled pilot study of carbamazepine in the treatment of alcohol dependence. *Alcoholism: Clinical and Experimental Research* 21, 86–92.

Oei, T.P.S. and Jackson, P.R. (1982) Social skills and cognitive behavioural approaches for the treatment of problem drinking. *Journal of Studies on Alcohol* 43, 532–47.

O'Farrell, T.J., Choquette, K.A., Cutter, H.S.G., Brown, E.D. and McCourt, W.F. (1993). Behavioural marital therapy with and without additional couples relapse prevention sessions for alcoholics and their wives. *Journal of Studies on Alcohol* 54, 652–66.

O'Malley, S., Jaffe, A.J., Chang, G., Schottenfeld, R.S., Meyer, R.E. and Rounsaville, B. (1992) Naltrexone and coping skills therapy for alcohol dependence, a controlled study. *Archives of General Psychiatry* 49, 881–7.

O'Malley, S.S., Jaffe, A.J., Chang, G. et al. (1996) Six-month follow-up of naltrexone and psychotherapy for alcohol dependence. *Archives of General Psychiatry* 53, 217–24.

Ouimette, P.C., Finney, J.W. and Moos, R.H. (1997) Twelve-step and cognitive–behavioural treatment for substance abuse: a comparison of treatment effectiveness. *Journal of Consulting and Clinical Psychology* 65, 230–40.

Paille, F.M., Guelf, J.D., Perkins, A.C., Royer, R.J., Steru, L. and Parot, P. (1995) Double-blind randomised multicentre trial of acamprosate in maintaining abstinence from alcohol. *Alcohol and Alcoholism* 30, 239–47.

Parks, G., Anderson, B.K. and Marlatt, G.A. (2001a) Relapse prevention therapy. In *International Handbook of Alcohol Problems and Dependence*, ed. Heather, N., Peters, T.J. and Stockwell, T. Chichester: John Wiley and Sons, 575–92.

Parks, G.A., Marlatt, G.A. and Anderson, B.K. (2001b) Cognitive behavioural alcohol treatment. In *International Handbook of Alcohol Problems and Dependence*, ed. Heather, N., Peters, T.J. and Stockwell, T. Chichester: John Wiley and Sons, 558–73.

Pelc, I., Verbanck, P., Le Bon, O., Gavrilovic, M., Lion, K. and Lehert, P. (1997) Efficacy and safety of acamprosate in the treatment of detoxified alcohol-dependent patients. *British Journal of Psychiatry* 171, 73–7.

Pettinati, H.M., Volpicelli, J.R., Kranzler, H.R., Luck, G., Rukstalis, M.R. and Cnaan, A. (2000) Sertraline treatment for alcohol dependence: interactive effects of medication and alcoholic subtype. *Alcoholism: Clinical and Experimental Research* 24, 1041–9.

Poldrugo, F. (1997) Acamprosate in a long-term community-based alcohol rehabilitation programme. *Addiction* 92, 1537–46.

Proschaska, J.O. and DiClemente, C.C. (1986) Towards a comprehensive model of change. In *Treating Addictive Behaviours: Processes of Change*, ed. Miller, W.R. and Heather, N. New York: Plenum Press, 3–27.

Prochaska, J.O., DiClemente, C.C. and Norcross, J.C. (1992) In search of how people change: applications to addictive behaviors. *American Psychologist* 7, 1102–14.

Project MATCH Research Group (1997a) Matching alcoholism treatments to client heterogeneity: Project MATCH post-treatment drinking outcomes. *Journal of Studies on Alcohol* 58, 7–29.

Project MATCH Research Group (1997b) Project MATCH secondary a priori hypotheses. *Addiction* 92, 1671–98.

Project MATCH Research Group (1998a) Matching alcoholism treatments to client heterogeneity: treatment main effects and matching effects on drinking during treatment. *Journal of Studies on Alcohol* 59, 631–9.

Project MATCH Research Group (1998b) Matching alcoholism treatments to client heterogeneity: Project MATCH three-year drinking outcomes. *Alcoholism: Clinical and Experimental Research* 22, 1300–11.

Project MATCH Research Group (1998c) Therapist effects in three treatments for alcohol problems. *Psychotherapy Research* 8, 455–74.

Rogers, C.R. (1957) The necessary and sufficient conditions for therapeutic personality change. *Journal of Consulting Psychology* 21, 95–103.

Rohsenow, D.J., Colby, S.M., Monti, P.M. et al. (2000) Predictors of compliance with naltrexone among alcoholics. *Alcoholism: Clinical and Experimental Research* 24, 1542–9.

Sass, H., Soyka, M., Mann, K. and Zieglgänsberger, W. (1996) Relapse prevention by acamprosate: results from a placebo controlled study on alcohol dependence. *Archives of General Psychiatry* 53, 673–80.

Shaw, G.K., Majumdar, S.K., Waller, S., MacGarvie, J. and Dunn, G. (1987) Tiapride in the long-term management of alcoholics of anxious or depressive temperament. *British Journal of Psychiatry* 150, 164–8.

Sutton, S. (1996) Can 'stages of change' provide guidance in the treatment of addictions? A critical examination of Prochaska and DiClemente's model. In *Psychotherapy, Psychological Treatments and the Addictions*, ed. Edwards, G. and Dare, C. Cambridge: Cambridge University Press, 189–205.

Tempesta, E., Janiri, L., Bignamini, A., Chabac, S. and Dotgieter, A. (2000). Acamposate and relapse prevention in the treatment of alcohol dependence: a placebo-controlled study. *Alcohol and Alcoholism* 35, 202–9.

Volpicelli, J.R., Alterman, A.I., Hayashida, M. and O'Brien, C.P. (1992) Naltrexone in the treatment of alcohol dependence. *Archives of General Psychiatry* 49, 876-80.

Volpicelli, J.R., Rhines, K.C., Rhines, J.S., Volpicelli, L.A., Alterman, A.I. and O'Brien, C.P. (1997) Naltrexone and alcohol dependence. *Archives of General Psychiatry* 54, 737–42.

Volpicelli, J.R., Watson, N.T., King, A.C., Sherman, C.E. and O'Brien, C.P. (1995) Effect of naltrexone on alcohol 'high' in alcoholics. *American Journal of Psychiatry* 152, 613–15.

Wanigaratne. S., Wallace, W., Pullin, J., Keaney, F. and Farmer, R. (1990) *Relapse Prevention for Addictive Behaviours. A Manual for Therapists*. Oxford: Blackwell Scientific Publications.

Weingardt, K.R. and Marlatt, G.A. (1998) Sustaining change: helping those who are still using. In *Treating Addictive Behaviours*, 2nd edn, ed. Miller, W.R. and Heather, N. New York: Plenum Press, 337–51.

Whitworth, A.B., Fischer, F., Lesch, O.M. et al. (1996) Comparison of acamprosate and placebo in long-term treatment of alcohol dependence. *Lancet* 347, 1438–42.

20

Working towards normal drinking

It is sensible to remember the varied nature of the population coming for help with drinking problems. Not everyone who turns for help because of drinking is suffering from alcohol dependence. With greater public understanding, people with earlier and lesser problems are increasingly asking for help and especially in the primary care or general hospital setting. To propose one exclusive goal for everyone, be it normal drinking or abstinence, is therefore not sensible (Heather and Robertson, 1981). We need, as always, to plan treatment in terms of flexible responses to multiple needs. To claim that no-one who has experienced trouble with drinking will ever be able to drink in a trouble-free way is mistaken (Sobell and Sobell, 1973, 1976, 1987). But it is unhelpful to make 'normal drinking' into a slogan or heedlessly to attack the position of Alcoholics Anonymous (AA). The probability of successful long-term, controlled drinking among the kind of patients who usually present to specialized centres is not high (Davies, 1962; Helzer et al., 1985; Edwards, 1985, 1994). A sense of balance is needed when considering these questions (Heather, 1995).

Much that was said in Chapter 17 about abstinence-oriented approaches is equally applicable to the normal drinking goal, for instance the relevance of the patient–therapist relationship, and those general points will not be repeated. The discussion of special techniques in Chapter 19 also bears on present considerations. In this chapter, the phrases 'normal drinking' and 'controlled drinking' are used synonymously.

What is 'normal' drinking?

If a patient or client is to aim for normal drinking, how is 'normality' to be defined in practical and recognizable terms? It is no good leaving the definition vague, for only when a goal is closely specified is goal-setting possible. The matter is made difficult by society's latitude in regard to what constitutes an ordinary way of using alcohol. Getting drunk once a month is to some people the expected way to drink, whereas for others even one episode of mild intoxication would transgress expectations. For goal-setting, normality must be considered in terms of at least two different criteria.

1. *Objectively normal drinking: quantity/frequency dimensions.* In a research report, American physicians defined 'light', 'moderate' and 'heavy' drinking as respectively averaging 1.2, 2.2 and 3.5 drinks a day (Abel et al., 1998). Canadian researchers proposed sex-specific guidelines for goal-setting when working towards 'moderate drinking': they suggested that men should limit themselves to 16 drinks in a week and not more than four drinks on any one day, whereas for women the respective limits should be 12 drinks a week and three on any day. The upper limit which is to be permitted needs to be agreed with the patient. As a simple working rule, we suggest that about 16–20 g of alcohol on any one drinking occasion (say 1 pint of beer, a double of spirits, two glasses of wine) is a reasonable ceiling for anyone, man or woman, who is working towards control of a drinking problem, but may perhaps initially be rather too high. As for frequency, it is wise to agree that drinking should not be reinstated on a fixed daily schedule and there should be breaks and variation, with probably not more than ten drinks taken in a week. Normality in these terms certainly implies avoidance of drunkenness.

2. *Subjectively normal drinking.* Someone who is drinking alcohol normally should be no more apprehensive about this activity than if they were drinking a fruit juice. They should know their usual intake level without having to monitor their drinking behaviour and without a sense of effort. If at a certain point they say: 'Not another, thank you', this should be without the conscious exertion of iron will. They should be able to think about the company and the conversation rather than their thoughts being preoccupied with drinking, the next drink, or not having the next drink. Such easiness in the relationship between drinkers and what they drink is characteristically lacking when moderate or severe alcohol dependence has been established. Patients who have progressed even to mild dependence will, when they have brought their drinking back to objective normality, often at first still experience subjective unease. Subjective normality usually, therefore, takes longer than objective normality to attain, and sometimes considerably longer. 'Normal' drinking in the true and complete sense has not been won until the two elements have come together, and when there has only been an objective change the patient's position remains precarious. This probable two-stage nature of recovery should be discussed with, and understood by, the patient (Edwards et al., 1986; Booth, 1990).

Other dimensions could also be added to provide a more complex definition of normality, for instance limitations on the speed of drinking, or limitations on the circumstances in which alcohol is taken.

Table 20.1 Factors relevant to the choice of a normal drinking goal

Factors unfavourable to a controlled drinking goal	Favourable factors in support of a controlled drinking goal
Severe dependence	Mild or absent signs of dependence
Previous failures at controlled drinking	Recent sustained normal drinking
Strong preference of the drinker for abstinence	Strong preference of the drinker for normal drinking
Commitment to the AA ethic	
Poorly developed capacity for self-control in other areas	Mature and determined person with evidence of strong self-control in other areas of life
Diagnosis of mental illness or drug misuse	No evidence of mental illness or drug misuse
Severe alcohol-related organ damage	Mild or no physical complications of alcohol misuse
Heavy-drinking family or friends	Supportive family and friends
Heavy drinking at work	
Social isolation	
Employment jeopardized by drinking problems at work	Drinking has not affected employment or work performance
Violent when drinking	Not violent when drinking

Who is a candidate for a normal drinking goal?

There are many patients for whom it is inappropriate to attempt such a goal. For those with a history of fully developed alcohol dependence, abstinence is the only feasible objective (Edwards et al., 1983). Equally, there are instances in which no-one could doubt that, for at least a trial period, it is sensible to go along with and support the patient's wish to ameliorate rather than abstain (Sanchez-Craig et al., 1984; Booth et al., 1992). This would often be true of the patient who has been drinking too heavily only recently and intermittently, and who is not manifesting significant dependence symptoms. The following considerations often contribute to the decision-making and are summarized in Table 20.1.

Degree of dependence

The importance of this factor has just been mentioned. In practical terms, if the patient has never experienced withdrawal symptoms of such severity as to demand morning relief drinking, then (other things being equal) normal drinking is an option. If the patient has experienced withdrawal symptoms and drunk intermittently in the morning but only for the last 6 months or less, normal drinking is possible but questionable. If for 6 months or longer the patient has not only experienced withdrawal symptoms but has repeatedly engaged in morning relief drinking, a return to normal drinking is unlikely to be achieved. These guidelines are to be read as ways in which the evidence may be examined, rather than as fixed rules. Some authorities regard a Severity of Alcohol Dependence Questionnaire (SADQ) score of greater than 30 on the 60-point scale as precluding normal drinking, but Heather et al. (2000) have questioned this assumption.

Evidence of recent sustained normal drinking

If within the last couple of years the patient has been able to drink in a relaxed and controlled manner continuously for 2–3 months, this may indicate that they retain a capacity for a normal style of drinking, and that this capacity may now, with due care, be strengthened and extended. The evidence must, however, be approached warily. Careful questioning may reveal that this previous period of 'sustained normal drinking' was less sustained and less normal than the patient at first suggested, and it may have been only a slide towards reinstatement of dependence.

The patient personally wishes to attempt a normal drinking goal

Patients who want to return to normal drinking may be deluding themselves, and it is then the therapist's responsibility to try to help them to accept abstinence rather than conniving in the delusion – the golden rule for the therapist when talking through these patient choices is to be open-minded but not gullible. Some patients will frankly declare that drinking other than for intoxication is for them a purposeless use of alcohol. However, others may be right in believing they can control their drinking, and be strongly committed to attempting that goal.

Personality

The mature and determined person who is good at exercising self-control is more likely to succeed in drinking normally than the person whose capacity for self-control is, in general, not well developed.

Underlying mental illness

The patient who is suffering from any type of mental illness and as a result uses alcohol to relieve unpleasant feelings, is not in a good position to attempt normal drinking. Whatever its nature, the underlying disorder has first to be treated, but there is always the danger that a relapse into the illness will precipitate loss of control over drinking, although equally it may overthrow an intention of complete abstinence. Underlying brain damage or learning disability usually suggests that normal drinking will not be possible, and a concurrent drug dependence which has not been dealt with successfully also rules out a return to the safe use of alcohol.

Pathological gambling may threaten the maintenance of control over drinking. The euphoria of the win, the depression of the loss, or the tension associated with continuous gambling rather easily invites a return to heavy use of alcohol.

Alcohol-related physical illness

The decision in this instance must be made in relation to the actual type and degree of illness, but alcohol-related physical illness usually suggests that the patient would be wise to avoid any further drinking and the risk of progressive tissue damage.

Social and family support

The client who is socially isolated and without a family will probably find it more difficult to drink normally again than the person whose behaviour is being monitored and influenced by close supports. However, a certain type of family network may positively encourage excessive drinking. Occupation has similarly to be taken into account. Someone who has no job, much time on their hands and no structure to their day may find it hard to control their drinking, and jobs which involve exposure to heavy drinking may make it difficult to pursue a controlled drinking goal.

The clinical skill thus lies in knowing how to weigh and integrate these and other factors when assessing the feasibility of a normal drinking goal, and in learning how to feed information to patients so as to help their own decision-making. However, whatever the therapist proposes, it is finally the patient who makes the decision.

An interval of sobriety as first step

For some patients, normal drinking emerges directly out of more chaotic drinking. Suddenly or gradually, the new pattern supersedes the old. To begin with there may be occasions when drinking is at a social level with frequent occasions where limits are broken, but after a few months the 'bad occasions' are averted. Alternatively, the story may be of a shorter or longer initial period of abstinence, followed by a tentative move towards moderate drinking. That move may have been planned at the outset as a step which would be taken after a certain interval of sobriety, or the patient may start to drink again while feeling anxious about breaking the rules. When drinking follows a period of sobriety, the therapist has the responsibility of working out with the patient whether this is a sadly familiar story of unguardedness and self-deception foreshadowing major relapse, or whether it is indeed the evolution of re-established control.

Whether the patient who is aiming at controlled drinking does best to do so directly or by the pathway of initial abstinence, is not an easy question to answer. Different strategies suit different people. However, if the drinking is chaotic and surrounded with problems, in general patients are likely to do better if they start out afresh from an abstinent base.

Techniques for establishing and maintaining control

Patients are themselves often very inventive in designing ways to keep their drinking within a limit, and it is always useful therefore to explore and encourage these personal strategies. The paragraphs below describe a variety of methods which may be employed (Marlatt and Gordon, 1985; Heather et al., 1987; Alden, 1988; Connors, 1993; Saunders, 1994).

Full initial discussion with the patient

The first step in setting a treatment programme for the individual patient who is aiming at controlled drinking must be to clarify what is being expected of treatment and the precise goal which is to be achieved, the methods of working and the mutual level of commitment.

Limiting the type of beverage

Shifting from one type of alcoholic drink to another is often dismissed as the typical strategy of the drinker who refuses to face up to the fact that their problem lies not in the specific drink but in their relationship with any sort of alcohol – the whisky drinker who believes that 'beer will be safe' is classically warned that alcohol is simply alcohol, whatever the label on the bottle. The therapist has to distinguish between self-delusion and sound strategy, but the patient who is going to effect a successful return to normal drinking may often spontaneously discover that a change of beverage is helpful. They choose what they may term a 'social drink' – beer instead of wine, perhaps, or wine instead of beer, but in any case a beverage free of old associations.

Limiting the quantity and frequency of intake

The importance of strictly defining with each patient what is to count as 'normal' has already been mentioned. If the patient is making their definition in terms of 'a single of...', or 'a glass of...', or other such familiar but often rather vague measures (a 'single' is a very uncertain quantity of alcohol if the patient is pouring their own drink), then properly objective measures have to be agreed.

Speed of drinking

A patient may learn to pace their drinking. This may be in terms of either not drinking faster than a slow-drinking companion or pacing against the clock.

Motivations for drinking

The patient may discover that it is unwise for them to drink in response to mood, for instance when they are angry, depressed or bored. They do better to drink only when they do not 'need' a drink.

Circumstances and company

Drinking is at first often best limited to situations in which that individual's previous experience has shown that control is more likely to be maintained, while drinking situations which can be identified as leading to loss of control are best avoided. For instance, the patient may decide that they will drink with their spouse on Tuesdays in the pub at the corner, but will 'avoid the Saturday night crowd'. They will never drink at work during the day, and will not drink when they are on business trips away from home. When guests come to dinner, control will mean no drink before dinner or after dinner, but only with the meal (and within explicit limits).

Identifying 'competing activities'

The client may usefully identify activities which can immediately be engaged in to prevent the risk of uncontrolled drinking. For instance, if a housewife knows that she is likely to start drinking in an uncontrolled fashion when she is alone in the middle of the afternoon, then she has to find and plan activities which can divert her from drinking at this time of the day. She may decide on a simple strategy such as doing some shopping in the afternoon or calling on a friend. If the dangerous circumstances which particularly invite uncontrolled drinking can thus be neutralized by competing activity, practice in normal drinking can then be restricted to occasions when the chances of success are more real.

Individual behavioural analysis

The headings above provide ideas about the kinds of strategies which might be suggested for any patient. Essentially, what is being learnt is self-control. It may in addition be useful to carry out an individual and more detailed behavioural analysis of the patient's drinking. The aim is to identify the circumstances in which a particular patient tends to drink excessively, using recent instances and the experiences which evolve during treatment. General statements such as 'I drink when I am bored' are not to be discounted, but are usually of far less value to the planning of treatment than minute analysis of the immediate antecedents and circumstances of, say, last Friday's drinking binge. The analysis identifies the *cues* which are related to excessive drinking, both in internal (mood) and external (event and situation) terms. It is necessary to form an idea of how such cues interact rather than seeing them only in isolation, and to understand the sort of *pathway* that the individual is apt to move along when indulging in excessive drinking. Such material is then used in planning the package of strategies which go to make up the individual drinking programme.

Formal cognitive–behavioural treatment protocols

Heather et al. (2000) have compared the efficacy of moderation-oriented cue exposure and behavioural self-control training and their report gives details of these approaches (there were no outcome differences). Marlatt et al. (1998) employed a focused, brief motivational approach with high-risk student drinkers, with some benefit. Substantial attention to the design of protocols has been given by Sanchez-Craig and her colleagues (e.g. Sanchez-Craig et al., 1984).

How testing should the programme be?

The patient must identify risky situations (Marlatt and Gordon, 1985; and see Chapter 19), although it may then be difficult for them to avoid many of these. They may, for instance, have to go away on business trips knowing that a lonely weekend in a hotel is particularly likely to invite heavy solitary drinking. However, not only may exposure to such a risky situation be unavoidable, but, for real effectiveness of treatment, such exposure to temptation may be highly desirable. The patient should not make impossible demands on their own strength and determination, but the essence of therapy is that they should experience some sense of struggle, of temptation, and perhaps of craving to drink excessively, *and that temptation and craving should then be successfully resisted.* It is the repeated exposure to the relevant cues and the repeated resistance to an excessive drinking response which will in the end extinguish the potency of those cues. Without experience of craving, there can be no long-term extinction of craving. In terms of a familiar analogy, a child who is afraid of dogs is unlikely to overcome that fear simply by avoiding all dogs. Such a normal fear is dealt with in terms of ordinary family wisdom by introducing a dog to the child, and then by praise and close support persuading the child on this occasion not to run away. The objective behaviour towards dogs changes and then, more slowly, the anxiety experienced at the approach of a dog begins to fade out.

In similar fashion, the patient who only avoids risk will probably only achieve an objective recovery. Their drinking will be objectively within acceptable social limits, but it will still be associated with subjective unease. Subjective recovery comes about when there has been repeated exposure to cues, and repeated resistance to an excessive drinking response. Yet treatment will suffer a reverse if on too many occasions the patient does, in fact, drink excessively; the potency of the risky cue is confirmed rather than extinguished.

Involving the spouse

The spouse has an important part to play in supporting the patient's work on their problem. They are often accepted as a direct and useful restraining influence, and as the person within whose company normal drinking may most safely be attempted. If, however, their help is effectively to be enlisted, their views should be taken into account. Therapy will be handicapped if the spouse's reservations about their partner's normal drinking goal have not been discussed.

Seeing it through

The patient who is aiming at normal drinking is likely to need close support over some months. Treatment which aims at a return to normal drinking is far from being a cheap option in terms of service costs and, if such a treatment is to be given, its place within the range of what is offered by a treatment service, it cannot be on a casual, unplanned and understaffed basis which fails to provide the proper follow-through of support and which risks irresponsibility.

Monitoring of progress must firstly involve the patient's own regular objective and subjective report at follow-up treatment sessions, and these sessions should probably be at not less than 2-weekly intervals. Verbal reports may usefully be supplemented by asking the patient to keep a drinking diary, and thus to engage in self-monitoring. Feedback of repeat laboratory test results may be helpful, with, it is to be hoped, gamma glutamyl transferase (GGT) and mean corpuscular volume (MCV) moving towards normal (Chapter 14). Spouses should also be seen regularly, both so that they can share in the discussion and planning of treatment and for their contribution to monitoring.

One of two alternative decisions will then at some point have to be made in the light of progress and monitoring.

Termination of successful treatment

A successful outcome may be assumed when, over about 12 months, the patient has achieved both objective and subjective normality in their drinking. Judgement of 'success' is, as ever, provisional, but at some point treatment and frequency of visits should be reduced. The patient may be left with an open invitation to return if they encounter further difficulties, or it may be wise to offer widely spaced (say 6-monthly) follow-up appointments and 'booster' discussions over the next year or two.

Termination of unsuccessful treatment

The patient who is failing to make progress should not immediately and without review be told to abandon the normal drinking goal. Lack of progress is to be taken in the first instance as a matter for careful analysis of the causes of the difficulty, and on that basis some planned shift in the strategy may be possible. But if the patient still fails in any way to progress, there comes a moment when there is no profit in encouraging them in a frustrating and perhaps damaging pursuit of normal drinking. They may now be persuaded by experience that it is better to opt instead for an abstinence goal, either as the short-term or longer-term solution.

Self-help groups which aim to support return to normal drinking

AA is usually not appropriate for the drinker who wants to moderate rather than stop drinking. The emphasis there is of an out-and-out commitment to not drinking. In the USA, a number of self-help groups have come into existence which specifically aim to support the normal drinking goal. These include Rational Recovery (Galanter et al., 1993; Trimpey 1996), Secular Organizations for Sobriety (Connors and Dermen, 1996) and Moderation Management (Kishline, 1999). The expansion of the self-help movement in this kind of direction may be helpful for some people and is unlikely to cut across the AA message, which is largely directed at a different and more extreme segment of the troubled drinking population.

Limits on goal choice which may be set by institutional ways of working

Some institutions such as Twelve Step facilities will restrict their work to helping patients towards abstinence, whereas other types of facility may take controlled drinking as their universal first choice (Donovan and Heather, 1997). Organizational cohesion may be vested in a rigid commitment to one or other narrow choice. The interests of the wide and varied range of people who experience drinking problems may in part be well served by narrow-range institutions with high levels of confidence in what they are doing, and people can often make their own choice as to which type of facility they attend. Within this market dangers do, however, also exist of patients becoming engaged in a narrow approach which is not optimal for them. The situation may be helped by more informed advice from referral agencies, by greater diversity of treatment facilities within a locality, and generally by an enhanced degree of open-mindedness.

A final word of caution

The decision to advise a patient to aim for total abstinence may sometimes result in that person alternating sobriety with explosive and damaging relapses, rather than learning how to control their drinking or attenuate relapse. Choice of the abstinence goal does not by itself guarantee anyone's safety. Treatment of every new case is an experiment which requires the patient's informed consent and professional and ethical decisions on the therapist's behalf, and that is so whatever the drinking goal.

That having been said, there are special problems which can attach to work towards normal drinking. What is to be done if, in the therapist's experienced judgement, normal drinking is for a particular patient likely to lead only to further postponement of the necessary decision to stop drinking? Depending on the circumstances, two different types of response can be envisaged.

1. *Supporting a normal drinking goal on an experimental basis and in the short term.* If there are no pressing dangers, it may be acceptable to work with the patient and let them determine whether normal drinking is attainable. In the process and one way or another, something useful will have been learnt.

2. *Stating firmly that abstinence is, for carefully explained reasons, probably the only feasible goal.* One is dealing here with probabilities rather than certainties, but the therapist may feel that, for this patient and on strong balance of probabilities, normal drinking is likely to be unattainable and dangerous in its pursuit. That then should be said. In the long term, it may be better for a patient, at least temporarily, to break contact, but take with them an unambiguous, honest and accurate message, rather than the therapist being drawn into a course of action which they see as against the patient's best interests. It may be the moment for challenge rather than connivance.

Twenty years ago, discussion of how treatment can assist a return to normal drinking might have been seen as heterodox. Today, with the growing awareness of the need to provide help for people whose drinking problems are of many different degrees and kinds, a discriminating ability to work with some patients or clients towards a normal drinking goal is a necessary therapeutic skill.

REFERENCES

Abel, E.L., Kruger, M.L. and Friedl, J. (1998) How do physicians define 'light', 'moderate' and 'heavy' drinking? *Alcoholism: Clinical and Experimental Research* 22, 979–84.

Alden, L. (1988) Behavioral self-management: controlled drinking strategies in a context of secondary prevention. *Journal of Consulting and Clinical Psychology* 56, 280–6.

Booth, P.G. (1990) Maintained controlled drinking following severe alcohol dependence – a case study. *British Journal of Addiction* 85, 315–22.

Booth, P.G., Dale, B., Slade, P.D. and Dewey M.E. (1992) A follow-up study of problem drinkers offered a goal choice option. *Journal of Studies on Alcohol* 53, 594–600.

Connors, G.J. (1993) Drinking moderation training as a contemporary therapeutic approach. In *Innovations in Alcoholism Treatment: State of the Art Reviews and their Implications for Clinical Practice*, ed. Connors, G.J. New York: Haworth Press, 117–34.

Connors, G.J. and Dermen, K.H. (1996) Characteristics of participants in Secular Organizations for Sobriety (SOS). *American Journal of Drug and Alcohol Abuse* 22, 281–95.

Davies, D.L. (1962) Normal drinking by recovered alcohol addicts. *Quarterly Journal of Studies on Alcohol* 23, 194–204.

Donovan, M. and Heather, N. (1997) Acceptability of the controlled-drinking goal among alcohol treatment agencies in New South Wales, Australia. *Journal of Studies on Alcohol* 58, 253–6.

Edwards, G. (1985) A later follow-up of a classic case series: D.L. Davies's 1962 report and its significance for the present. *Journal of Studies on Alcohol* 46, 181–90.

Edwards, G. (1994) D.L. Davies and 'Normal drinking in recovered alcohol addicts': the genesis of a paper. *Drug and Alcohol Dependence* 35, 249–59.

Edwards, G., Brown, D., Duckitt, A., Oppenheimer, E., Sheehan, M. and Taylor, C. (1986) Normal drinking in a recovering alcohol addict. *British Journal of Addiction* 81, 127–37.

Edwards, G., Duckett, A., Oppenheimer, E., Sheehan, M. and Taylor, C. (1983) What happens to alcoholics? *Lancet* ii, 269–71.

Galanter, M., Egelkos, S. and Edwards, H. (1993) Rational recovery: alternatives to AA for addiction? *American Journal of Alcohol and Drug Abuse* 19, 499–510.

Heather, N. (1995) The great controlled drinking consensus: is it premature? *Addiction* 90, 1160–2.

Heather, N., Brodie, J., Wale, S. et al. (2000) A randomized controlled trial of moderation-oriented cue exposure. *Journal of Studies on Alcohol* 61, 561–70.

Heather, N. and Robertson, I. (1981) *Controlled Drinking*. London: Methuen.

Heather, N., Robertson, I., Macpherson, B., Allsop, S. and Fulton, A. (1987) Effectiveness of a controlled drinking self-help manual: one year follow-up results. *British Journal of Clinical Psychology* 26, 279–87.

Helzer, J.E., Robins, L.N., Taylor, J.R. et al. (1985) The extent of long-term moderate drinking among alcoholics discharged from medical and psychiatric facilities. *New England Journal of Medicine* 312, 1678–82.

Kishline, A. (1999) *Moderate Drinking: the Moderation Management Guide for People who Want to Reduce their Drinking*. New York: Three Rivers Press.

Marlatt, G.A., Baer, J.S., Kivlahan, D.R. et al. (1998) Screening and brief intervention for high-risk college student drinkers: results from a 2-year follow-up assessment. *Journal of Consulting and Clinical Psychology* 66, 604–15.

Marlatt, G. and Gordon, J. (1985) *Relapse Prevention*. New York: Guilford Press.

Sanchez-Craig, M., Annis, H.M., Bornet, R. and MacDonald, K.R. (1984) Random assignment to abstinence and controlled drinking. Evaluation of a cognitive–behavioral program for problem drinkers. *Journal of Consulting and Clinical Psychology* 52, 390–403.

Sanchez-Craig, M., Wilkinson, A. and Davila, R. (1995) Empirically based guidelines for moderate drinking: 1-year results from three studies with problem drinkers. *American Journal of Public Health* 85, 823–8.

Saunders, B. (1994) The cognitive–behavioural approach to the management of addictive behaviour. In *Seminars on Alcohol and Drug Misuse*, ed. Chick, J. and Cantwell, R. London: Gaskell, 154–73.

Sobell, M.B. and Sobell, L.C. (1973) Individualized behavior therapy for alcoholics. *Behavior Research and Therapy* 4, 49–72.

Sobell, M.B. and Sobell, L.C. (1976) Second year treatment outcome of alcoholics treated by individualized behavior therapy: results. *Behavior Research and Therapy* 14, 195–215.

Sobell, M.B. and Sobell, L.C. (eds) (1987) *Moderation as a Goal or Outcome of Treatment for Alcohol Problems: a Dialogue.* New York: Haworth Press.

Trimpey, J. (1996) *Rational Recovery: the New Cure for Substance Addiction.* New York: Pocket Books.

21

When things go wrong, and putting them right

Every attempt has been made in previous chapters of this book to present a perspective which avoids an idealized view of the therapeutic process as an operation smoothly and inevitably moving forward to success, as each patient responds to our wise and well-planned interventions. This chapter seeks further to correct any such caricature, and considers some problematic workaday situations.

Going wrong

People who wish to treat alcohol problems must develop an appreciation of the ways in which treatment can go wrong. They must train their eyes quickly to recognize these situations, and must be aware of the familiar patterns of events against which to interpret the latest instance of something going wrong. They must learn to examine the extent to which the therapist is going wrong, and the extent to which it is the patient, and most particularly to analyse what is amiss in the interaction. They must learn not to be discouraged or defeated by such events, but to turn them so far as possible to good therapeutic advantage. One cannot treat alcohol dependence without things very often going wrong, and the essence of treatment is usually a series of trials and errors rather than a straight-line advance. Such a statement is not to be read as a licence for complacency. True, things will go wrong and we must not be too flustered by that fact, but equally true is the insistence that the situation must be recognized and an effort made to put it right.

This chapter does not attempt a consideration of all possible eventualities. Anyone who has experience of this field will see ways in which the list might be extended, and a personal listing of cases in which therapy went wrong (a list kept, as it were, on mental file) is a valuable working tool.

Losing the balances

Much of therapy is a matter of finding balances (and of readily shifting balances), and things often go wrong because balance has been lost. Let us give this statement meaning by considering balance in terms of a number of different paired factors.

Emphasizing the drinking/emphasizing all else

It is possible to go wrong because the treatment has become so exclusively focused on the individual's drinking that the man or woman doing that drinking in a complex personal and social setting is overlooked: the drinking is everything. The complementary imbalance is a sensitive awareness of that individual's total life situation, but with the reality of alcohol as a destructively pervasive aspect of that situation discounted: the drinking is hardly anything. This problem has already been noted in an earlier chapter (Chapter 12). To set the balance right is often difficult, and at a certain stage of learning and experience it is particularly the sensitive, open-minded therapist who is apt to fall into the trap of underestimating the seriousness of the drinking problem. However, the admirable desire to see the whole person and to respect the complexities of that individual's life should not be put in opposition to awareness of the true threat of the drinking.

A man aged 44 had experienced a deprived and troubled childhood. Despite this, he managed to contract a seemingly happy marriage and for 16 years all had appeared to go well. Then his wife had an affair, and his world fell to pieces. All his fearful beliefs as to the inevitability of rejection were proved to be well founded. His feelings towards his wife were unforgiving. He determined that an unhappy episode should be the occasion for catastrophe and he divorced, threw in his job, sold his house, gave up his friends and moved to a new city. A couple of years later he overdosed and consequently came under the care of a psychotherapist, who spent a year exploring with this patient problems relating to his mother. He frequently turned up for interviews drunk, and this was duly interpreted. He was then admitted to hospital for a further and more serious suicidal attempt. The psychiatrist who saw him forthwith instituted a course of electroconvulsive therapy (ECT) for what he diagnosed as a severe and untreated depressive illness. He noted that the patient had 'recently engaged in some secondary relief drinking'. The evening following the first ECT, the patient developed an acute confusional state: it was one of the night nurses who made the diagnosis of delirium tremens.

Both the psychotherapist and the psychiatrist had focused on important aspects of this man's condition, but both had over-focused, and seen things comfortably in terms of their own predilections. Neither had bothered to take a drinking history. It seems likely that the patient was not so much covering up the seriousness of his drinking, as that those who came in contact with him were almost wilfully turning a deaf ear to what he was telling them. A careful reconstruction of the history later suggested a drinking problem going back to the early days of marriage, a marriage much affected by drinking, and a wife who finally moved out because she could no longer tolerate the drinking and the violence. The next move must not be the substitution of an exclusive alcohol focus and a new imbalance for old, but ensuring that treatment of this man's alcohol dependence is accorded its balanced place within the total strategy of his treatment.

There are many different ways of falling into error through seeing the patient as 'an alcoholic' and believing therefore that all their problems are to be understood and treated within that definition alone. A short extract from another case history should correct any notion that the error is always in one direction.

A 33-year-old building worker had been admitted to an alcohol treatment unit, where a diagnosis of alcoholic hallucinosis was made. It was noted that he had previously been admitted to another hospital with what was now deemed to be the mistaken diagnosis of schizophrenia; the case notes were not borrowed. He was put into the ward therapeutic group, but seemed to spend more time listening to imaginary voices than participating. After 6 weeks or so, he was thought to be 'somewhat improved', and was discharged to a hostel for people with drinking problems which was run on intensive therapeutic community lines. He was put into a challenging group on the evening of his arrival, and shortly thereafter again developed florid schizophrenic symptoms, and was re-admitted to the first hospital rather than to the alcohol unit. The case notes recorded an initial attack of schizophrenia at the age of 17, in a man who did fairly well provided he was not too stressed and could find a supportive environment. But this was certainly a patient who, over recent years, had begun to over-medicate himself with alcohol.

The staff of the alcohol treatment unit had so specialized a perspective that when a case of schizophrenia presented to them they reacted in terms of a predetermined psychological set, and the consequent diagnosis led to a package of group therapy and confrontation for a man whose needs were quite otherwise.

So much for two rather extreme cases to illustrate the poles of imbalance which can occur. The errors are usually on a smaller scale and more subtle. Perhaps the mass of general agencies tend to underrate the importance of the drinking, and the specialized alcohol agencies run the risk of being too alcohol focused.

Too ambitious/too unambitious goals

Sometimes things go wrong because the therapist (and the patient) has got the balance wrong with regard to reasonable expectation of what changes may be achieved, or the pace of such change. This dilemma can occur at any stage of treatment. The mistake may be that too great a therapeutic pace is being set, which can readily force the patient into breaking contact, but equally the problem may be in the direction of inertia.

A 60-year-old man stopped drinking but continued to treat his wife in a curmudgeonly fashion, was at cross-purposes with his grown-up children, and had no leisure activities other than watching television and grumbling about the quality of the entertainment provided. At the end of a further year he was still sober and still regarding the world with unrelenting enmity.

What is the community psychiatric nurse (CPN) to do next time they call round on this family and the man purposely turns up the volume on the television, while otherwise angrily staring ahead and not acknowledging the caller's presence? The wife offers a cup of tea in the kitchen and says, 'He's always been that way and I suppose he won't change – a real old misery I call him'. What is the right balance of treatment ambition?

The reality may indeed be that a man of 60 who has for most of his existence defined the world as antagonistic and who has built up his self-image largely in terms of afflicted righteousness, is unlikely radically to change his ways. His wife's assessment of the situation may be just about right, and she does not seem too put out by his ill-grace. Her father was much like that anyhow, and this husband's behaviour is in accord with what she expects of men. She is happy enough that he is no longer running her short of money.

Yet it seems sad to leave it at that. There is the lingering feeling that the goal is being set too low, that more happiness for two people should be possible than is seen here. The answer is perhaps for the CPN to try setting a moderately more ambitious goal on a trial basis. The goal had better be expressed concretely, and the starting point must be the identification of something which the patient and his wife at least half hint at being wanted. In this particular instance the wife let drop 'and he never takes me on holiday of course'. The 'of course' was an important part of the statement; it was clear that the wife's communication with her husband often carried the implication that she expected his response to be negative. A modestly realistic goal in these circumstances was to see if this couple could go away for a week's holiday together and come home with the feeling that they had enjoyed themselves. Working at first through the wife and suggesting that she might for once expect the answer 'yes' from her husband, the holiday was booked. The couple went for a week to the seaside, and although the holiday provided much cause for grumbling, in sum the week provided a real sense of shared reward. Beyond the immediate happening, a small shake-up had occurred in negative patterns of interaction, and the basis was established for the possibility of further small changes.

Too indulgent/too hard

There is a balance to be struck regarding the degree to which the relationship offered by the therapist to the patient or client is to be supportive and non-judgemental, as contrasted with one which emphasizes elements of tough-minded expectation and hard confrontation. To put the matter in terms of absolutes and contradictions is an oversimplification, but it may be useful to examine this particular idea in terms of two contrasting examples – firstly, imbalance in the direction of indulgence.

A social worker of relatively little professional experience became highly committed to helping a family. The 30-year-old man was not alcohol dependent, but seemed to use drink to enhance his passivity and incompetence. He seldom worked. He borrowed, pawned and stole. The wife, who was faced with this chronically difficult situation, tried to prop up the family as best she might. When the social worker arrived on the scene, she soon became no more than a provider of gifts, and she protected the husband from the consequence of his having cheated on welfare payments. She found him good second-hand clothes so that he could go for a job interview, and when he sold the clothes and did not go to the interview she treated him as an amusingly naughty child.

The social worker was operating on the hypothesis that this patient was emotionally deprived and was testing out her 'goodness'; she believed that she 'must not reject him'. Where she may have gone wrong is in her assumption that the opposite to rejection is indulgence.

As an example of the tough-minded imbalance, the following case is illustrative. It relates to consequences of a stance which is quite commonly taken by helping agencies in their attempt to screen-out the 'unmotivated' patient.

A man with a drinking problem was to be discharged from prison and it had been agreed that he should then be admitted to hospital. He was homeless. However, the decision was made 'to test this man's sincerity'. The consultant in charge of the treatment unit decided that the man would not be admitted straightaway, but should find himself lodgings, go to Alcoholics Anonymous (AA), and then present at a ward group for assessment by the other patients. Coming out of prison after 4 years, the man was anxious, a little bit elated, very lost, and immediately made his way to old friends. He was drinking again within hours, and within days had once more committed his familiar offence of breaking and entering. The consultant was confirmed in his sense of wisdom, and took these events as evidence that the patient was 'insufficiently motivated'.

There are occasions when it is therapeutically useful to be nurturing and others on which it is kind and constructive openly to challenge.

Too directive/too afraid of a position

The alternative to forcing one's opinion on a client is not necessarily the pretence of having no opinions at all. A therapist may have difficulty in treating drinking problems because they give their clients the impression of lacking confidence at a time when the client badly needs to borrow some certainties. An orthodox therapeutic detachment is, for instance, inappropriate in a situation in which someone needs very practically to be helped by the therapist's knowledge of how to deal with a drinking crisis, whereas a dictatorial attitude will be equally counter-productive. Here is an example which bears on this particular and difficult aspect of balance.

A 40-year-old woman who, over a 2-year period, had begun to move towards severe alcohol dependence in the setting of a depressive illness was visited on the ward by her husband. The husband made himself unpopular with the staff by his unsympathetic and scolding attitude towards his wife. One of the junior nurses exclaimed to the patient, 'I don't see how living with that man you could ever stay sober – you should go and live with that son of yours who seems so fond of you.'

In the treatment of drinking problems more than in the treatment of many other conditions, the therapist is faced with the problem of directiveness. It often appears glaringly obvious that the patient is engaging in wrong-headed and self-destructive behaviour, is revealing a chaotic inability to make good decisions and order their life well, and manifestly does not know what is best for their own good. This area of practice seems, therefore, to pose a specially acute challenge to the orthodox notion of the therapist's need to maintain neutrality. The nurse felt that she knew what was good for the patient, and said what she thought. Discussion of this incident in the staff group would usefully bring into the open wider issues related to the limits of directiveness, but the conclusion in this particular instance could only be that the balance had gone wrong. The nurse knew too little about the marriage to give directive advice and she certainly knew too little about that patient's son.

Defeated by defences

That the patient's defences have to be identified, their utility for the patient under-stood, and their existence adequately dealt with are ideas common to the treatment of many conditions other than a drinking problem, and the defences which the drinker may deploy are by no means specific to their particular condition. The therapist who is going to work with drinking problems will, however, do well to cultivate a lively awareness of how defences can manifest themselves on this scene. An inadequate response to the patient's defences is one of the more common reasons for things going wrong.

Denial in pure or mixed form

By *denial* is meant a defence against the threat of reality which is based on a refusal to admit the existence of that reality; it is oneself rather than others who have to be deceived. In pure form, the mechanism is pictured as operating at a subconscious level, with denial thus differentiated from a conscious untruth which is aimed at the deception of other people. Often, the patient's difficulty in facing up to the threat posed by their drinking is a manifestation both of denial in the classic sense and of prevarication. In practice, it is often difficult to determine the extent to which the two different elements are contributing to a given presentation, and conscious and unconscious processes commonly seem to merge.

In the popular image, 'alcoholics' are frequently pictured as people who insist on drinking themselves to death while maintaining that no drop of alcohol ever passes their lips. Such crude and primitive defensiveness is relatively uncommon, but when it reaches extreme proportions it can be baffling and a block to all progress, despite every therapeutic stratagem. Here is a case abstract which shows the kind of problems that can be set by entrenched denial.

A 50-year-old accountant was brought to a psychiatric clinic by his business partner, who said that unless something was done his colleague would have to be pensioned off. The patient's breath smelled heavily of drink, his liver was mildly enlarged and he had bruises from several recent falls. He charmingly acknowledged his gratitude to the partner for taking this trouble, but said that the poor man was overworked, worried and getting things out of proportion. The patient admitted to having an occasional beer at lunchtime, but that was the limit of his drinking. He was then seen with his wife, who said that he was permanently intoxicated, that he was frequently incontinent, that he had recently fallen down stairs when drunk and that empty bottles were falling out of every cupboard. He said that his wife was a dear woman but a terrible worrier, that of course he was often tired at the end of the day (who wasn't?), and as for falling down those steps, there had been a loose stair rod.

Given that one does not at this point surrender hope entirely, the best approach might first be to try to get some insight into the reasons which could lead a patient to engage in this stonewalling. Usually, there are several reasons rather than one. For instance, some people make lifelong use of certain favoured defensive mechanisms (in sickness and in health), and this man may, under stress, be reaching for his personally most available coping mechanism out of a limited repertoire. Another explanation may be that this stance is a passive–aggressive response to what he conceives as an attack on his integrity. He sees his partner and his wife (his father and mother) as out to dominate him, and he reacts with angry and childish stubbornness.

With these guesses in mind, the therapist might then sit down alone with the patient, with the other actors out of the room. With no implication of attack, the therapist will start a discussion on the basis of an openly stated assumption that both he and the patient know that reality is being denied. The therapist will furthermore immediately lay ground rules for the interaction by stating that the interview will not be allowed to degenerate into a useless cross-examination which could offer no fruitful result but only further entrenchment. The aim is thus not frontal assault on the defensive position, but to get behind the defence. It can be put to the patient that a lot of people find difficulty in talking openly about the degree of worry and trouble which their drinking is causing – they may be afraid of attack and afraid of being demeaned – and, in such circumstances, to try to insist that the worrying facts do not exist can be a natural response. The therapist might try to convey that he or she sees this situation from the patient's point of view, and then offer possible alternative solutions. It can be put to the patient that if a man drives his car off the road and someone comes up and asks questions, the driver may well respond defensively if they think that it is a policeman who is questioning them, but it will make no sense to treat the person who is offering first-aid as if they were a policeman, and hence bleed to death.

The defensiveness may still remain absolute. The patient may take the line that the therapist is a nice person whom it is a privilege to meet, but that the clinic's valuable time is being wasted on the basis of a most unfortunate mistake – everyone is getting hold of absolutely the wrong end of the stick. What to do next?

It may be possible as a temporary measure to go on leaving the defence in place, as it were, but to take no notice of it – to allow the patient to hold to the assumption that he has no drinking problem, while the therapist works on the assumption that there is a serious problem which has to be treated. Such a peculiar agreement to differ is unlikely to continue happily for long; either the patient will slide into accepting the therapist's definition of reality or contact will be unprofitable. Another and rather simple approach which may sometimes be promising is to concentrate for the time being on the patient's physical health. He may find it acceptable that he is in need of advice on his physical health (an alcohol-free diet for his liver's sake), without any of the loss of face which he fears will result from fully admitting his dependence on alcohol.

If none of these approaches pays dividends, the only course may be to leave the patient with an unambiguous message as to the need for him to open his eyes, and a factual warning of the dangers which will stem from the denial and prevarication continuing, and then not to make any offer to see the patient again for a period of some months, unless he so asks. The wife, meanwhile, may well need help or support in her own right.

The occasional baffling intractableness of deeply entrenched denial should not itself be denied. The temptation is almost literally to raise one's voice in the hope that the patient will actually hear, or to confront them with every sort of proof positive and hope that the high walls of their defences will then dramatically collapse. The temptation is, in short, to resort to the battering ram. Sadly, the consequences of that attack will probably only be the patient strengthening their wall of defence.

The defence of sickness

Sometimes, a client will claim that they continue to drink because they are indeed 'an alcoholic'. They are suffering from an illness which is the explanation of their behaviour, and the responsibility for curing this illness rests with the therapist. The client may then continue their drinking, with the position nicely established that the therapist is to blame. Things go wrong if this position is accepted, but they go equally wrong if the therapist automatically assumes that this person is playing games or working some kind of intentional trickery. They may be taking up this particular version of the sick role because they truly believe that they are sick, damaged and no longer able to control their own behaviour. They are not then so much displaying a defence as manifesting symptoms of learned helplessness. The two different possible meanings of outwardly similar presentations have therefore to be distinguished. In the wrong circumstances, cutting the drinker down with an aggressively neat analysis of the game they are playing is likely to result in the therapist being rid of a difficult client, but nothing else. It may be more useful to try to move this person towards a realization that they can indeed start to take responsibility for not drinking, that they have more resources than they supposed, and that it would be misleading if anyone else were to pretend to be able to take over their responsibilities for them. The job is to work for increased self-efficacy and strengthening of motivation.

Absolution

A patient may be able to defend themselves from the pain which would otherwise force them to change their behaviour, if they can find a doctor or counsellor who can be persuaded to offer regular absolution. They may present a picture of pseudo-insight. Intellectually they know what suffering they are causing to themselves and others, but they are able to divorce this insight from any deep feelings provided they are given regular doses of forgiveness. They are, in fact, seeking the therapist's connivance as actor in a repetitive and unproductive play. Here is a case extract which illustrates one such presentation.

The patient settled into a chair and said that he knew he was an 'alcoholic', had been going to AA for years, and knew that all he now had to do was to get through one day without drink. His wife was threatening to leave him, and after this last 'slip' and all that she had been through, he entirely saw her point of view and did not blame her in the least. He was most dreadfully sorry and knew that he had behaved to her like a swine. Furthermore, he had let the doctor down again, and was thoroughly ashamed of himself. He had said exactly the same thing on many occasions, with a similar show of contrition coupled with detachment from real feeling.

Things go wrong if the therapist falls into the position of aiding and abetting this cycle of behaviour. Such a story is not uncommon and the patient may sometimes be a long-term AA attender who has managed to get little out of AA. One may suspect that they have used the AA meetings in much the same way as they would employ the interview with the therapist, and they are nowhere near grasping the real AA message. For the therapist to continue contact on this non-therapeutic or anti-therapeutic basis is useless. It is more helpful to throw the responsibility back on the patient and refuse to be the confessor. An element of challenge and confrontation may produce new possibilities, but there is always the risk that the patient will instead go off and find another therapist who will, at least temporarily, provide the absolution.

The romantic defence

Drinking peculiarly lends itself to a romantic defence, an identification with famous drinking poets and playwrights. The following is an abstract from a referral letter.

This lady is a successful artist and you will certainly know of her husband who is the novelist. She has led a truly amazing life, and if she gets round to telling you about her years in Paris you will find it fascinating. Everyone in her set drinks, and I think one has to accept that drinking is for her essential to the creative life. Recently she has been hitting the bottle and she was seen by someone last year who rather annoyed her by calling her an alcoholic. She cannot accept help which is conditional upon her giving up drinking.

In this instance, the patient's defence has overwhelmed the judgement of an experienced physician, who had been seduced into accepting drinking as symbolizing 'the creative life'. That the drinking was profoundly affecting this woman's ability to work and threatened to destroy her was being screened out.

If this position is accepted, things will certainly go wrong, with the patient continuing to drink and the therapist effectively neutralized as an amused and admiring spectator of a fascinating way of life, but with the therapeutic position lost. At the start of the contact, the therapist has therefore to hold to the position that drinking must be de-symbolized and seen in its reality. The patient may have an immediate sense of relief if they find that they can discard the pretence that self-destruction is romantic fun.

Endless argument

The problems set by intellectual defence are familiar in any area of psychotherapy. In work with drinking problems, the intellectualization is likely to go off in certain special directions – the patient will divert the discussion away from any real therapeutic content towards making the interview a symposium either on the definition of alcohol dependence or on the determinants of drinking behaviour, or both. The therapeutic response should be to steer the patient away from consideration of generalities and back to the immediacy of their own position. Otherwise, the therapist may become engaged in a lengthy analysis of 'the disease concept', while the patient continues to drink.

The patient who knows someone who drinks much more

A block to treatment – which can be no more than a minor distraction but which may sometimes be employed as a major stratagem to escape the reality of the threat which drink poses – is the claim made by the patient that they knew someone who drank much more than they ever did themselves, or who drank a great deal and never came to harm.

All right, I drink my share. But I'll tell you this, my old father died at 86 and he drank much more heavily than I have ever done. Absolutely routine, he'd never go outside the house without putting a bottle of whisky in his pocket, just like picking up his tin of tobacco.

To enter a debate with such a patient as to whether their drinking is more or less than the father's is bound to be defeating. The data on the patient's drinking are probably at that stage uncertain and the data on the father's drinking much falsified, so the patient is in a position to prop up their defence by revising all elements of the comparison at will. If one agrees to enter this debate, one gets involved in a kind of pub conversation, with wildly unlikely but incontrovertible assertions being heaped one on the other. 'Look at Winston Churchill. He had the best part of a bottle of brandy every morning before he got out of bed. Greatest Englishman who ever lived . . .'. The best way to avoid entanglement in this unproductive argument is to say that it is not the patient's father or Winston Churchill who has come for the consultation, and they will be left outside the room.

Medical negligence

Sadly, it is not unknown for a doctor treating a drinking problem to find themselves facing an action for negligence. At the extreme there may be risk of action for medical manslaughter. This is a difficult area of practice, but that does not excuse practitioners from the inalienable responsibility of delivering a high quality of care. As ever, the practitioners' best defence is to ensure that their treatment is of a kind and quality which would be seen as reasonably good practice by their peers. Scrupulous attention to note keeping and letter writing is important. When a patient poses a danger of self-harm or harm to others, it may be good medico-legal as well as good medical practice to consult with another professional and fully record the consultation on file.

Here is a list of the kind of problems which good practice in this arena will seek most strenuously to avoid.

- Over-prescribing of benzodiazepines to a drinking patient with consequent instatement of benzodiazepine dependence is a not uncommon cause for legal action.
- In the UK, long-term prescribing by a GP of chlormethiazole to a patient who is still drinking is probably legally indefensible.
- Failure of an accident and emergency department doctor to diagnose and immediately treat incipient Wernicke's encephalopathy may lead to tragic brain damage for the patient and enormously expensive damages against the hospital and doctor.
- Careless use of an intravenous chlormethiazole drip for sedation during a hospital-based detoxification can lead to overdose or death.
- Failure of a general hospital ward to deal adequately with withdrawal and to maintain a safe environment may see staff held responsible for a very expensive tragedy.
- Careless prescribing of disulfiram can lead to repeated confusional episodes.

None of these types of accident should ever be allowed to happen, but unfortunately they still continue to occur, thus bearing witness to the fact that, in every medical setting, enhanced alertness and better training regarding drinking problems are much required.

When everything goes wrong

In Box 21.1, some ideas are set out concerning ways of getting a therapeutic block unstuck. There are times in treating drinking problems when everything seems to go wrong at once, and this is not just in terms of happenings relating to one particular patient, but also with several patients getting into serious difficulties over the same few weeks. One's most hopeful patient relapses, another seems bent on destroying themselves with their continued drinking, and a patient for whom the therapist had especially warm feelings dies and there is an element of self-blame. These periods occur, and it is necessary for the therapist who runs into such a patch of trouble to remind themselves (or be reminded by their colleagues) that this kind of practice will inevitably at times be a fraught and perplexing business. Sometimes, a therapist may have been selecting for themselves all the more difficult cases, and there is the possibility that they have become overstretched, overtired or careless. However, it is more likely that events have randomly clustered and that the therapist needs their self-confidence supported, more than being invited to blame themselves. Sometimes, things go wrong because of forgetfulness and oversight: the need for a physical examination is overlooked, the spouse is not seen, what the patient is trying to say is not heard. Perhaps more dangerously, things go amiss when the therapist becomes over-confident, fails to entertain doubts and assumes that they know all, and that if the patient fails to respond, what is needed is more medicine of the same kind. On occasions, the way in which the treatment system is working may also need to be scrutinized and it may, for instance, be evident that difficulties stem from staff liaison being in poor repair or from personal tensions between staff members.

BOX 21.1 **When things go wrong: the positive therapeutic response to case problems**

- Problems should be shared: talk through the situation with a colleague.
- Problems can be two way: try to understand your own behaviour, attitudes and expectations as well as those of the patient.
- Identify blocks: in particular the therapeutic approach losing its balance or the unhelpful defence mechanisms which the patient may be using to negate progress.
- Motivation is essential to change: does further work need to be done on readiness to change?
- Check back on the original assessment and formulation, review the case, and get a purposive plan in place with the patient participating; recover the therapeutic motivation.
- Remember, no-one is omnipotent and therapists have rightful needs.

Treating the person with a drinking problem is about moving that individual by every available strategy towards alliance with his or her own recovery. The richest arena for learning is the actuality of contact, the experience of things sometimes going wrong, and the discovery that, with patience, flexibility and mutual effort, things often very happily come right.

Every individual and team should explore the question of how, within their practice circumstances, they are going to address such problems positively and effectively, so as to help the patient through and themselves learn in the process. Younger and more experienced therapists equally have needs in this regard, and male and female staff members may at times have different kinds of support needs. Sharing of problems rather than a drift to isolation is vital, and the availability for staff support of an experienced therapist from outside the team can be valuable. There should be an open and unashamed willingness to see oneself as needy, rather than yielding to the destructive belief that one can endlessly give without being given.

22

Treatment settings, professional roles and the organization of treatment services

Treatment is provided for people with drinking problems in varied settings, by diverse professionals and by non-professionals. Many of the organizations and individuals that provide this treatment have different goals as well as different conceptions of the underlying problem, and they aim to help the problem drinker in different ways. This diversity offers advantages and pitfalls which need to be understood both by helping agencies and treatment purchasers and by the people who are seeking help.

This chapter considers the way in which different settings and different professional roles contribute to the treatment of the problem drinker, as well as the ways in which treatment services can be integrated and organized. All of these considerations vary internationally, with differences being related to varying conceptions of alcohol-related problems, varying drinking cultures and varying economic stability. However, across a broad band, the overall wealth of a country seems to make relatively little difference to its provision of services for people with drinking problems. Klingemann et al. (1992, 1993) give an international perspective on alcohol treatment systems in 16 countries.

Treatment settings

Help may be offered to the drinker in an almost infinite variety of settings by a wide range of people. Such help is given by the spouse who encourages a partner to seek help, the employer who counsels an employee regarding drunkenness in the workplace, the barman who refuses to serve a customer who has already had too much to drink, and the policeman who arrests someone who is 'drunk and disorderly'. The home, the workplace, premises on which alcohol is served and even a public space may all, therefore, be settings in which help is provided. The primary care physician or social worker may identify evidence of a drinking problem when visiting the home to see another member of the family.

Internationally, there has been a move away from institutional care towards out-patient treatment, as well as a decentralization of care, although some countries (such as Hungary and Russia) still rely on compulsory in-patient treatment. In many countries, care for people with drinking problems is now provided within the overall framework of health care services, but mutual help groups, notably Alcoholics Anonymous (AA), have been very influential upon the treatment services in Nordic and English-speaking countries (Klingemann et al., 1993).

It is helpful to identify some of the more formal settings in which professionals are likely to work on a day-to-day basis (see Box 22.1). Each of these settings has its own particular opportunities, as well as certain drawbacks, for the provision of help to the problem drinker. Each will be more or less prominent in any national context, depending upon the degree of medicalization of alcohol treatment service provision, the extent of influence of AA and the Twelve Step philosophy, and the degree to which decentralization and de-institutionalization have resulted in a move away from in-patient treatments towards out-patient treatment and care in the community.

BOX 22.1 **Treatment settings**
- Primary care
- Community alcohol team
- Specialist alcohol treatment unit
- Residential rehabilitation
- Self-help groups
- General hospitals
- Psychiatric hospitals
- Criminal justice system
- Workplace

Primary care

The provision of primary medical care varies considerably around the world. In some countries it may include the provision of care by staff with minimal training. The traditional healer, or the priest or shaman, and a belief in folk medicine may play a more significant role than that of orthodox Western medicine. However, primary care will be taken here to refer principally to the non-specialist provision of medical care in the community by a physician and a variable team of professionals drawn from a background of psychology, nursing, social work, occupational therapy, counselling and other disciplines.

The doctor working in primary care has a unique perspective which accommodates both the family and long-term context, as well as a good overall medical history of his or her patients. This offers the opportunity for early detection of a range of alcohol-related problems that might not be obvious to others or that might not warrant specialist referral. It also offers opportunities for interventions, including brief counselling, support and education, in a setting which is non-stigmatizing. The effectiveness of early interventions offered in primary care has been demonstrated by research (Wallace et al., 1988; Edwards et al., 1994; Deehan et al., 1998).

Where specialist referral is required, the physician working in primary care is in a good position to know what resources are available, and which ones might be most appropriate for a given patient. It is increasingly clear that the role of many specialist agencies, such as community alcohol teams, should be to support the management of problem drinkers within the primary care setting. Thus they may offer advice and support to the primary health care team, or arrange clinics to be held within the buildings of the health centre or surgery. Furthermore, there is evidence that the majority of patients can be treated as effectively in primary care as by a specialist service, in respect of improvements in both drinking behaviour and alcohol-related problems (Drummond et al., 1990). However, it is important that the primary health care team is provided with adequate support by the specialist agency. Primary care staff often feel unconfident about, and inadequately trained for, the detection and management of alcohol misuse, and recognize their need for training and support offered by local alcohol services (Deehan et al., 1997, 1999; Marshall and Deehan, 1998).

For clinical guidelines on working with people with drinking problems in a primary care setting, the UK Alcohol Forum (2001) is helpful.

The community alcohol team

In recent years, in many countries, there has been a trend towards providing substance misuse services in the community rather than in a residential or 'in-patient' setting. This partly stems from the economic benefits of such an approach to treatment, but it also reflects a realization that, in many cases, in-patient treatment is no more effective than out-patient treatment. There is much research evidence to support this approach. A large proportion, if not the great majority, of alcohol dependent patients can be detoxified safely, economically and successfully in the community (Hayashida et al., 1989; Collins et al., 1990; Stockwell et al., 1991). There is evidence that out-patient treatment for drinking problems is as effective as in-patient treatment (Edwards and Guthrie, 1967) and even that brief advice is as effective as intensive (Edwards et al., 1977) or extended treatment (Chick et al., 1988) for many patients. Furthermore, treatment in the community avoids some of the stigma associated with admission for 'drying out'.

To some, it may seem that the community alcohol team is simply a relocated out-patient clinic, and in certain cases this may be true. However, at its best, the community team is far more flexible in its ability to liaise with the primary health care team, as well as the community mental health team and other agencies. It is also able to provide services in a series of geographically convenient locations and, where necessary, conduct domiciliary assessments.

The range of treatments offered by the community alcohol team is likely to vary depending upon contractual obligations, local need, and the experience and interests of staff. In principle, most patients with drinking problems can be offered most treatments in this setting. Brief and longer-term counselling, relapse prevention and cognitive–behavioural treatments, individual and group psychotherapy, pharmacotherapy and detoxification can all be provided by this route. A day programme may be available.

The specialist alcohol treatment centre

This kind of facility may take many forms. In some cases it will be difficult to distinguish the therapeutic environment from that found in non-medical therapeutic communities or other forms of residential rehabilitation (see below). The 'specialist alcohol treatment centre' will be taken here to refer to the facility which has a multidisciplinary staff, including medical and other professionals, with or without an in-patient unit, a day centre, an out-patient clinic, and possibly a community team (see above). It may be able to offer urgent assessment or treatment in any of these settings.

The function of such a unit is the diagnosis or management of the difficult case, including, where necessary, specialist physical, psychological or psychiatric investigation and management. The centre is also likely to offer support and advice to other services, and may offer a teaching or educational programme. Liaison with primary care (see above), the general hospital (Glass-Crome et al., 1994) and mental health services may be an important function of the specialist alcohol treatment centre. It may also offer assessment or management of patients awaiting trial for, or convicted of, criminal offences (see below).

In many communities, a facility of this sort may not be available at all. Where it is available, it may or may not offer in-patient care. In-patient facilities are particularly expensive to run and, as mentioned earlier, there is reason to believe that out-patient services may be equally effective for many patients. However, the in-patient unit offers certain advantages where it is available. Some patients cannot be safely detoxified in the community (see Chapter 16), and others may require admission for the assessment or treatment of co-morbid psychiatric disorders. It is also recognized that many patients fail to respond to out-patient interventions and, in a minority of cases, it appears reasonable to attempt a period of in-patient treatment when all else has failed. An in-patient unit offers access to more intensive psychotherapy, occupational therapy and medical care than is available in the community.

The specialist alcohol centre is not associated with the stigma that discourages patients from attending psychiatric services. It is also important to maintain and develop expertise in a field which is still often not popular with, or well understood by, generic staff in medical or psychiatric facilities (Potamianos et al., 1985).

Residential rehabilitation

Residential rehabilitation usually occurs in a non-medical setting, and the form that it takes reflects the underlying philosophy of the particular organization. Such settings are extremely varied, both in respect of the particular programme that is offered and also in the underlying beliefs concerning alcohol-related problems. Most offer some sort of therapeutic community approach (Kennard, 1983), with counselling or psychotherapy seen as an important part of the rehabilitative process. Staff are often, although not invariably, drawn from recovering alcoholics or addicts who have graduated from the programme. The therapeutic goal is almost always towards total abstinence, and this is usually taken to include abstinence from all addictive substances, not just alcohol.

In the USA and, to a lesser extent, in many parts of Europe, most of these centres are based upon the Twelve Step programme of AA. In these facilities, problem drinking (or 'alcoholism') is treated alongside other forms of substance misuse (or 'chemical dependency') using a common approach to treatment often known as the 'Minnesota Model' (Cook, 1988a, 1988b). This form of treatment is discussed further in Chapter 18. In some countries (e.g. Austria and Poland), it is not currently available (Mäkelä et al., 1996).

On a worldwide basis, the next most frequently encountered type of residential rehabilitation would probably be that based upon a religious philosophy. In most cases, such centres operate from a Christian foundation, and the Salvation Army is particularly active in this area of work. These centres are much less homogeneous in terms of programme content than the Minnesota Model facilities. Group work is less central and contribution to the running of the community through practical chores is more frequently emphasized. In some cases, religious devotions may also be given priority, although most such communities do not demand adherence to the Christian faith as a prerequisite for residents.

Self-help groups

The role of AA and related organizations is discussed in Chapter 18. Although the self-help model strictly excludes consideration of this as a 'treatment' setting, it is still a very important source of help to many people with drinking problems. It also provides a reminder that people with drinking problems receive help in many settings other than those which involve interaction with treatment professionals. Patients staying on alcohol treatment units, or in residential rehabilitation, may be encouraged to travel to attend such meetings off site. Many people in the community will attend such groups in addition to any other professional help they are receiving. For others, AA will provide their only source of help, and large numbers have achieved abstinence through this route alone, with no professional help at all. The willingness of professionals to refer patients to AA varies from one country to another.

General hospitals

Alcohol-related problems are encountered in every department of the district general hospital, and there is evidence that they contribute a significant proportion of the morbidity seen in many accident and emergency (A & E) departments, wards and clinics (Persson and Magnusson, 1987; Canning et al., 1999; Working Party of the Royal College of Physicians, 2001). Physicians and surgeons are thus in an excellent position to advise their patients about sensible drinking limits, and about the effects that alcohol consumption is having upon their physical health. Nurses also have an important role to play in counselling problem drinkers in this setting, the potential efficacy of which has been demonstrated by research (Chick et al., 1985). It may be difficult to offer counselling amidst the hectic activity of a busy A & E department, and therefore liaison with specialist services is particularly important here.

Strategic recommendations, and examples of good practice, for the management of alcohol-related problems in the general hospital are provided by the Working Party of the Royal College of Physicians (2001).

The opportunities for helping problem drinkers in the general hospital setting will be lost unless steps are taken to identify who these patients are. It is thus vital that an alcohol history becomes a routine part of medical and nursing assessments in this setting. It is to be hoped that stories such as the following will become increasingly rare.

In the course of an epidemiological study of a general medical award, a consultant physician declared that 'he never saw alcoholism'. There was on that day a patient on his ward, admitted for treatment of a bleeding ulcer, who was rapidly going into delirium tremens. The notes showed no evidence whatsoever of enquiry into the patient's drinking history, and a look at further case notes showed that on that treatment service it was quite exceptional to ask about a patient's drinking.

At least one recent study, looking at patients who had taken an overdose, has revealed that an alcohol history is still often neglected by medical staff (Shepherd et al., 1995).

Psychiatric hospitals

In many areas, there may not be specialist in-patient alcohol facilities and often there is an expectation that patients with drinking problems will be admitted to the general psychiatric ward instead. This setting offers certain advantages for patients who suffer from co-morbid psychiatric disorders in addition to their drinking problem. It should also provide opportunities for pharmacotherapy, counselling, psychotherapy and occupational therapy. However, many general psychiatric wards are now reserved for acutely psychotic or suicidal patients, and such an environment is particularly unsuitable for the management of patients with drinking problems. Clinical guidelines for working with patients with drinking problems in a community psychiatric setting are provided by UK Alcohol Forum (2001).

Criminal justice system

The association between crime and alcohol is discussed in Chapter 6. The large number of alcohol-related offences committed each year indicates an opportunity to identify, and intervene in, drinking problems amongst offenders.

Treatment as an alternative to sentencing

It has long been recognized that neither society nor the offender benefits from the repeated fines or custodial sentences that result from a long series of drunkenness offences. Various systems have been operated, in different countries, in an effort to avoid this scenario. The police may take the street drunk to a detoxification centre rather than to a police cell, and possibly thus avoid a court appearance altogether. Alternatively, the courts may impose treatment in place of or in addition to a punitive sentence.

Treatment imposed by courts

Having recognized the existence of a drinking problem, and having found a person guilty of a crime, a court may decide to impose treatment as a condition of probation, or as an alternative to a punitive sentence, or else in addition to any other sentence that is imposed. Alternatively, the court may take into consideration treatments which are being undertaken on a voluntary basis. All of these arrangements offer the opportunity for people to enter treatment when they might not otherwise have done so. However, this can also create difficulties.

Some patients may enter treatment purely as a means of attracting a more sympathetic response from the courts. Other patients may be reluctantly referred for treatments with which they do not want to engage. Surprisingly, it seems that these instances do not necessarily prejudice treatment outcome (Laundergan et al., 1979). Occasionally, a patient may be compulsorily admitted to hospital in order to protect the public from violence or other serious crime. It is rarely, if ever, appropriate that admissions of this sort should be made to an alcohol treatment centre.

Drink driving offenders

Drink driving is itself an important alcohol-related problem, and drink-drivers will include many who have also experienced other alcohol-related problems. Yet, it is a feature of the 'prevention paradox' (see Chapter 2) that many drink-drivers will not be very heavy drinkers or experience other alcohol-related problems. Two drink driving convictions are much more likely to be indicative of a serious underlying drinking problem (McMillen et al., 1992).

Educational and therapeutic interventions should be made available for those who have been convicted of drink driving offences, and in many countries (e.g. France, Italy, New Zealand, Switzerland and the USA) participation of offenders in such programmes is required by law (Klingemann et al., 1993). Increasingly, in some parts of the world, these programmes are being offered by courts as an alternative to punitive sentences. The research evidence for the benefits of such programmes is modest, and it would seem best that they are offered in addition to, rather than instead of, punitive measures such as fines, licensing restrictions and prison sentences (Peacock, 1992; Edwards et al., 1994).

Treatment in prison

Many people in prison – on a worldwide basis, probably most people in prison – receive no help for their drinking problem. A few prisons have provided special facilities for problem drinkers and AA groups may hold meetings in prisons. In some places individual counselling is available and the prison doctor or chaplain is in a position both to identify the need for such interventions and to ensure that they are provided.

Prison provides a most unusual environment in so far as it generally (although not always) ensures enforced abstinence for the duration of a sentence. Although this may appear to offer advantages to the problem drinker in the short term, in the longer-term perspective it denies the opportunity to learn coping skills which are relevant to an environment in which alcohol is freely available. Furthermore, release from prison is in itself a stressful life event, which may easily precipitate relapse. This is, therefore, a treatment setting in which relapse prevention work is especially appropriate.

Workplace

The workplace provides particularly good opportunities for preventive measures to combat problem drinking, combined with opportunities for early detection and intervention for problems that do arise. Whereas the interface between employment

and health care poses ethical and policy dilemmas, the need to maintain employment also provides a strong incentive for the problem drinker actively to engage in
treatment.

Workplace alcohol programmes are often combined with programmes to address
drug misuse and other health or welfare needs. In North America, and increasingly
in Europe, such programmes are referred to as Employee Assistance Programmes
(or EAPs). As with other treatment programmes, EAPs may be strongly influenced
by a particular approach to treatment, such as the Twelve Steps of AA.

There are a number of issues which all such programmes need to address if they
are to be effective.

Policy

It is vital that workplace alcohol policies should be established through a written
policy agreed by employers and unions in order to clarify what is and is not allowed
in respect of drinking and work. In some cases this will need to be very strict,
particularly where public or employee safety is concerned.

A written workplace alcohol policy will be needed to document the procedures
for identifying and managing the employee with an alcohol problem, and it may
specify the implementation of an alcohol screening programme (see Chapter 14).

Provision of help

Large organizations may have their own services through which help may be offered
to the employee with an identified drinking problem. In smaller organizations,
arrangements may be made for help to be provided by local primary care services
or specialist alcohol agencies. Whatever the size of the organization, a separation
of medical treatment provision from occupational health will, in any case, usually
be necessary for ethical reasons (British Medical Association, 1998).

Confidentiality and ethical issues

The occupational physician, counsellor or nurse is in an unusual position in comparison with others of their profession. Whereas confidentiality of information
divulged by a client or patient would normally be absolute, in the occupational setting there is also a duty to the welfare of the entire workforce, and possibly also to
the general public, as well as to the employer. These dual allegiances can sometimes
lead to ethical dilemmas. Staff are unlikely to confide in a nurse or counsellor who
will 'tell all' to the employer. Neither do employers have a right to expect that all information obtained through such channels should be made available to them. In so
far as information is obtained which affects safety in the workplace, confidentiality
may be over-ridden. It must be made clear at the outset that this is the case, and
written agreement should be obtained from employees for the passing of medical
information to the employer.

The occupational physician should also not usually offer treatment to an employee, but this should be arranged by, or in consultation with, the patient's own general practitioner (British Medical Association, 1998).

An example

A patient was referred by an occupational physician to a specialist alcohol unit for assessment and advice. He had for several years shown evidence of minor liver damage attributable to drinking, which was above the recommended limits (see Chapter 10). The company policy indicated that his continued employment would not be allowed unless he had received a period of in-patient treatment for his alcohol problem. This hard line had been taken because of the risk to public safety that was involved. But it was clear to the specialist that this employee's alcohol problem was relatively minor, that it had never impaired his performance at work, and that in-patient treatment would never normally be considered appropriate for such a patient. The occupational physician was able to provide continued monitoring of the problem on an out-patient basis, the correct treatment was offered to the patient for his drinking problem, public safety was ensured, and the patient retained his job.

Professional roles

It was suggested above that the broader context of treatment involves diverse individuals operating in diverse settings. Many of those who may significantly influence the treatment of a problem drinker are not themselves treatment professionals. Thus, the important roles of the spouse, the friend, the AA sponsor and others should not be underestimated. In this section, we focus primarily upon the roles of different professionals involved in the treatment of problem drinkers (see Box 22.2).

BOX 22.2 **Professional roles**
- Medical
- Nursing
- Social work
- Occupational therapy
- Psychology
- Counselling
- Psychotherapy
- Teamwork

The provision of a comprehensive service for people with alcohol-related problems requires a range of skills and experience which is beyond the boundaries of any one profession and arguably beyond the capacity of any individual. It is therefore

essential that treatment is seen in the context of a multidisciplinary team provision, albeit some relatively isolated professionals may find themselves working
outside any formal team structure. The relative prominence of particular professions within any given national treatment context will reflect a variety of factors,
including particularly the degree of medicalization of treatment services and the
extent of influence of AA.

Medical

There will be few doctors who do not encounter alcohol-related problems in their
day-to-day clinical practice. Medical advice is taken seriously by most patients,
and doctors are therefore in a strong position to influence their patients' alcohol
consumption. Simple advice on the adverse effects of alcohol consumption upon
liver function, intellectual capacity, mental state, heart disease and hypertension
can be very effective in persuading a patient to cut down or discontinue alcohol
consumption.

In addition to providing education and care for patients with alcohol-related
physical or psychiatric disorders, doctors have other important roles to play in the
treatment of alcohol dependence and alcohol misuse. A range of pharmacotherapies has been shown to influence alcohol consumption or reduce relapse rates
(see Chapter 19). Alcohol withdrawal is a potentially serious medical condition
which requires appropriate medical treatment and supervision (see Chapter 16).
Psychiatrists specializing in various forms of psychotherapy can contribute usefully
to the psychological management of patients with drinking problems.

Nursing

Almost all nurses will have opportunities to offer education, advice and counselling
to their patients regarding alcohol consumption and alcohol-related problems.
Some patients may feel more able to speak freely to a nurse than to a doctor, and
more time may be available for them to do this.

The practice nurse working in the primary care setting has an especially important role to play in the detection of harmful, or potentially harmful, drinking and
alcohol-related problems as well as in offering brief interventions. Such nurses are
often presented with a good opportunity to engage in such work by virtue of their
role in screening and assessing new patients as they register with the primary health
care team. Community psychiatric nurses, working as part of a community mental
health team, have a similar role to play in the secondary care setting. By definition,
it is probable that most (or all) of their patients will have a dual diagnosis of a
drinking problem and a co-morbid psychiatric disorder (see Chapter 8), and it is
therefore likely that they will need to liaise closely with the local community alcohol
team.

On an in-patient alcohol unit, nurses will fulfil the traditional nursing roles of dispensing medication, observing and recording clinical signs (such as severity of withdrawal, pulse and blood pressure, etc.) and planning and providing 24-hour care. As with most other areas of psychiatric nursing, these traditional functions are a relatively small part of the task that the nurse faces. A nurse working with this group of patients, particularly, requires skills in counselling and psychotherapy.

Much of the counselling and psychotherapeutic work associated with specialist alcohol work, in the community or in a residential setting, is ideally suited to the appropriately trained nurse. Thus, community alcohol teams, hospital liaison services, specialist alcohol units and even non-medical alcohol agencies may all find that nurses comprise a large proportion of their staff.

Social work

Social workers and probation officers are well equipped to engage the problem drinker in appropriate counselling and psychotherapeutic work, especially in the family context, as well as to offer help with the practical issues of housing, benefits, employment and legal matters. Their training offers a different perspective on these activities from that provided by most nursing and other medical staff. Yet it is important that their expertise is not diverted solely towards the adverse social consequences of alcohol misuse, whilst denying the opportunity to address the drinking itself.

Alongside their other responsibilities, social workers in some countries are entrusted with statutory duties in respect of matters such as child care and mental health legislation. Although these duties may have only an indirect relevance to working with problem drinkers, they can assume great importance in individual cases. For example, the suitability of a parent with drinking problems to care for children may be in serious doubt (see Chapter 5), or co-morbid psychotic illness may necessitate assessment of the need for formal admission to a psychiatric unit under the terms of national mental health legislation.

Occupational therapy

Although occupational therapy offers a vital contribution to general psychiatric and medical services, it is disappointing that this discipline is often neglected in specialist alcohol treatment services. Occupational therapists help individuals to learn or relearn behaviours necessary in daily life, including social skills (Royal College of Psychiatrists and College of Occupational Therapists, 1992).

A dependent drinker who becomes abstinent will find that they have to fill time which was previously spent drinking. The occupational therapist should play a part in the assessments and treatments offered by any comprehensive alcohol treatment service. However, it is important that other members of staff do not see the role of the occupational therapist as 'simply filling time'. The concern of the occupational therapist is with the occupational and therapeutic purpose of activity, and not simply activity for its own sake.

Occupational therapists, along with most of the other disciplines described here, also have a contribution to make to a broad spectrum of counselling and psychotherapeutic work, especially in the group context.

Psychology

If alcohol misuse is viewed as a learned behaviour, then the clinical psychologist would appear to be a very important player. Many of the psychotherapeutic methods employed in this field have a behavioural psychological basis, and ultimately the focus of all such work is on a behavioural outcome – the context, quantity and pattern of alcohol consumption. A comprehensive behavioural analysis of the context of alcohol consumption can provide a valuable basis for further counselling and treatment. Many psychologists are also interested in cognitive or dynamic therapeutic methods and these can also have a part to play.

Most psychologists would be quick to recognize that they cannot personally conduct all psychological treatments within any department, and the alcohol unit is no exception. The clinical psychologist must therefore expect to play a role in the training of other members of the multidisciplinary team in psychological treatment methods.

The assessment of alcohol-induced brain damage is also an area in which the skills of the clinical psychologist are required. In addition, the occupational psychologist may make a contribution to identifying alcohol-related problems in the workplace, and the educational psychologist may encounter the adverse effects of parental drinking upon children and teenagers.

Counselling and psychotherapy

A contribution to counselling and psychotherapy is a role for all of the professional groups listed above. Counselling in this sphere of activity also attracts counsellors of a type not seen in many other areas of work. These are the addicts and 'alcoholics' who have themselves achieved sobriety and who have felt a calling to help others who suffer as they did. In many cases, these people have found help through AA and Narcotics Anonymous (NA) and their principles of working thus draw much from the Twelve Steps and the Minnesota Model. Their experience is varied, and their training even more so. However, standards of training and practice are improving, and many of these individuals now combine a sound theoretical knowledge with the insights of their personal experience. However, in one study of eight countries, only the USA was found to provide officially recognized formal courses for AA counsellors (Mäkelä et al., 1996). In most centres, a mandatory minimum period of abstinence (usually 2 years or more) is expected before such a counsellor will be employed on the staff team.

The advantages and disadvantages associated with the employment of 'ex-alcoholic' counsellors in a treatment team have been discussed in detail elsewhere, and the idea of employing such staff is not new (Anderson, 1944). Although they offer a sound role model to patients, personal experience of the problems associated with drinking and a thorough understanding of the AA programme, there may also be problems associated with their employment. Competition and conflict with other staff can arise. Such counsellors may also over-identify with clients. On balance, there is more to be gained than lost from the incorporation of this kind of experience within the multidisciplinary team.

Teamwork

In planning an alcohol treatment service, thought should be given to the composition of the multidisciplinary team. If 20 nurses are employed alongside a single occupational therapist, it is likely that the latter individual will become either de-skilled or isolated. In any setting, individuals should be chosen who display an ability to work with and learn from, rather than fight against, the different perspective of other professions.

The appointment of the right individuals will not in itself ensure a happy outcome. Good communication must be built into the working week in the form of business meetings, clinical reviews (or 'ward rounds'), staff groups and individual staff supervision. The final ingredient is clinical leadership and management, without which even the best team can become inefficient and lose sight of its objectives.

Planning, integration and organization of services

Often, the different treatment settings described above are planned and operated separately. Funding may come from the health service, social services, insurance and charitable or private sources. However, at some level, an overview of these different services is required in order to ensure that they provide for the total needs of the community and that they work efficiently together. This overall perspective of treatment provision should be seen in the broader context of a public health policy in which prevention plays the major role (Edwards et al., 1994). Depending upon the national and local setting, this overview may be achieved by political authorities, by purchasing authorities or by health service planners. In every case, the research evidence base would ideally be the prime factor determining local and national policy and service planning. Raistrick et al. (1999) provide a review of the evidence base related to UK alcohol policy considerations, and Alcohol Concern (1999) gives a national alcohol strategy for England.

Context of treatment services

The overall context within which treatment is offered is that of a community which is a complex, dynamic and adaptive system. Health care and social services should be considered as one component of a 'social, economic and health consequences subsystem', which is in interaction with a variety of other subsystems, including consumption, social norms and legal sanctions (Holder, 1998). Because of this, we must be wary of expecting simple benefits of the kind 'Treatment service T' will reduce the number (n) of alcoholics in the community by proportion P. Short-term reductions of this kind are likely to be swamped as other components of the overall system compensate and produce yet more individuals who are at risk, or who experience alcohol-related problems.

Assessment of need

In an ideal world, the planning of alcohol services would always start with an assessment of need (Marshall, 2001). Sadly, this is often neglected or given a lower priority than it deserves. In many countries, the true prevalence of alcohol-related problems is still unknown and, even in a relatively small community, research into the true extent of the problem may be costly and time consuming. However, in most cases, at least some information may be obtained relatively easily.

Purchasing decisions

Whether or not a detailed assessment of need is available, it is inevitable that treatment resources will be limited, and that decisions must be made as to purchasing priorities. The good news for purchasers and planners of services is that brief interventions are cheap and effective (Bien et al., 1993; Freemantle et al., 1993), and the good news for health departments is that there are also cost-effective means of prevention of alcohol-related problems (Edwards et al., 1994). A cornerstone of planning should therefore be to introduce such measures. This should adopt an integrative approach, which targets individual patients and practitioners, health care settings and health systems, and whole communities and the general population (Babor and Higgins-Biddle, 2000).

There are significant numbers of individuals who do not readily respond to simple interventions. These people, and their families, suffer considerably as a result of their drinking and cannot be ignored. What treatments should be purchased for this group of problem drinkers?

It would seem sensible, on an economic basis, to purchase shorter, less intensive, out-patient treatments for as many problem drinkers as possible and there is research to support the efficacy of such an approach. However, some studies have provided evidence of superior efficacy for in-patient programmes (see, for example,

Walsh et al., 1991; Bunn et al., 1994), and a recent review has suggested that there may be a need to re-evaluate the evidence concerning the influence of treatment setting on outcome (Finney et al., 1996). Other reviewers have also pointed out that, although many may benefit from cheap and brief interventions, the need for intensive in-patient services for a minority must still be recognized (Godfrey, 1992; Heather, 1996). It is therefore important that in-patient services are retained for those problem drinkers with serious medical and psychiatric conditions, those with few social resources, those whose environments are not conducive to recovery in the community, and possibly also those with severe dependence or other severe alcohol-related problems.

Managed care

In settings in which treatment decisions are primarily determined by service providers and consumers (e.g. where most treatments are funded via health insurance), anomalies and inefficiencies may arise. In the USA, this has led to the introduction of 'managed care' as a means of ensuring that organizational and management practices reflect financial as well as clinical considerations.

Managed care utilizes one or more of four strategies in order to achieve its objectives (Subcommittee on Health Services Research; National Advisory Council on Alcohol Abuse and Alcoholism, 1997). In *utilization management*, individual cases are reviewed prior to, and during, treatment in order to ensure appropriate care and to control costs. By means of *selective contracting*, consumers are offered incentives to choose providers who maintain good practice with respect to cost control. *Financial incentives for providers* are offered to those providers who control costs, and *guidelines for clinical decision-making* ensure that the referral and treatment of individual cases are governed by pre-determined criteria.

In the USA, managed care has reduced the costs of services and the numbers of service providers, and has reduced the length of stay in residential facilities by 50%. The debate continues as to whether access to services, effectiveness and quality of services have been maintained or impaired (Subcommittee on Health Services Research; National Advisory Council on Alcohol Abuse and Alcoholism, 1997; Weisner et al., 1999). Managed care has also altered the balance of service provision, such that in-patient care has declined and short-term and group care have increased. Most importantly, it is a system in which the business of treatment provision is influenced not only by clinicians and research developments, but also by administrative, economic and political considerations (Sosin and D'Aunno, 2001).

Diversity of services: choice, competition and co-operation

In many countries, there is a combination of provision by the state, by private organizations and by voluntary organizations or charities. The extent to which each of these sectors provides help will vary considerably from place to place. For example, in the UK, voluntary treatment agencies play a vital part in the overall provision of services and are financed, indirectly, by local authorities through community care provision. In a number of countries (notably the USA, France and Canada), alcohol treatment funding as a whole has been subsumed within mainstream health care provision (Klingemann et al., 1993).

This diversity of provision should be seen as a strength rather than as a problem, and efforts should be made to try to match drinkers with the most appropriate source of help. Unfortunately, although research suggests some benefits in patient–treatment matching (Lindström, 1992), there can be no universal guidance as to which are the most important patient characteristics upon which such selections should be made. An important US clinical trial known as Project MATCH, which compared three different psychological treatments, was able to reveal only very minor evidence for any matching between baseline patient characteristics and treatment that would optimize outcome (Project MATCH Summary, 1999). The clinician has therefore to make matching decisions on the basis of experience, intuition, trial and error and the patient's own preferences, and this cannot be substituted by a rule book. Professionals working in the field need to be willing to recognize the limitations of their own services and to be ready to refer to other sources of help when this seems appropriate.

Training

Effective services clearly depend upon the quality of training that their staff receive. In many cases, this training will be provided and funded through a variety of professional and educational pathways. Medical and nursing education has often been deficient in this respect, with doctors and nurses feeling inadequately prepared for the task they face once qualified (Deehan et al., 1999). Furthermore, this is not simply a matter for medical education, because a range of professionals, including counsellors, psychologists, social workers, occupational therapists and others, require training in this field. Within each profession there will also be those who require only a basic level of skills and knowledge, whereas others will specialize and require a higher level of proficiency. It is therefore inevitable that training will need to be offered in a multidisciplinary context, at a number of educational levels, with relevance to vocational and professional accreditation processes, and in such a way as to be responsive to service needs and cognisant of the evidence base for treatment. In order to achieve this, a consensus is required as to the required knowledge and skills for each professional group, and co-ordination is required among the different service, commissioning, professional and educational bodies concerned (Raistrick et al., 1999).

Audit and research

In view of the limited knowledge concerning how to choose the best treatment for any given patient and the limited funding available for services, it is important that all alcohol services are subject to audit and research. At the same time, the self-sufficiency of AA, which accepts no outside financial support, may be seen as an impressive form of cost-efficiency.

Any comprehensive assessment of outcomes should seek to address at least some items from each of the three dimensions of alcohol consumption, alcohol-related problems and level of dependence. A quantitative estimate of the actual levels of consumption, problems and dependence is to be preferred. These assessments should be conducted before, and at intervals after, any intervention or treatment that is offered. Assessments of change can be useful.

An independent assessment of outcome, based upon the account of a spouse or repeated measures of a suitable laboratory test, adds valuable corroboration to the account of the patient or client.

More detail on outcome studies is provided in a review (Plinius Maior Society, 1994). However, it should not be imagined that good outcome data are easily obtained. A comprehensive and valid assessment is both expensive and time consuming.

Treatment services: the responsibility to get them right

No-one would doubt that the individual therapist, whatever their profession, will be committed to doing their very best possible to assist the person who comes to them for help. However, they all operate within a context of service structure. Ensuring that services are designed as the very best possible to provide help to meet the needs of a vastly varied client population is a further responsibility in which we must also expect to share. Services which only treat a small sector of the true community need and which deploy methods only suitable for a small subset of the totality of troubled drinkers, may contribute to the sum of good. However, they are not the model for the modern treatment service response to drinking problems. That response must be based on a much broader vision.

REFERENCES

Alcohol Concern (1999) *Proposals for a National Alcohol Strategy for England.* London: Alcohol Concern.

Anderson, D. (1944) The place of the lay therapist in the treatment of alcoholics. *Quarterly Journal of Studies on Alcohol* 5, 257–66.

Babor, T.F. and Higgins-Biddle, J.C. (2000) Alcohol screening and brief intervention: dissemination strategies for medical practice and public health. *Addiction* 95, 677–86.

Bien, T.H., Miller, W.R. and Tonigan, J.S. (1993) Brief interventions for alcohol problems: a review. *Addiction* 88, 315–36.

British Medical Association (1998) *Medical Ethics Today.* London: British Medical Association.

Bunn, J.Y., Booth, B.M., Loveland Cook, C.A., Blow, F.C. and Fortney, J.C. (1994) The relationship between mortality and intensity of in-patient alcoholism treatment. *American Journal of Public Health* 84, 211–14.

Canning, U.P., Kennell-Webb, S.A., Marshall, E.J., Wessely, S.C. and Peters, T.J. (1999) Substance misuse in acute general medical admissions. *Quarterly Journal of Medicine* 92, 319–26.

Chick, J., Lloyd, G. and Crombie, E. (1985) Counselling problem drinkers in medical wards: a controlled study. *British Medical Journal* 290, 965–7.

Chick, J., Ritson, B., Connaughton, J., Stewart, A. and Chick, J. (1988) Advice versus extended treatment for alcoholism: a controlled study. *British Journal of Addiction* 83, 159–70.

Collins, M.N., Burns, T., Van den Berk, P.A.H. and Tubman, G.F. (1990) A structured programme for out-patient alcohol detoxification. *British Journal of Psychiatry* 156, 871–4.

Cook, C.C.H. (1988a) The Minnesota model in the management of drug and alcohol dependency: miracle method or myth? Part I. The philosophy and the programme. *British Journal of Addiction* 83, 625–34.

Cook, C.C.H. (1988b) The Minnesota model in the management of drug and alcohol dependency: miracle method or myth? Part II. Evidence and conclusions. *British Journal of Addiction* 83, 735–48.

Deehan, A., Marshall, E.J. and Strang, J. (1998) Tackling alcohol misuse: opportunities and obstacles in primary care. *British Journal of General Practice* 48, 1779–82.

Deehan, A., Marshall, E.J. and Strang, J. (1999) Who in the primary health care team can tackle alcohol misuse? *Journal of Substance Use* 4, 51–6.

Deehan, A., Taylor, C. and Strang, J. (1997) The general practitioner, the drug misuser, and the alcohol misuser: major differences in general practitioner activity, therapeutic commitment, and 'shared care' proposals. *British Journal of General Practice* 47, 705–9.

Drummond, D.C., Thom, B., Brown, C., Edwards, G. and Mullan, M.J. (1990) Specialist versus general practitioner treatment of problem drinkers. *Lancet* 336, 915–18.

Edwards, G., Anderson, P., Babor, T.F. et al. (1994) *Alcohol Policy and the Public Good.* Oxford: Oxford University Press.

Edwards, G. and Guthrie, S. (1967) A controlled trial of in-patient and out-patient treatment of alcohol dependency. *Lancet* 1, 555–9.

Edwards, G., Orford, J., Egert, S. et al. (1977) Alcoholism: a controlled trial of 'treatment' and 'advice'. *Journal of Studies on Alcohol* 38, 1004–31.

Finney, J.W., Hahn, A.C. and Moos, R.H. (1996) The effectiveness of in-patient and out-patient treatment for alcohol abuse: the need to focus on mediators and moderators of treatment settings. *Addiction* 91, 1773–96.

Freemantle, N., Gill, P., Godfrey, C. et al. (1993) Brief interventions and alcohol use. *Effective Health Care*, Number 7, University of Leeds.

Glass-Crome, I.B., Jones, P. and Peters, T.J. (1994) A joint problem drinking clinic: the King's College and Maudsley hospitals initiative. *Alcohol and Alcoholism* 29, 549–54.

Godfrey, C. (1992) *The Cost Effectiveness of Alcohol Services: Lessons for Contracting?* YARTIC Occasional Paper, 2. York: Centre for Health Economics, University of York.

Hayashida, M., Alterman, A.I., McLellan, A.T. et al. (1989) Comparative effectiveness and costs of in-patient and out-patient detoxification of patients with mild-to-moderate alcohol withdrawal syndrome. *New England Journal of Medicine* 320, 358–65.

Heather, N. (1996) *Treatment Approaches for Alcohol Problems.* Copenhagen: World Health Organization, Regional Office for Europe.

Holder, H.D. (1998) *Alcohol and the Community: a Systems Approach to Prevention.* International Research Monographs in the Addictions, Series ed. Edwards, G. Cambridge: Cambridge University Press.

Kennard, D. (1983) *An Introduction to Therapeutic Communities.* London: Routledge and Kegan Paul.

Klingemann, H., Takala, J.-P. and Hunt, G. (eds) (1992) *Cure, Care, or Control: Alcoholism Treatment in Sixteen Countries.* New York: State University of New York Press.

Klingemann, H., Takala, J.-P. and Hunt, G. (1993) The development of alcohol treatment systems. *Alcohol Health and Research World* 17, 221–7.

Laundergan, J.C., Spicer, J.W. and Kammeier, M.L. (1979) *Are Court Referrals Effective? Judicial Commitment for Chemical Dependency in Washington County Minnesota.* MN, Center City: Hazelden.

Lindström, L. (1992) *Managing Alcoholism: Matching Clients to Treatments.* Oxford: Oxford University Press.

Mäkelä, K., Arminen, I., Bloomfield, K. et al. (1996) *Alcoholics Anonymous as a Mutual-help Movement: a Study in Eight Societies.* Wisconsin: University of Wisconsin Press.

Marshall, E.J. (2001) Needs assessment – alcohol. In *Measuring Mental Health Needs,* 2nd edn, ed. Thornicroft, G., Brewin, C. and Wing, J. London: Gaskell, 486–512.

Marshall, E.J. and Deehan, A. (1998) Needs of special groups: drug and alcohol problems. *International Review of Psychiatry* 10, 136–8.

McMillen, D.L., Adams, M.S., Wells-Parker, E., Pang, M.G. and Anderson, B.J. (1992) Personality traits and behaviors of alcohol-impaired drivers: a comparison of first and multiple offenders. *Addictive Behaviors* 17, 407–14.

Peacock, C. (1992) International policies on alcohol-impaired driving: a review. *International Journal of the Addictions* 27, 187–208.

Persson, J. and Magnusson, P.-H. (1987) Prevalence of excessive or problem drinkers among patients attending somatic out-patient clinics: a study of alcohol related medical care. *British Medical Journal* 295, 467–72.

Plinius Maior Society (1994) Guidelines on evaluation of treatment of alcohol dependence. *Alcoholism* 30 (Suppl.).

Potamianos, G., Winter, D., Duffy, S.W., Gorman, D.M. and Peters, T.J. (1985) The perception of problem drinkers by general hospital staff, general practitioners, and alcoholic patients. *Alcohol* 2, 563–6.

Project MATCH Summary (and Editor's Introduction) (1999) *Addiction* 94, 31–4.

Raistrick, D., Hodgson, R. and Ritson, B. (eds) (1999) *Tackling Alcohol Together*. London: Free Association.

Royal College of Psychiatrists and College of Occupational Therapists (1992) *Occupational Therapy and Mental Disorders*. London: Royal College of Psychiatrists and College of Occupational Therapists.

Shepherd, R.M., Dent, T.H.S., Alexander, G.J.M. and London, M. (1995) Prevalence of alcohol histories in medical and nursing notes of patients admitted with self poisoning. *British Medical Journal* 311, 847.

Sosin, M.R. and D'Aunno, T. (2001) The organization of substance abuse managed care. In *Services Research in the Era of Managed Care: Organization, Access, Economics, Outcome*, ed. Galanter, Recent Developments in Alcoholism, 15, series ed. Galanter, M. New York: Kluwer, 27–49.

Stockwell, T., Bolt, L., Milner, I., Russell, G., Bolderston, H. and Pugh, P. (1991) Home detoxification from alcohol: its safety and efficacy in comparison with in-patient care. *Alcohol and Alcoholism* 26, 645–50.

Subcommittee on Health Services Research National Advisory Council on Alcohol Abuse and Alcoholism (1997) *Improving the Delivery of Alcohol Treatment and Prevention Services*. Bethesda, MD: National Institute on Alcohol Abuse and Alcoholism.

UK Alcohol Forum (2001) *Guidelines for the Management of Alcohol Problems in Primary Care and General Psychiatry*, 2nd edn. London: UK Alcohol Forum.

Wallace, P., Cutler, S. and Haines, A. (1988) Randomised controlled trial of general practitioner intervention in patients with excessive alcohol consumption. *British Medical Journal* 297, 663–8.

Walsh, D.C., Hingson, R.W., Merrigan, D.M. et al. (1991) A randomized trial of treatment options for alcohol-abusing workers. *New England Journal of Medicine* 325, 775–82.

Weisner, C., McCarty, D. and Schmidt, L. (1999) New directions in alcohol and drug treatment under managed care. *The American Journal of Managed Care* 5, SP57–69.

Working Party of the Royal College of Physicians (2001) *Alcohol – Can the NHS Afford it? Recommendations for a Coherent Alcohol Strategy for Hospitals*. London: Royal College of Physicians.

Author index

Subject index

Numbers in italics refer to *tables*.